THE WASHINGTON MANUAL®
OF PATIENT SAFETY AND
QUALITY IMPROVEMENT

T0200222

THE WASHINGTON MANUAL® OF PATIENT SAFETY AND QUALITY IMPROVEMENT

Editors

Emily Fondahn, MD
Assistant Professor of Medicine
Associate Program Director, Internal Medicine Residency
BJH Patient Safety and Quality Physician Liaison
Division of Medical Education
Washington University School of Medicine
St. Louis, Missouri

Michael Lane, MD, MPHS
Assistant Professor of Medicine
Division of Infectious Diseases
Washington University School of Medicine
Outcomes Physician, Center for Clinical Excellence
BJC HealthCare
St. Louis, Missouri

Andrea Vannucci, MD, DEAA
Associate Professor
Patient Safety Officer
Department of Anesthesiology
Washington University School of Medicine
St. Louis, Missouri

Series Editor

Thomas M. De Fer, MD
Professor of Medicine
Director, Internal Medicine Clerkship and the ACES Program
Division of Medical Education
Washington University School of Medicine
St. Louis, Missouri

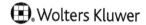

Philadelphia • Baltimore • New York • London
Buenos Aires • Hong Kong • Sydney • Tokyo

Executive Editor: Rebecca Gaertner
Senior Product Development Editor: Kristina Oberle
Senior Production Project Manager: Alicia Jackson
Design Coordinator: Teresa Mallon
Senior Manufacturing Coordinator: Beth Welsh
Editorial Coordinator: Katie Sharp
Prepress Vendor: SPi Global

Copyright © 2016 by Department of Medicine, Washington University School of Medicine

9 8 7 6 5

Printed in the United States of America

Library of Congress Cataloging-in-Publication Data
  Names: Fondahn, Emily, editor. | Lane, Michael (Michael Andrew), editor. | Vannucci, Andrea, 1964- , editor.
  Title: The Washington manual of patient safety and quality improvement / editors, Emily Fondahn, Michael Lane, Andrea Vannucci.
  Other titles: Manual of patient safety and quality improvement
  Description: Philadelphia : Wolters Kluwer, [2016] | Includes bibliographical references and index.
  Identifiers: LCCN 2015049525 | ISBN 9781451193558
  Subjects: | MESH: Patient Safety | Quality Improvement Classification: LCC R729.8 | NLM WX 185 | DDC 610.28/9—dc23 LC record available at http://lccn.loc.gov/2015049525

LWW.com

We dedicate this work to our patients.
Thank you for allowing us to take care of you and
inspiring us to constantly work to
improve health care for all.

And to Kate Mitchell,
a very capable, professional, and
dedicated colleague. She will be sorely missed
by her patients, colleagues, friends, and family.

Contributors

Kathleen S. Bandt, MD
Resident
Department of Neurological Surgery
Washington University School of Medicine
St. Louis, Missouri

Andrew Bierhals, MD, MPH
Assistant Professor
Mallinckrodt Institute of Radiology
Washington University School of Medicine
St. Louis, Missouri

Melvin Blanchard, MD, FACP
Associate Professor
Chief, Division of Medical Education
Director, Internal Medicine Residency Program
Department of Medicine
Washington University School of Medicine
St. Louis, Missouri

Bernard C. Camins, MD, MSc
Associate Professor
Division of Infectious Diseases
University of Alabama at Birmingham
Birmingham, Alabama

Adam Carlisle, MD
Resident
Division of Medical Education
Department of Internal Medicine
Washington University School of Medicine
St. Louis, Missouri

Christopher Carpenter, MD, MSc
Associate Professor
Division of Emergency Medicine
Washington University School of Medicine
St. Louis, Missouri

Laura F. Cavallone, MD
Assistant Professor
Department of Anesthesiology
Washington University School of Medicine
St. Louis, Missouri

Thomas Ciesielski, MD
Patient Safety and Quality Fellow
Instructor of Medicine
Division of Medical Education
Department of Internal Medicine
Washington University School of Medicine
St. Louis, Missouri

Rosalyn Corcoran, RN
Director, Patient Safety and Clinical Performance Improvement
Barnes Jewish Hospital
St. Louis, Missouri

Thomas M. De Fer, MD
Professor of Medicine
Director, Internal Medicine Clerkship and the ACES Program
Division of Medical Education
Washington University School of Medicine
St. Louis, Missouri

Tina Doshi, MD
Resident
Department of Anesthesiology
Washington University School of Medicine
St. Louis, Missouri

James R. Duncan, MD, PhD
Professor
Chief Quality and Safety Officer
Mallinckrodt Institute of Radiology
Washington University School of Medicine
St. Louis, Missouri

Charles S. Eby, MD
Professor
Department of Pathology and Immunology
Washington University School of Medicine
St. Louis, Missouri

Alex S. Evers, MD
Henry E. Mallinckrodt Professor and Chairman
Department of Anesthesiology
Washington University School of Medicine
St. Louis, Missouri

James J. Fehr, MD
Professor
Director of Saigh Pediatric Simulation Center
Washington University School of Medicine
St. Louis, Missouri

Emily Fondahn, MD
Assistant Professor of Medicine
Associate Program Director, Internal Medicine Residency
BJH Patient Safety and Quality Physician Liaison
Division of Medical Education
Washington University School of Medicine
St. Louis, Missouri

Victoria J. Fraser, MD
Adolphus Busch Professor and Chairman
Department of Medicine
Washington University School of Medicine
St. Louis, Missouri

Hiram Gay, MD
Associate Professor of Radiation Oncology
Radiation Oncology–Clinical Divisions
Washington University School of Medicine
St. Louis, Missouri

Anne L. Glowinski, MD, MPE
Professor
Department of Psychiatry
Washington University School of Medicine
St. Louis, Missouri

Matthew I. Goldsmith, MD
Associate Professor
Division of Pediatric Critical Care Medicine
Washington University School of Medicine
St. Louis, Missouri

Richard T. Griffey, MD, MPH
Associate Professor
Division of Emergency Medicine
Washington University School of Medicine
St. Louis, Missouri

Katherine E. Henderson, MD
Assistant Chief Medical Officer
Director, Graduate Medical Education & Medical Staff Services
Barnes-Jewish Hospital
St. Louis, Missouri

Laureen L. Hill, MD, MBA
Professor and Chair
Department of Anesthesiology
Emory University School of Medicine
Atlanta, Georgia

Bryan Kane, MD
Director of Research and Assistant Program Director
Department of Emergency Medicine
Lehigh Valley Hospital and Health Network
Allentown, Pennsylvania

Ivan Kangrga, MD, PhD
Professor
Department of Anesthesiology
Washington University School of Medicine
St. Louis, Missouri

Kara Kniska, PharmD
St. Louis Children's Hospital
St. Louis, Missouri

Nikoleta S. Kolovos, MD
Assistant Professor
Department of Pediatrics
Washington University School of Medicine
Medical Director
Pediatric Intensive Care Unit
St. Louis Children's Hospital
St. Louis, Missouri

Gokul Kumar, MD, MBA
Clinical Instructor
Chief Resident
Department of Ophthalmology and Visual Sciences
Washington University School of Medicine
St. Louis, Missouri

Michael Lane, MD, MPHS
Assistant Professor of Medicine
Division of Infectious Diseases
Washington University School of Medicine
Outcomes Physician, Center for Clinical Excellence
BJC HealthCare
St. Louis, Missouri

Rachael A. Lee, MD
Fellow
Division of Infectious Diseases
University of Alabama at Birmingham
Birmingham, Alabama

Stephen Y. Liang, MD
Assistant Professor
Divisions of Infectious Diseases and Emergency Medicine
Washington University School of Medicine
St. Louis, Missouri

Ellen M. Lockhart, MD
Vice Chairman and Professor
Department of Anesthesiology
Washington University School of Medicine
St. Louis, Missouri

George A. Macones, MD
Professor and Chair
Department of Obstetrics and Gynecology
Washington University School of Medicine
St. Louis, Missouri

Robert J. Mahoney, MD
Assistant Professor
Division of Hospitalist Medicine
Department of Medicine
Washington University School of Medicine
St. Louis, Missouri

Jonas Marschall, MD
Adjunct Assistant Professor
Division of Infectious Diseases
Washington University School of Medicine
St. Louis, Missouri

Kate Mitchell, RNC, WHNP*
Patient Safety Coordinator
Department of Obstetrics and Gynecology
Washington University in St. Louis
St. Louis, Missouri

Denise M. Murphy, RN, BSN, MPH, CIC
Vice President, Quality and Patient Safety
Main Line Health
Bryn Mawr, Pennsylvania

Sasa Mutic, PhD
Professor of Radiation Oncology
Radiation Oncology–Physics Division
Washington University School of Medicine
St. Louis, Missouri

Elna Nagasako, MD, PhD, MPH
Instructor of Medicine
Division of General Medical Sciences
Department of Medicine
Washington University School of Medicine
St. Louis, Missouri

Aaron J. Norris, MD, PhD
Resident
Department of Anesthesiology
Washington University School of Medicine
St. Louis, Missouri

Brian Nussenbaum, MD, FACS
Christy J. and Richard S. Hawes III Professor
Vice Chair for Clinical Affairs
Division Chief, Head and Neck Surgery
Patient Safety Officer
Department of Otolaryngology–Head and Neck Surgery
Washington University School of Medicine
St. Louis, Missouri

*deceased

Robert F. Poirier, MD
Assistant Professor
Division of Emergency Medicine
Washington University School of Medicine
St. Louis, Missouri

Myra Rubio, MD
Associate Professor
Division of Hospital Medicine
Department of Medicine
Washington University School of Medicine
St. Louis, Missouri

Ahmed S. Said, MD, PhD
Instructor
Division of Pediatric Critical Care Medicine
Washington University School of Medicine
St. Louis, Missouri

Paul Santiago, MD
Associate Professor
Patient Safety Officer
Department of Neurological Surgery
Washington University School of Medicine
St. Louis, Missouri

Richard A. Santos, MD, PhD
Assistant Professor
Division of Hospital Medicine
Department of Medicine
Washington University School of Medicine
St. Louis, Missouri

Ryan Schneider, ACNP-BC
Patient Safety and Quality Coordinator for Emergency Medicine
Division of Emergency Medicine
Washington University School of Medicine
St. Louis, Missouri

Noah Schoenberg, MD
Division of Hospital Medicine
Department of Medicine
Washington University School of Medicine
St. Louis, Missouri

Douglas J. E. Schuerer, MD, FACS
Director of Trauma
Associate Professor
Director, Surgical Critical Care Fellowship
Section of Acute and Critical Care Surgery
Washington University School of Medicine
St. Louis, Missouri

Anshuman Sharma, MD, MBA
Professor
Division of Anesthesiology
Washington University School of Medicine
St. Louis, Missouri

Binjon Sriratana, MD
Resident
Department of Anesthesiology
Washington University School of Medicine
St. Louis, Missouri

Michael Stock, MD
Resident
Department of Ophthalmology and Visual Sciences
Washington University School of Medicine
St. Louis, Missouri

Melissa Sum, MD
Resident
Division of Medical Education
Department of Medicine
Washington University School of Medicine
St. Louis, Missouri

Mary Taylor, JD
Director, Patient Safety, Washington University Physicians
Washington University School of Medicine
St. Louis, Missouri

Sergio E. Trevino, MD
Fellow
Division of Infectious Diseases
Department of Medicine
Washington University School of Medicine
St. Louis, Missouri

Andrea Vannucci, MD, DEAA
Associate Professor
Patient Safety Officer
Department of Anesthesiology
Washington University School of Medicine
St. Louis, Missouri

Peter Vila, MD
Resident
Department of Otolaryngology–Head and Neck Surgery
Washington University School of Medicine
St. Louis, Missouri

David Vollman, MD, MBA
Assistant Professor
Department of Ophthalmology and Visual Sciences
Washington University School of Medicine
St. Louis, Missouri

Jason C. Wagner, MD
Assistant Professor
Associate Residency Program Director
Director of Augmented Learning
Washington University School of Medicine
St. Louis, Missouri

Michael H. Wall, MD, FCCM
JJ Buckley Professor and Chairman
Department of Anesthesiology
University of Minnesota
Minneapolis, Minnesota

Amy D. Waterman, PhD
Associate Professor
Division of Nephrology
David Geffen School of Medicine at UCLA
Los Angeles, California

Charl de Wet, MD
Associate Professor
Medical Director, Cardiothoracic Intensive Care Unit
Washington University School of Medicine
St. Louis, Missouri

Keith F. Woeltje, MD, PhD
Director, Healthcare Informatics
BJC Center for Clinical Excellence
Professor of Medicine
Division of Infectious Diseases
Department of Medicine
Washington University School of Medicine
St. Louis, Missouri

Laurie Wolf, MS, CPE
Performance Improvement Engineer
Barnes-Jewish Hospital
St. Louis, Missouri

Feliciano B. Yu Jr., MD, MSHI, MSPH
Associate Professor
Chief Medical Information Officer, St. Louis Children's Hospital
Washington University School of Medicine
St. Louis Children's Hospital
St. Louis, Missouri

Preface

Health care providers around the world are dedicated to improving the health and lives of their patients. Sometimes, despite our best efforts, we are not able to accomplish these goals. At times, we may even harm patients. For too long these mistakes and errors have been hidden from other health care workers, hospitals, patients, and the public. The patient safety and quality improvement movement has worked to improve systems and processes, prevent errors, and promote transparency when harm occurs.

We hope this manual provides a broad overview for the fundamentals of patient safety and quality improvement, as well as insight into how these principles apply to clinical settings. Each chapter of the manual starts with a clinical vignette and discussion questions meant to show how patient safety and quality improvement principles apply in the clinical setting. We also list additional resources at the end of each chapter, which provide more information about a particular topic. This manual was a joint effort of many faculty members from multiple departments at Washington University. This cooperation among professionals with different professional priorities and backgrounds supports the principle that, in modern health care systems, effective patient safety and quality improvement needs a multidisciplinary team approach.

This manual was designed to be a resource for anyone working in health care and to be applicable to those new to safety and quality improvement and those with years of experience. The manual can be carried in the pocket of a lab coat or can be a reference for online access and reading. We hope that it will become an invaluable tool to support health care providers in acquiring the knowledge and skills to develop a proactive approach to patient safety and quality improvement.

We have many people to thank for the creation of the first *Patient Safety and Quality Improvement Manual.* First, Dr. Victoria Fraser and Dr. Alex Evers, the chairs of our departments, motivate us to provide excellent care to our patients and serve as exemplary role models. Dr. Melvin Blanchard, Dr. William Powderly, and Dr. Rene' Tempelhoff, our respective division chiefs, have been instrumental to our success. Dr. Tom De Fer, the series editor, provided great insight and guidance from the conception of the manual to the final product. Katie Sharp has kept us on track for our deadlines and been a wonderful resource.

Last, we would each like to thank our families: Emily—to Andy and Caroline Rowe for being patient while I spent many nights editing chapters, and Dr. Dean Fondahn, who taught me what it means to be a great doctor. Mike—to Laura, Sara, and Alex Lane for their support and understanding for the many days and nights I spent away trying to improve the lives of others, and my parents, Hal and Julie, who were role models for the ideals of fairness and justice. Andrea—to my wife and colleague Laura, who has rebuilt the life of our family in St. Louis; my encouraging and far-sighted parents, Ornella and Rodolfo, who, many years ago in Italy, paid for my first *Washington Manual*®; and my brother Enrico and my children Bianca, Pietro, and Angelica for the many insights they give me.

Emily Fondahn, Mike Lane, and Andrea Vannucci

Chairman's Note

Colleagues, it is with great pleasure that we are publishing our first edition of the *Washington Manual® of Patient Safety and Quality Improvement*. The Washington Manual® series has long focused on providing regular updates for medical students, house officers, fellows, and practicing physicians in internal medicine and various subspecialties.

This new manual provides access to important practical information on patient safety and quality improvement methods, tools, and competencies for physicians, medical trainees, and other health professionals. Patient safety and quality improvement are essential skills for all medical providers. The literature on patient safety and quality improvement has expanded dramatically over the past decade and exists in many different formats and venues. This manual provides key patient safety and quality improvement information in a concise format so that health professionals can increase their understanding of basic principles of patient safety and quality improvement and develop additional skills so that they may apply patient safety and quality improvement principles into their daily medical practice.

This manual also serves as a useful resource to address the Graduate Medical Education initiatives requiring medical training programs to develop and provide curriculum and real-world experiences in patient safety and quality improvement, thereby ensuring that future generations of providers develop competencies in patient safety and quality improvement. We look forward to your feedback.

Sincerely,
Victoria Fraser, MD
Adolphus Busch Professor and Chairman
Department of Medicine
Washington University School of Medicine
St. Louis, Missouri

Contents

1 Introduction to Patient Safety and Quality Improvement   1

Thomas Ciesielski and Victoria J. Fraser

SECTION 1 • QUALITY   10

2 Introduction to Quality Improvement   10

Adam Carlisle and Melvin Blanchard

3 Building High Reliability in the Health Care System   24

Ellen M. Lockhart, Laureen L. Hill, and Alex S. Evers

27 Patient Safety Issues Specific to Psychiatry 311

Anne L. Glowinski

28 Laboratory, Transfusion Medicine, and Pathology Services 321

Charles S. Eby

29 Medication Safety 337

Thomas M. De Fer

30 Transitions in Care and Readmissions 357

Emily Fondahn and Elna Nagasako

31 Patient Safety in Radiation Oncology 367

Hiram Gay and Sasa Mutic

Glossary: Introduction to Patient Safety Terminology G-1

Tina Doshi, Aaron J. Norris, and Andrea Vannucci

1 Introduction to Patient Safety and Quality Improvement

Thomas Ciesielski and Victoria J. Fraser

INTRODUCTION

"First, do no harm" should serve as the basic foundation for all interactions between patients and physicians, health care practitioners, and health care organizations. The science of medicine has progressed exponentially in the past century with the evolution of new technology, devices, medications, and the subspecialization of care. The increasingly complex health care system leads to fragmented care and an increased risk of medical errors that may result in harm to patients. The magnitude of patient harm was brought to the forefront of the nation's attention in 1999 when the *Institute of Medicine* (IOM) published the seminal report, *To Err is Human: Building a Safer Health System*, that highlighted the risk and impact of medical errors. The report estimated that there were between 44,000 and 98,000 deaths occurring each year from preventable errors. If these estimates are indeed accurate, medical errors would be the eighth leading cause of death.[1] A more recent study using the Institute for Healthcare Improvement (IHI) Global Trigger Tool estimates that there are between 210,000 and 400,000 patient deaths from preventable medical errors.[2] These two estimates vary widely, and the true number of patient deaths due to medical error will likely never be known. However, clearly, too many patients are being harmed by medical errors, and improvements are needed for the health care system.

In 2001, an equally important report, *Crossing the Quality Chasm: A new Health System for the 21st Century,* the IOM noted that health care was in need of significant changes and discussed specific recommendations to improve the quality of health care.[3] The argument put forth in *Crossing the Quality Chasm* is that the "care delivered is not…the care we should receive…[and] health care…harms too frequently and routinely fails to deliver its potential benefits."[3] The authors established goals for developing a 21st-century health care system and proposed six aims for health care (Table 1-1).[3]

These two reports helped lay the groundwork to promote the new fields of patient safety and quality improvement (QI) in medical schools, hospitals, and health care systems. While patient safety and QI are often talked about in unison, they are actually two distinct fields. The most straightforward way to think about these two disciplines is like medicine—patient safety is the diagnostic arm, figuring out what the errors were and what contributed to the errors, and QI is the treatment arm, fixing the system to prevent the errors from occurring again.[4] The IOM reports challenged hospital leaders and health care workers to develop new educational programs to change the culture and processes of health care delivery to ensure that safety and quality became priorities for the health care system as a whole.

TABLE 1-1	IOM's Six Aims of Quality Health Care
Aim	Definition
Safe	Health care systems never harm patients
Effective	Using scientific evidence to guide evaluation and treatment decisions
Patient centered	Provides the patient control in the care delivered, requiring a partnership that facilitates shared decision making
Timely	Patients are evaluated and treated quickly after a need is identified
Efficient	Care minimizes waste and utilizes resources in a cost-effective manner
Equitable	Care minimizes disparities across socioeconomic strata

(Data from: Institute of Medicine. *Crossing the Quality Chasm: A New Health System for the 21st Century.* Washington, DC: The National Academies Press; 2001.)

PATIENT SAFETY

Patient safety is, by itself, a nebulous term. *To Err is Human* defined patient safety as "freedom from accidental injury."[1] With that serving as a foundation, the field was further defined by patient safety thought leaders, including Linda Emanuel, Don Berwick, and Lucian Leape, as "a discipline in the health care professions that applies safety science methods toward the goal of achieving a trustworthy system of healthcare delivery...[and] an attribute of health care systems that minimizes the incidence and impact of adverse events and maximizes from such events."[5] This manual will introduce safety science methodologies and discuss strategies to mitigate errors and how health care systems can learn from errors that occur.

QUALITY IMPROVEMENT

Quality and QI are broad terms that need to be understood in the context of health care. Quality is roughly defined as "[t]he degree to which health services for individuals and populations increase the likelihood of desired health outcomes which are consistent with current professional knowledge."[6] Thus, the health care system and outcomes are inextricably linked. With quality broadly defined by the IOM, the U.S. Health Resources and Services Administration (HRSA) refined the definition to include how an organization currently operates and the organization's performance as measured by efficiency, the outcome of care, and patient satisfaction. QI means achieving a better performance level by changing the current system/operation; thus, quality is linked to the system, and to improve quality, the current system needs to change.[7] To do so, the HRSA feels that a QI program must include the following four areas:

1. QI work is performed on systems and processes.
2. Focus on patients.
3. Focus on being part of a team.
4. Focus on the use of data.[7]

The QI section of this manual will focus on how hospitals can become highly reliable organizations, QI methodologies, and the future of QI for health care systems.

HISTORY OF PATIENT SAFETY AND QUALITY IMPROVEMENT

Although the development of many patient safety and quality initiatives are often linked to the *To Err is Human* report,[8] other notable events that predate the report have influenced the evolution of the patient safety and quality movements in health care. The case of Libby Zion is one such event that had a profound impact on medical education and house staff training. Libby Zion was an 18-year-old college freshman who was admitted to a major New York academic hospital in 1984 with fever, agitation, and jerking movements of her limbs. She died in the hospital approximately 8 hours after presenting to the emergency room. She likely died from serotonin syndrome that was not recognized by the intern and second-year resident who took care of her. Her father, Sidney Zion, fiercely campaigned for changes in medical training to improve patient safety. This case was one of the first to garner national attention and put the spotlight on errors occurring in the hospital. The subsequent litigation from this case eventually led to the convening of the Bell Commission, whose report advocated for resident work hour restrictions and eventually led to national resident work hour restrictions.[9,10] Other important cases that influenced the patient safety and quality movement include the Betsy Lehman and Josie King cases. In 1994, Betsy Lehman, a Boston Globe reporter, died after receiving a massive overdose of cyclophosphamide while she was being treated for breast cancer at the Dana-Farber Cancer Institute. The medication error was missed by multiple providers and multiple departments before reaching the patient.[11] As a result of her death in 2004, the Commonwealth of Massachusetts founded the Betsy Lehman Center for Patient Safety and Medical Error Reduction, which focuses on improving patient safety through education and legislation.[12] Josie King, an 18-month-old girl admitted to Johns Hopkins Medical Center in 2001, died from a combination of preventable medical errors. After her death, Josie's mother, Sorrel King, founded the Josie King Foundation, which has advanced patient safety through legislation, formation of patient safety groups, and partnering with institutions.[13]

In addition to the IOM reports, many other important developments have prompted activity from multiple different organizations to improve safety and quality.

- **2001:** the Agency for Healthcare Research and Quality (AHRQ) received $50 million in funding from Congress to fund research in patient safety.
- **2002:** the Joint Commission (JC, formerly JCAHO) published its own patient safety goals, and the National Quality Forum (NQF) began publishing its Serious Reportable Events (SREs) list, which is commonly referred to as the "never events" list.
- **2003:** Minnesota became the first state to create a statewide error reporting system. Twenty-six more states have developed error reporting systems since.
- **2004:** the US government created the Office of the National Coordinator for Health Information Technology (IT) and the World Health Organization (WHO) developed a patient safety organization.
- **2005:** the IHI launched its first national campaign to improve patient safety and congress authorized the creation of patient safety organizations (the implementation was delayed until 2008).
- **2008:** Medicare launched a "no pay for errors" initiative.

- **2009:** the US congress approved $19 billion for implementation of electronic health records,[8] which was part of the federal stimulus package.
- **2010:** the Affordable Care Act was enacted by the US legislature, which contains provisions for patient safety and quality, specifically aimed at reducing hospital readmissions, which was followed by the Centers for Medicare and Medicaid Services (CMS) enacting policies to reduce readmissions for four major diagnoses: acute myocardial infarction (MI), congestive heart failure (CHF), pneumonia, and chronic obstructive pulmonary disease (COPD).[14,15]

LEARNING FROM INDUSTRY

Regrettably, medicine as a whole has been late in implementing QI tools compared to other industries, such as aviation and chemical manufacturing. That many of the IOM aims have yet to be achieved means that we in health care can and need to borrow the tools and concepts used by industry to create a safer environment for our patients. A paragon of safety is the aviation industry, and many lessons can be gleaned to make health care safer.

Safety in the aviation industry is based on a multifactorial approach, which includes a comprehensive reporting system, programs for setting and enforcing policies, accident investigation, research to foster new improvements, team training, the use of simulation, and the development of standard operating procedures, manuals, and checklists.[1,8,16] The comprehensive Aviation Safety Reporting System (ASRS) is a voluntary system that is designed to evaluate near misses and other incidents and quickly disseminates information on these issues to the industry and the Federal Aviation Administration (FAA).[1,8] Another major component of aviation safety is the use of checklists. The development of checklists in aviation can be traced back to an Army test flight of a Boeing Model 299, which was a large plane that was complicated to fly. On October 30, 1935, one of the first test flights ended in tragedy when shortly after takeoff, the plane stalled and crashed, killing two of the five crew members aboard. After review, the crash was deemed to be due to pilot error. The plane was felt to be too complicated to fly and the crash nearly doomed the Boeing Company. However, a few determined Army test pilots created short checklists on index cards documenting the essential steps for taxiing, takeoff, and landing. Subsequent test flights of the Model 299 using these checklists demonstrated an impeccable safety record making the Boeing plane a viable option for the military. Following the improved safety with the checklists, the Army purchased approximately 13,000 of the Model 299 planes and changed the name to the B-17 bomber, which played a significant role in World War II.[17] Checklists continue to be a major factor in aviation safety and remain in daily use today.

Chemical manufacturing is another potentially dangerous industry that has been on the forefront of safety and quality. The DuPont Company, one of the largest chemical and materials manufacturers in the world, has fostered a culture of safety within the company since the 1800s leading to an outstanding safety record.[1] DuPont has established a culture of safety principles among its core values that all employees must abide. Furthermore, the company has a nonpunitive incident-reporting system so employees can report safety issues, near misses, and incidents.[1] This reporting system allows the company to investigate and learn from near-miss incidents without an employee fearing punishment. Applying the lessons learned from these industries will be central to improving the safety and quality of health care going forward.

TRANSFORMING MEDICINE INTO A HIGH RELIABILITY ORGANIZATIONS

The industries described above are high-risk, high-stakes industries that have improved their safety records and so are described as high reliability organizations (HRO).[18] HRO share the following characteristics:

* Constant awareness among everyone in the organization about the risk of errors.
* A willingness to shift decision making to knowledgeable experts to respond quickly to errors.
* The organization is unwilling to explain away errors.
* The organization will invest in ways to empower employees to learn from experience.[19]

The patient safety and QI fields aim to transform health care into a HRO by focusing on ensuring predictable and effective results in an industry that does have the chance for errors and harm.[19] The theory behind HROs has already been applied to medicine with significant results. Peter Pronovost, MD, a leader in patient safety, used five features of HROs in designing his seminal study to decrease catheter-associated bloodstream infections in the ICU. The five features Pronovost used include the following:

* Identifying evidence-based interventions that will improve the health outcome
* Selecting an intervention that will have the most impact on the desired health outcomes and converting these interventions to behaviors
* Measuring baseline performance
* Developing measures to evaluate the intervention
* Finally, ensuring patients receive the evidence-based interventions[18]

Certain specialties, including anesthesiology, transfusion medicine, and infection prevention, have applied principles of HROs to improve care of patients.

An important feature of a safe organization is the creation of a "just culture." A just culture allows frontline employees or personnel to feel comfortable disclosing errors, even one's own error. The initial report of a just culture in medicine was in transfusion medicine and was published after *To Err is Human* and *Crossing the Quality Chasm*.[1,3] A just culture takes into account system failings, but has no tolerance for negligence or conscious disregard of established safety guidelines or reckless behavior.[20] Creating a just culture is an important step in creating a safe health care system.

ERROR IDENTIFICATION AND CLASSIFICATION

One of the first steps to improve safety and quality in health care settings is to understand the epidemiology and causality of safety events and appropriately classify events. Initial patient safety initiatives established standard definitions and terminology for errors and adverse events to use in surveillance, reporting, and research. Medical errors are events that lead to a negative outcome or have potential for a negative outcome.[21] An adverse event is defined as an unintended injury or complication due to management or medical care that affects the patient. A near miss is a medical error that was identified and caught prior to it reaching or harming the patient.[22] Classification and identification of errors, adverse events, and near misses allow health care systems to analyze events, track trends, and make improvements to prevent future errors.

Errors can be active or latent. Active errors occur in close relationship to the activity, and the effects of the error are usually noted immediately, such as a pilot error that leads to an airplane crash. Latent errors do not usually occur in close proximity to the activity and so the effects are delayed. Latent errors are much more difficult to catch and mitigate since their effects are distant from the action.[23] Additional types of errors have been described for health care. Diagnostic errors include delays in diagnosis, failure to use indicated tests, or failure to act on results. Treatment errors can be related to procedures, administering treatments, dosing errors, delays in acting on tests results, or delays in care. Preventive errors result from failure to provide indicated prophylaxis or failure of follow-up. There is also a general category for "other" types of errors that includes communication errors, equipment/device failures, and systems failures.[1]

The JC created a list of sentinel events, which are events that should never occur and need to be investigated to prevent their reoccurrence. Examples of sentinel events include death or permanent injury from a medication error, wrong-site surgery or procedure, hemolytic transfusion reactions due to blood group incompatibility, and unintended retained surgical objects. There are also specific lists of sentinel events for inpatient hospital care, ambulatory care, behavioral health care, critical access hospitals, laboratory medicine, office-based surgery, long-term care, and disease-specific care.[24] The JC allows individual health care systems to define additional sentinel events on their own and report these events voluntarily to the JC.[25] After a sentinel event has occurred, it is imperative to perform a root cause analysis (RCA) to understand the origins of the error and determine how the error propagated and reached a patient and how to prevent such errors in the future. RCAs were originally developed to analyze industrial accidents and seek to answer three fundamental questions, "what happened, why did it happen, and what can be done to prevent it from happening again?"[25]

THE FUTURE OF SAFETY AND QUALITY

Quality and safety measures are becoming a part of payment models and facing increased scrutiny by the public. The AHRQ developed Patient Safety Indicators (PSIs) in 2003, as a way to measure, track, and compare major complications and adverse events related to hospital admissions. Hospitals are monitored on a range of complications, including central line–associated bloodstream infections, pressure ulcers, and postoperative deep venous thrombosis (DVTs). The PSIs are available to the public, although the raw data remains difficult to locate efficiently, and thus, the distribution of comparative data is likely limited.[26] Several organizations are now using the PSIs to compare the quality of hospitals within a region as well as incorporating the indicators into a pay-for-performance (P4P) model.[27] In 2002, the CMS partnered with AHRQ and developed the Hospital Consumer Assessment of Healthcare Providers and Systems (HCAHPS) tool.[28] HCAHPS is a 27-point survey provided to patients to measure their perceptions of their hospital care, the results of which are now published online with the goal of enhancing accountability in health care.[28] In 2002, the NQF began tracking SREs list with the goal of creating a uniform reporting system of major adverse events. These events are serious, largely preventable, and harmful clinical events that should not occur; the list includes wrong-site surgery, events due to medical devices, deaths associated with introduction of a metallic object into a magnetic resonance imaging (MRI) area, and stage III to IV pressure ulcers acquired after admission.[29] The government and private payers acquire and track major safety and quality data. The public is now able to access this data and can use this information to select health care providers

Health care is an exceedingly expensive endeavor currently, with the US spending on medical care in 2010 reaching $2.6 trillion.[30] Preventable adverse events lead to unnecessary costs. Zhan et al. examined Medicare discharge data from an AHRQ database and linked it to five PSIs (decubitus ulcer, pneumothorax, post-op hematoma or hemorrhage, post-op deep vein thrombosis or pulmonary embolism, and post-op sepsis). The study found that Medicare paid approximately $300 million dollars in 2002 for these five adverse events.[31] This huge number only reflects the cost for five conditions over 1 year in one payer group. There is potential for huge cost savings by reducing preventable adverse events, decreasing complication rates, and limiting unnecessary or overutilized care and services.

CONCLUSION

The importance of safety and quality cannot be overstated in medicine. First and foremost, our duty as health care providers is to protect patients from harm, and we must strive to provide safe, effective, patient-centered, timely, efficient, and equitable care to individual patients and to populations. We must challenge ourselves to continuously improve the health care delivery system as a whole to ensure the safest and highest quality care possible. We must learn from medical errors to prevent them from reoccurring in the future. HRO engender a culture and environment that is dedicated to safety and improvement at all levels including leadership, frontline caregivers, and all staff. Furthermore, health care is becoming more and more accountable with publicly reported quality metrics, meaning that practitioners, hospitals, and health care systems will likely be judged by their outcomes, quality, and safety by the public and by the payers.

This manual was created with these principles in mind. This book is designed to provide important and useful information on patient safety and quality for current and future generations of health care workers including physicians, nurses, pharmacists, and anyone involved in patient care. The manual will introduce and broadly define key topics related to ensuring quality in health care and introduce major QI tools as well as introduce patient safety principles, describe methods to enhance patient safety, and provide necessary information on creating a culture of safety in hospitals and health care systems. The topics covered in this manual are wide ranging, and the manual is organized into three sections, QI, patient safety, and safety issues for specific areas. The QI section addresses high reliability QI tools, models for quality, accountability and reporting, health care IT, preventable harm, health care–associated infections, and coding and documentation. The patient safety section addresses creating a culture of safety, event analysis, disclosure of adverse events and errors, teamwork and communication, the role of human factors to improve safety and quality, cognition and decision making, and tools to improve safety.

The section on specific areas is written by experts in specific clinical fields and addresses how a safety and QI program can be designed and implemented in anesthesia, intensive care units, the emergency department, pediatrics, radiology, psychiatry, ambulatory care, and laboratory and pathology services. In addition, there are specific chapters on medication safety and safety and quality issues related to hospital readmissions and transfers of care that address issues common to several clinical disciplines. Finally, there is a glossary of important terms located at the end of the manual, and cases, methods, and tools are described to facilitate readers' engagement in patient safety and quality activities.

Although there are many important comprehensive textbooks on individual aspects of patient safety and quality, we believe that this manual provides the readers with an overview of current knowledge in patient safety and quality in an easy to understand and retain format. Furthermore, we are confident that it provides an introduction and a guide to the methods and tools that can be implemented into your own practice and help you to become a patient safety and quality champion in your institution.

REFERENCES

1. Kohn LT, Corrigan JM, Donaldson MS, eds. *To Err is Human: Building a Safer Health System*. Washington, DC: The National Academies Press; 1999.
2. James J. A new, evidence-based estimate of patient harms associated with hospital care. *J Patient Saf.* 2013;9(3):7.
3. *Crossing the Quality Chasm: A New Health System for the 21st Century*. Washington, DC: The National Academies Press; 2001.
4. Luther K, Buchert A. *Healthcare quality*. In *GME: Focusing on Quality and Safety in a Clinical Learning environment*. Chicago, IL.
5. Emanuel LBD, Conway J, et al. What exactly is patient safety? In: Battles J, Henriksen K, Keyes MA, Grady ML, eds. *New Directions and Alternative Approaches*. Rockville, MD: Agency for Healthcare Research and Quality; 2008.
6. *Crossing the Quality Chasm: The IOM Health Care Quality Initiative*. May 8, 2013 8:22 AM [cited June 2013]; Available from: http://www.iom.edu/Global/News%20Announcements/Crossing-the-Quality-Chasm-The-IOM-Health-Care-Quality-Initiative.aspx
7. HRSA Administration, ed. *Quality Improvement*. Rockville, MD: HRSA Administration; 2011:1–17.
8. Wachter R. Patient safety at ten: unmistakable progress, troubling gaps. *Health Aff.* 2010;29(1):165–73.
9. Lerner B. A case that shook medicine: how one man's rage over his daughter's death sped reform of doctor training. *The Washington Post*, Washington, DC, 2006.
10. Brody J. A mix of medicines that can be lethal. *The New York Times*, New York, NY, 2007.
11. Altman L. Big doses of chemotherapy drug killed patient, Hurt 2d. *The New York Times*, New York, NY, 1995.
12. *Betsy Lehman Center for Patient Safety and Medical Error Reduction*. 2013 [cited November 16, 2015]; Available from: http://www.chiamass.gov/betsy-lehman-center/
13. King S. Our story. *Pediatric Radiol.* 2006;36(4):284–6.
14. *Readmissions Reduction Program*. April 26, 2013 [cited June 25, 2013]; Available from: https://www.cms.gov/Medicare/Medicare-Fee-for-Service-Payment/AcuteInpatientPPS/Readmissions-Reduction-Program.html
15. *Provisions in the Affordable Care Act that Relate to PSOs and Reducing Unnecessary Readmissions*. Rockville, MD: Agency for Healthcare Research and Quality; 2010.
16. Toff NJ. Human factors in anaesthesia: lessons from aviation. *Br J Anaesth.* 2010;105(1):21–5.
17. Gawande A. *The Checklist Manifesto*. New York, NY: Metropolitan Books; 2009:279.
18. Pronovost PJ, et al. Creating high reliability in health care organizations. *Health Services Res.* 2006;41(4p2):1599–617.
19. Carroll JS, Rudolph JW. Design of high reliability organizations in health care. *Qual Safety Health Care.* 2006;15(suppl 1):i4–9.
20. Marx D. *Patient Safety and the "Just Culture:" A Primer For Health Care Executives*. New York, NY: Columbia University; 2001.
21. *AHRQ PSN Glossary*. 2013 [cited July 29, 2013]; Available from: http://www.psnet.ahrq.gov/popup_glossary.aspx?name=error

22. Friedman S, et al. Errors, near misses and adverse events in the emergency department: What can patients tell us? *CJEM.* 2008;10(5):421–7.

23. Reason J. *Human Error.* Cambridge, UK: Cambridge University Press; 1990.

24. *Sentinel Event Policy and Procedures.* 2013 [cited June 26, 2013]; Available from: http://www.jointcommission.org/Sentinel_Event_Policy_and_Procedures/

25. Wu AW, Lipshutz AKM, Pronovost PJ. Effectiveness and efficiency of root cause analysis in medicine. *JAMA.* 2008;299(6):685–7.

26. H.a.H. Services, ed. *Patient Safety Indicators A Tool To Help Assess Quality and Safety of Care to Adults in the Hospital.* Rockville, MD: Agency for Healthcare Research and Quality; 2010.

27. *AHRQ Quality Indicators—Guide to Patient Safety Indicators.* Rockville, MD: Agency for Healthcare Research and Quality; 2003.

28. *HCAHPS Fact Sheet.* 2012 [cited June 2013]; Available from: http://www.hcahpsonline.org/files/HCAHPS%20Fact%20Sheet%20May%202012.pdf

29. NQF. *Serious Reportable Events In Healthcare—2011 Update: A Consensus Report.* Washington, DC: NQF; 2011.

30. CDC. *Health Expenditures.* May 30, 2013 [cited August 28, 2013]; Available from: http://www.cdc.gov/nchs/fastats/hexpense.htm

31. Zhan C, et al. Medicare payment for selected adverse events: building the business case for investing in patient safety. *Health Affairs* 2006;25(5):1386–93.

2 Introduction to Quality Improvement

Adam Carlisle and Melvin Blanchard

CLINICAL VIGNETTE

As part of her Internal Medicine residency program, Emily receives quarterly reports regarding the quality of care she provides her patients with diabetes. Her last report showed that the majority of her patients with diabetes were not at goal for screening of neuropathy. By evaluating the process for screening patients, she determined that she often forgot to do a foot exam and the monofilaments were not readily available. She created a new process where nurses would put a monofilament on the front of all patients with diabetes charts as a reminder to perform the neuropathy screen. After instituting this process, her screening for neuropathy improved to 95%.

• Why is quality improvement important in health care?
• What are the first steps in starting a quality improvement project?

Health care systems routinely fail to deliver high-quality, evidence-based care to patients. Quality improvement (QI) work strives to remove gaps between the care provided and the care that should have been provided. Practitioners need a brief and practical guide to information about effective QI and interventions. The modern health care "systems" evolved out of necessity, not intentional design.[1] While patients are individuals and each presents with different clinical challenges, they often share the same systems and encounter the same obstacles to care. QI methods seek not to limit the freedom or dictate the terms of the patient–provider relationship but to ensure the care plan is carried out as intended—especially with regard to those elements that are most critical and common. QI methods seek to increase health care value by focusing on what helps patients the most and how we can do those things better.[2,3]

Quality health care has been defined in numerous different ways; perhaps, the most commonly used definition was composed by the Institute of Medicine and is framed by six central aims (Table 2-1). Poor quality in health care leads to poor patient outcomes and costs the health care system limited resources. Three types of poor quality in health care are overuse, underuse, and errors.[4] An example of overuse is repeating a chest x-ray because the initial x-ray was not available in the electronic medical record (EMR). Underuse includes not performing a colonoscopy for colorectal cancer screening on an appropriate patient. Opportunities to provide effective, timely, and patient-centered care are often missed (Table 2-2).

TABLE 2-1	IOM's Six Aims of Quality Health Care
Aim	Definition
Safe	Health care systems never harm patients
Effective	Using scientific evidence to guide evaluation and treatment decisions
Patient centered	Provides the patient control in the care delivered, requiring a partnership that facilitates shared decision making
Timely	Patients are evaluated and treated quickly after a need is identified
Efficient	Care minimizes waste and utilizes resources in a cost-effective manner
Equitable	Care minimizes disparities across socioeconomic strata

(Data from: Institute of Medicine. *Crossing the Quality Chasm: A New Health System for the 21st Century.* Washington, DC: The National Academies Press; 2001.)

SYSTEM OF PROFOUND KNOWLEDGE

Edward W. Deming created the idea of improvement known as the "System of Profound Knowledge." The concept of profound knowledge refers to the understanding that will lead to improvement, rather than simply the knowledge about a process from a subject matter expert. The four components of Deming's System of Profound Knowledge are shown in Figure 2-1. When considering ways to improve some component of health care, one must recognize and consider these four concepts before initiating a QI project.

IMPROVING QUALITY IN HEALTH CARE

Many health care providers are currently striving to provide quality patient care but are failing to do so. The problem facing health care is a failure of execution, not effort. Edward Deming famously illustrated this principle in his "red bead experiment."

TABLE 2-2	Opportunities to Provide Effective, Timely, Patient-Centered Care
Measures	Examples of Opportunities for Improvement
Effective	Only 59% of 50- to 75-year-olds received colon cancer screening in 2010, despite known benefits
Timely	One-third of emergency medicine patients in the 18- to 64-year-old age group wait an hour or more for care
Patient centered	Over 15% of patients reported that their usual care provider did not ask for their help in treatment decisions

(Data from: 2012 National Healthcare Quality Report. Agency for Healthcare Research and Quality. Rockville, MD; 2013. http://www.ahrq.gov/research/findings/nFhqrdr/nhqr12/index.html)

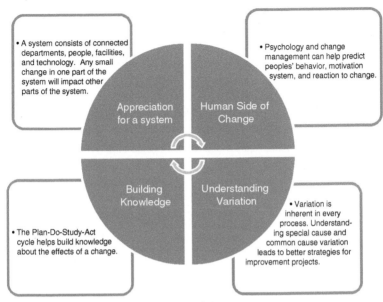

• A system consists of connected departments, people, facilities, and technology. Any small change in one part of the system will impact other parts of the system.

Appreciation for a system

• Psychology and change management can help predict peoples' behavior, motivation system, and reaction to change.

Human Side of Change

Building Knowledge

Understanding Variation

• The Plan-Do-Study-Act cycle helps build knowledge about the effects of a change.

• Variation is inherent in every process. Understanding special cause and common cause variation leads to better strategies for improvement projects.

Figure 2-1. Deming's system of profound knowledge.

When asked by industry leaders how processes could be improved, Deming filled a bowl with red and white beads, stating red beads represented a poor outcome and white beads represented the desired outcome. He would explain to the employees that "the goal is to pick the white beads." Then, he would blindfold employees and asked them to choose a bead from the bowl at random. When employees chose white beads, they were praised, and when they chose red beads, they were berated. In this example, the employees are doomed to fail by picking a red bead because of the design of the process. This experiment illustrates that workers are often blamed for defects in the system, even though they have no control over the system.

When processes are complex and poorly understood, managers commonly attribute errors to the performance of individual employees, while the root cause of errors is systemic and process related.[5] Health care delivery cannot be improved solely by culling out providers performing under the mean. Instead, interventions need to improve the mean performance of existing health care providers by changing the underlying system and process. This improvement requires an understanding of systems, data collection, implementation of changes, and measuring the effect of system alterations. Interventions must focus on the most common, most dangerous, most rate limiting, most costly problems in health care.

Resources used to produce health care are limited, including time. The concept of opportunity cost dictates that the cost of consuming these resources is not simply the value of the resource if left unconsumed but is instead the total value of the resource if used in the next best possible way. For example, if a doctor spends one additional hour per day manually writing prescriptions that could potentially be printed from an electronic medical record, then a hospital system must consider the daily cost of the current system as the hourly salary of that doctor but also the potential revenue foregone by an additional hour of patient evaluation, assuming there are patients available and in need of physician evaluation during that hour.

Furthermore, the theory of constraints can be extremely helpful when considering complex process occurring both in series and in parallel as with patient care to maximize or minimize a given outcome. The theory of constraints states that scarce resources should be devoted toward improving the significant bottleneck in a production process.[6] Continuing our example from above, if a health care system leadership is determining whether to use their limited resources to enable prescription printing from their electronic medical record, *or* to integrate the currently separate inpatient and outpatient electronic medical records with the goal of improving patient throughput time, then leadership should determine which steps in patient care represent the greatest bottleneck to throughput and which of the two above interventions would address this most effectively. The theory of constraints could also be applied to these scenarios with intent to maximize revenue or even minimize errors. This is accomplished by measuring the degree to which each of the multiple steps of patient care is most critical to the desired outcome.

METHODS OF QUALITY IMPROVEMENT USED IN HEALTH CARE

There are several different methods on QI currently used in health care:

- **Six Sigma** is an "improvement approach that seeks to find and eliminate the causes of mistakes or defects in business processes by focusing on outputs that are of critical importance to the customer."[7]
- Six Sigma seeks to eliminate defects by using the DMAIC (Define, Measure, Analyze, Improve, Control) methodology of process improvement. A set of process improvement tools developed by Motorola 1985, the name is derived from sigma, the statistic designation for standard deviation with the goal of manufacturing processes yielding six standard deviations of defect-free production. This is equivalent to 99.99966% of products being defect free or 3.4 defects per million opportunities.[8]
- **Lean**, termed by John Krafcik in 1988, was originally developed in the automobile manufacturing industry as an outgrowth of Toyota Production Systems. Lean focuses on removing unnecessary waste from a process, increasing efficiency and improving workflow, while preserving value. Specifically, lean mythologies seek to remove waste or "muda" in seven areas (Table 2-3).

TABLE 2-3	LEAN: Seven Areas of Waste
Overproduction	
Inventory	
Rejected/repaired product	
Motion	
Transport	
Processing	
Waiting	

- The **Plan, Do, Study, Act (PDSA) cycle** is practical, simple, and thus commonly used. The PDSA cycle mirrors the natural iterative process of trial-and-error problem solving. It is most effective when addressing a singular care process and must be repeated multiple times as the first cycle often uncovers new process problems that should be addressed in the next cycle (see Chapter 4, Quality Improvement Tools).
- **Continuous quality improvement** as a management strategy was first widely implemented in Japanese manufacturing where it was termed "Kaizen."[9] It is implemented broadly in many forms throughout health care.

While originally distinct in design, these methodologies are often used in combination. A single QI project should only use methods and tools as needed. Each may be applied to many types of QI interventions including rationing, education, feedback, incentives, penalties, organization, checklist utilization, EMR, human factor process reform, and team training.

COMPONENTS OF A QUALITY IMPROVEMENT PROJECT

A project charter is useful to communicate and confirm agreement between the problem-solving team and management. The project charter should include the goal, project background scope, measures, business case, team members, required resources, projected cost and saving, planned initial activities, and estimated time of completion. An aim statement should be included as part of the goal. It should be specific, measurable, appropriate, result oriented, and time scheduled. An example might be "The medicine clinic aims to increase monofilament testing and documentation on patients with diabetes from 60% to 80% by December 31, 2016." The measures should be connected with the goals and outcomes of the charter. Generally, most projects have three to eight measures, which are a mix of process, outcome, and balancing measures. A driver diagram is a structured logic tree to visually display the aim, the primary drivers that contribute to the aim, the secondary drivers that influence the primary drivers, and specific change ideas to test[10] (Fig. 2-2).

A vital component to any successful QI project is a good team. Important roles to fill on the team include a team leader with authority to make change, an executive sponsor to help overcome organizational roadblocks, subject matter experts and/or frontline workers (e.g., nurses, medical assistants, physicians), and an improvement expert to guide the team and patients or customers.

CONDUCTING A QUALITY IMPROVEMENT PROJECT

There are four basic steps to conducting a QI project: develop a change, test a change, implement a change, and spread a change.

Developing a Change

All improvement requires change, but not all change is an improvement (Improvement Guide). There are two types of change. *Reactive change* or first-order change consists of doing more or less of an existing process. This is reversible and requires minimal new learning. *Fundamental change* or second-order change represents a fundamentally different process that is not reversible and requires new learning to execute.[11] Determining what type of change to make requires understanding the system and the theory behind the change. A driver diagram is one tool to help organize the theory of the system, helps the team understand how factors are connected, and facilitates the process of identifying factors to address.

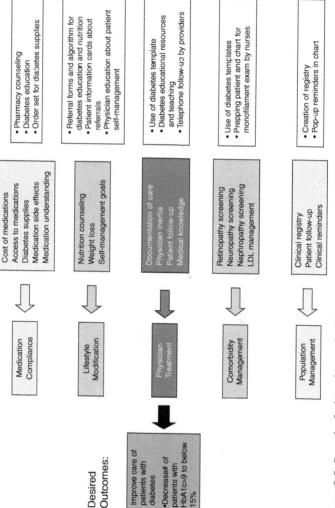

Figure 2-2. Example of a driver diagram for diabetes care.

Deciding what change to make is not always easy. People often perseverate on a few common ideas. For example, many thoughts start with "more of the same," meaning more physicians, more exam rooms, or more money would fix the problem. Rather, the system would likely benefit from an overall redesign. Another common pitfall is searching for the perfect change. A team may spend hours, weeks, or months debating what type of change to make and attempt to map out all the details of the change, leading to a paralysis of action. There are five approaches to assist teams with developing a change:

1. Logical thinking about the current system
   a. Often, mapping out a process with a flow diagram and bringing together a multidisciplinary group can lead to good ideas for change.
2. Learning from others
   a. Across the world, other teams are probably struggling with the same problems and some may have shown improvement through their changes. Reaching out to other health care systems and reviewing the literature can provide tested ideas for change. Additionally, as mentioned in previous chapters, health care can look at other industries for change concepts.
3. Using technology
   a. Technology, if tested and implemented appropriately, can improve a system. However, automating a bad system or having a technology that is inconsistent may only make things worse.
4. Creative thinking
   a. Creative thinking can help a team obtain new ideas. Provocative thinking exercises and brainstorming can spur creative thinking.
5. Using change concepts
   a. A change concept is "a general notion or approach to change that has been found to be useful in developing specific ideas for changes that lead to improvement"[12] (Table 2-4).

TABLE 2-4	Examples of Change Concepts
Change Concepts	Description
Improve workflow	Change the workflow so that the process is less reactive and more planned
Optimize inventory	Use of inventory pull systems such as "just-in-time" is one way to minimize inventory
Change the work environment	Examples include physical renovation of facilities and developing a "just culture"
Producer/customer interface	Improving communication, expectations, and thus satisfaction between producers and customers
Manage time	Lead time, cycle time, and waiting times can all be decreased
Error proofing	Redesigning the system to make it less likely for people in the system to make errors
Eliminate waste	See lean

Testing a Change

Testing change helps build knowledge about a system and teaching if a change will result in an improvement. Often, testing is done through PDSA cycles. Begin by testing on a small scale, and use the testing to build knowledge over time. The first test may just be on 1 patient. This strategy builds buy-in and prevents large-scale failure. The scale of the testing should be proportional to the current commitment to change within the organization, the degree of belief that the change will lead to improvement, and the cost of failure (Table 2-5).

Repeated small changes are often better than large changes as each change has the potential of unintended effects on other patient care processes. Unintended effects can be identified and negative effects remedied with minimal harm if changes are small and improved with each repeated iteration. With each test, collect data on the system and evaluate if the predictions made were correct. Testing should be done under a wide range of conditions. This strategy will help build buy-in that the change will lead to improvement and help the team identify problems with the improvement idea.

Implementing a Change

Implementation of a change is making the change an integral part of the system. It may require a broad and permanent change to the routine operations of the organization. During the implementation process, all other interacting systems also need to be evaluated to help support the change. Implementation must not ignore portions of the organization involved in documentation, hiring, training, and compensation. Failure of implementation can often be traced to inadequate preliminary testing. The same PDSA cycles used for testing can be used for implementation. There are several key implementation areas a team should consider:

1. Standardization— policies and procedures
2. Documentation—job descriptions
3. Training—staff education
4. Measurement—information flow
5. Resourcing—equipment

TABLE 2-5	Scale of Testing			
Current Situation		**Resistant**	**Indifferent**	**Ready**
Low confidence that current change idea will lead to improvement	Cost of failure large	Very small scale test	Very small scale test	Very small scale test
	Cost of failure small	Very small scale test	Very small scale test	Small scale test
High confidence that current change idea will lead to improvement	Cost of failure large	Very small scale test	Small scale test	Large scale test
	Cost of failure small	Small scale test	Large scale test	Implement

(Adapted from: Langley GL, Moen R, Nolan KM, et al. *The Improvement Guide: A Practical Approach to Enhancing Organizational Performance.* 2nd ed. San Francisco, CA: Jossey-Bass Publishers; 2009.)

TABLE 2-6	Human Response to Change
Resistance	Emotional or behavioral response to real or imagined threats to the work routine
Apathy	Feeling or showing little or no interest
Compliance	Publicly acting in accord with social pressure while privately disagreeing
Conformance	A change in behavior or belief as a result of real or imagined group pressure
Commitment	A state of being emotionally or intellectually bound to a course of action

(Data from: www.ihi.org/resources/Pages/Changes/UsingChangeConceptsforImprovement.aspx)

The human side of change is another important consideration when implementing a change. The human response to change follows a bell-shaped curve with a few innovators, some early adopters, and a few laggards, while most people will either be in the early or late majority. People will often have a strong emotional reaction to change (Table 2-6).

These reactions may be due to feeling of change in autonomy, programmed behavior, and stability with the current routine, real or perceived limits on resources, and a limited focus. Strategies to mitigate these barriers include creating the will among the staff for the change, providing information about why the change is being made and how it will affect staff, publicizing the change, allowing time for adequate training, and maintaining a feedback loop.

Spreading a Change

Spreading a change is implementing a good idea beyond the initial location. The positive effects of a change are determined not only by the fundamental improvement offered by the change itself but also the degree to with the change is used successfully throughout the organization. For example, if an intensive care unit develops a bundle that decreases central line–associated infection rates, this bundle should be spread to other hospital units. The IHI developed a framework for spread, which includes:

1. Strong leadership
2. Better ideas
3. Setup
4. Social systems
5. Measurement and feedback systems

Sustaining a Change

After a change has been made, continuing to monitor the system is critical. Often, a team may focus on measuring before the intervention and after the intervention. However, the focus should be on measuring continually to evaluate data over time. This monitoring can be done with run charts and control charts (discussed in Chapter 4).

MEASURING QUALITY

Measurement is an integral part of continuous QI.[13] Measuring quality in health care has been more difficult than in other industries due to the difficulty in determining whether patient outcomes are attributable to the quality of health care delivery or to patients' baseline health status, which can vary widely. However, quality can now be measured reliably in the health care industry by a variety of methods.[14] While measuring quality care is traditionally viewed as distinctly separate from providing quality care, there is mounting evidence to show that the two are inextricably linked.[15] It serves two critical purposes: first, to determine which of multiple processes within a system yield the best health outcomes and second, to determine how often known best practices are being applied to appropriate patients. Measurement can vary widely by type, assessment method, source, and scope.

Health care quality can be measured on the basis of structure, process, and outcome (Table 2-7)[16]:

1. *Structural measures* quantify the available resources of health care systems, such as number of nurses, hospital beds, or phlebotomy supplies.
2. *Process measures* quantify of the diagnostic and therapeutic processes that occur while caring for the patient, such as the number of patient with heart failure that were discharged with a β-blocker prescribed.
3. *Outcome measures* quantify the health status of patients after they received health care; mortally, morbid and even quality-of-life measures are examples.
4. *Balancing measures* quantify any of the changes during a QI project other than the primary outcome of the QI project to ensure that other systems or processes are not disrupted negatively. For example, if a project were designed to improve diagnosis of pulmonary embolism with the introduction of different imaging protocols, kidney function could be a balancing measure. A balancing measure can be a structural, process, or outcome measure.

TABLE 2-7   Types of Measurements to Assess Quality

Measurement Types	General Description	Health Care Examples
Structural	Quantify available resources	Number of nurses or number of hospital beds
Process	Quantify the steps that are necessary to achieve the desired outcome	Number of patients with heart failure discharged on a β-blocker
Outcome	Quantify the degree to which consumer specifications are met	Mortality or morbidity or quality of life
Balancing	Quantify if changes intended to improve one measure cause another measure to worsen	Kidney injury after interventions to screen for pulmonary embolism

(Data from: Donabedian A. *Explorations in Quality Assessment and Monitoring. Vol. 1: The Definition of Quality and Approaches to its Assessment.* Ann Arbor, MI: Health Administration Press; 1980.)

Each of these different measures has respective strengths and weaknesses that are important to consider. Structural and process measures are useful if proven to correlate with outcomes and are often easier to obtain than outcome measures. Process data can be more sensitive than outcome data as every process error does not lead to a poor outcome. However, the reliability of process measures is dependent on the degree that a process is known to influence outcomes, since poor patient outcomes are often not apparent until sometime after the measured health care is provided. When comparing outcomes data, it is important to measure baseline health. If differences in baseline health are not accounted for properly, then outcomes represent only the final state of health, not improvement associated with the care delivered. Most QI projects will have a variety of outcome, process, and balancing measures that are tracked over time.

Data for the measurement of quality in health care can be obtained from multiple sources including the clinical medical record, billing/insurance records, survey, or direct observation. The best source of data depends on the purpose for which the data will be used.[13] For example, educational counseling regarding diet for patients with diabetes could be measured by patient survey, medical record, or direct audio/video recording. Which source is best depends on whether quality care is linked to physicians completing the counseling, patients' memory of the counseling, or counseling being documented so other therapies are considered appropriately in the future.

Data must be measured in units appropriately scoped to the QI project at hand. For example, if a hospital wishes to reduce the average time to initial evaluation after arriving in the emergency department by 40 minutes but can only measure these times in hours, a new measurement system must be created. Data collection should not be a separate labor-intensive process demanding the time of providers at the opportunity cost of actually providing patient care. Systems should support efforts of frontline providers to measure their performance daily and adjust accordingly.

Data collected differently under different circumstances become unreliable and will be insufficient to determine whether changes are due to the interventions tested or from inconsistencies in data collection. Developing an operational definition of measurement is necessary to insure collected data are reliable and useful. An operational definition requires (1) agreement on a measuring device, (2) a degree of measurement precision, and (3) a criteria for judgment. For example, when trying to measure if decubitus ulcers have improved, one must determine the measuring device (visual estimation or tape measure or caliper), the degree of measurement precision (units of one centimeter or one-tenth of a centimeter), and the criteria for judgment (what is a decubitus ulcer and at what points of the skin lesion do you measure).

Measurement allows for identification of poor quality care; however, the further into the care process that this poor quality is identified, the more dangerous it is to the patient and the more costly it is to remedy.[17] For example, if an intravenous antibiotic is compounded incorrectly by a pharmacist, this will result in decreased quality of care, but the magnitude is dependent on how early or late in the care process this error is identified. If the error is detected by the pharmacist, the cost is only minimal wasted materials and one provider's time. If the error is detected by a nurse at bedside, more staff members' time was wasted and the patient's outcome could be worse due to delay in appropriate treatment. If a patient receives antibiotic before the error is detected, he or she may suffer kidney injury or much worse, as well as incur greater cost for further care related to the error. Fortunately, multiple tools are available to measure quality of care effectively[18] (see Chapter 4, Quality Improvement Tools).

QUALITY IMPROVEMENT VERSUS CLINICAL RESEARCH

QI and clinical research share the common goal of seeking to improve patient care by the combined application of intervention and repeated measurement. Clinical research requires approval from a board of ethics, the institutional review board (IRB) in the US, whose oversight is meant to insure the safety of patients. QI efforts are currently exempt from required IRB approval. It can be difficult to determine if a given project is primarily categorized as QI or clinical research; thus, the key characteristic of each is reviewed here (Table 2-8).[19,20] Of note, projects involving vulnerable population could benefit from the oversight of an ethical review committee. Vulnerable populations include students, employees, children, pregnant women, prisoners, active military personnel, individuals who have impaired decision-making capacity, or those who are educationally or economically disadvantaged.

TABLE 2-8	Difference in QI and Research
Quality Improvement	**Clinical Research**
Describes or improves a specific gap of health care delivery locally	Identifies a deficit in scientific knowledge from literature or proposes a hypothesis to develop new generalizable knowledge
An iterative intervention changes over time in response to ongoing feedback	Intervention protocol remains constant, often using randomization of individuals
Intervention within usual clinician–patient therapeutic relationship	Novel therapy
Known benefits to participants and local institution	Intended potential societal benefit, with unknown individual benefit
Primary risk is privacy or confidentiality of health information, and risk may be higher for patients not participating	Risks include physical, psychological, emotional, social, or financial risks and are described to participants during the informed consent process, who individually volunteer or IRB grants a waiver of consent
Review of results occurs throughout the process for continuous ongoing improvement	Analysis is periodic and will primarily be used to inform further investigations
The main intent of the activity is local system–level processes refinement by sharing results local with process participants	Results are intended to be generalized beyond the study population, often by peer-reviewed publication outside the institution

(Data from: US Dept of Health and Human Services. Protection of Human Subjects: 45CFR 46. 2005, www.hhs.gov/ohrp/humansubjects/guidance/45cfr46.html; Davidoff F, Batalden P, Stevens D, et al. Publication guidelines for quality improvement in health care: evolution of the SQUIRE project. *Qual Saf Health Care*. 2008;17[Supplement 1]:i3–9, www.squire-statement.org)

THE BUSINESS CASE FOR QUALITY IMPROVEMENT

As described in the text "Quality is Free," improving quality should not cost and, in fact, may reduce cost as "quality is the price of nonconformance."[21] A process that produces defective products leads to costs from (1) screening to identify defective product, (2) rework of detected defects, and (3) costs related to defects that reach customers. Joseph Juran terms this phenomenon "the cost of poor quality."[22] A process designed to produce products that consistently conform to specifications eliminates these costs. In 2004, the American Society for Quality released a white paper report entitled "Making the Economic Case for Quality," which summarizes a large body of empiric evidence of the economic impact of an organizational focus on QI. It concludes that the impact of quality management practice on bottom-line measures, market measures, and internal operating measures of profit is significantly positive.[23] Correspondingly, health care payors are beginning to demand more value for each dollar they spend. Health care cost could potentially be decreased while maintaining the same health outcomes with appropriate use of preventative medicine and providing treatments in a less resource-intensive setting, such as a primary care clinic.

KEY POINTS

- Quality improvement aims to make health care safe, effective, patient centered, timely, efficient, and equitable.
- Components of a quality improvement project include a charter; an aim statement; a driver diagram, outcome, process, and balancing measures; methods to display data; and a high-functioning team.
- Testing a change can be done through a series of PDSA cycles, which should start small then be scaled up.

ONLINE RESOURCES

1. Institute for Healthcare Improvement: www.ihi.org
2. Agency for Healthcare Research and Quality: www.ahrq.gov
3. American Society for Quality: www.asq.org

REFERENCES

1. Bohmer R. *Designing Care: Aligning the Nature and Management of Health Care*. Boston, MA: Harvard Business Press; 2009.
2. Porter ME. What is value in health care? *N Engl J Med*. 2010;363:26.
3. Gwande A. *Better: A Surgeon's Notes on Performance*. New York, NY: Henry Holt and Company; 2007.
4. McGlynn EA, Asch SM, Adams J, et al. The quality of health care delivered to adults in the United States. *N Engl J Med*. 2003;348:2635–45.
5. Deming EW. *Out of Crisis*. Cambridge, MA: MIT Center for Advanced Engineering Study Publishing; 1982.
6. Goldratt E. *The Goal: A Process of Ongoing Improvement*. Great Barrington, MA: North River Press; 1984.
7. Snee RD. Why should statisticians pay attention to six sigma? *Qual Prog*. 1999;32(9):100–3.

8. Wortman M, Pearson T, Patel JP, Carlson DR. *The Certified Six Sigma Black Belt Primer*. 3rd ed. West Terre Haute, Indiana: Quality Council of Indiana; 2012.

9. Imai M. *Gemba Kaizen: A Commonsense, Low-Cost Approach to Management*. New York, NY: McGraw-Hill; 1997.

10. http://www.institute.nhs.uk/quality_and_service_improvement_tools/quality_and_service_improvement_tools/driver_diagrams.html

11. www.thenationalacademy.org/ready/change.html

12. Langley GJ, Nolan KM, Nolan TW, et al. *The Improvement Guide*. San Francisco, CA: Jossey-Bass Publishers, Inc.; 2009.

13. Berwick DM. Continuous improvement as an ideal in health. *N Engl J Med*. 1989;320:53–6.

14. Brook R, McGlynn E, Cleary P. Measuring quality of care. *N Engl J Med*. 1996;335:966–70.

15. Berwick DM. Developing and testing changes in delivery of care. *Ann Intern Med*. 1998;128:651–6.

16. Donabedian A. *Explorations in Quality Assessment and Monitoring. Vol. 1: The Definition of Quality and Approaches to its Assessment*. Ann Arbor, MI: Health Administration Press; 1980.

17. Shewhart WA. *Economic Control of Quality of Manufactured Product*. New York, NY: D. Van Nostrand Co.; 1931.

18. Brook RH. Quality of care: do we care? *Ann Intern Med*. 1991;115:486–90.

19. US Dept of Health and Human Services. *Protection of Human Subjects: 45CFR 46*. 2005. http://www.hhs.gov/ohrp/humansubjects/guidance/45cfr46.html

20. Davidoff F, Batalden P, Stevens D, et al. Publication guidelines for quality improvement in health care: evolution of the SQUIRE project. *Qual Saf Health Care*. 2008;17[Supplement 1]:i3–9. www.squire-statement.org

21. Crosby PB. *Quality is Free: The Art of Making Quality Certain*. New York, NY: McGraw-Hill; 1979.

22. Juran J, Godfrey AB. *Juran's Quality Handbook*. New York, NY: McGraw Hill; 1999.

23. Ryan J. *Making the Economic Case for Quality: An American Society for Quality White Paper*. Milwaukee, WI. 2004. http://rube.asq.org/pdf/economic-case/economic-case.pdf

3 Building High Reliability in the Health Care System

Ellen M. Lockhart, Laureen L. Hill, and Alex S. Evers

CLINICAL VIGNETTE

You are an Anesthesiology attending supervising two resident cases in the operating room (OR) today and the fellow will be arriving late.

Case #1 is a thoracic aortic aneurysm repair and general anesthesia has been induced, with invasive monitors are in place, the patient is stable, and the surgical procedure is underway. You are called to start Case #2, which was delayed due to multiple transplants all night, resulting in extra time needed to properly restock your supplies. Case #1 is going well, and you ask the resident to send a blood gas sample to the lab. Point-of-care testing in the OR is not currently available because the analyzer was out for repair so the specimen goes to the central laboratory along with samples from several ORs.

While you are in Case #2, the lab calls with a critical lab value for Case #1. The circulating nurse is busy getting a new instrument for the surgeon who is encountering some bleeding and quickly shouts to your resident that the hemoglobin is 6.3 before going to retrieve the new clamp. The patient becomes hypotensive at this point in the case and requires frequent doses of vasopressors to maintain adequate blood pressure. When the resident hears the hemoglobin is 6.3 with hypotension and acute blood loss, the patient is transfused two units of packed red blood cells for presumed hemorrhagic shock.

At about that time, the OR tech arrives with the lab result slip and the hemoglobin value is 10.8. You call the lab to inquire about the discrepancy and they tell you they realized they called the wrong room because they had multiple critical values and they were too busy dispensing blood for bleeding patients at that moment to remedy the error. The surgical bleeding has now ended and your patient has received an unnecessary transfusion of two units of blood.

- What are the definitions and characteristics of a high reliability organization?
- Describe other types of complex system theory that may be applied to the health care industry.

INTRODUCTION

Hospitals today provide increasingly acute and complex care to sicker patients than ever before. The potential for hazard is constant, and prospect of failure can have tragic outcomes. There is increasing pressure to provide safer care to our patients. Whether it is the wake-up call of the Institute of Medicine report,[1] the desire to more rapidly and seamlessly implement clinical evidence into practice, new regulatory and reimbursement realities, or the public reporting of safety and quality indices, the health care industry is now motivated to make clinical processes more reliable and safe in this high-stakes environment. Other industries such as the commercial airline industry and the nuclear power industry have functioned with high reliability in such a high-stakes environment for many years. Recent study of these high-risk industries has led to identification of features and characteristics that could be employed by the health care industry in its quest to move toward high reliability.[2]

HIGH RELIABILITY ORGANIZATIONS

A high reliability organization (HRO) is one that has succeeded in avoiding catastrophes in an environment where normal accidents can be expected due to constant risk and complexity. HROs maintain a high degree of safety despite functioning in hazardous conditions.[3] Also implicit in this definition is consistency over time. There are varying philosophies and definitions of an HRO; however, several characteristics emerge as common principles. First and foremost, HROs maintain a culture of safety. Not simply a company motto but a defining atmosphere at every level of the organization. Weick and Sutcliffe refer to this as collective mindfulness[3] and further describe the characteristics that are essential. These organizations are preoccupied with failure,[3,4] demonstrate a passionate commitment to excellence,[5] and strive for a zero-defect environment.[6] In such an environment, everyone is keenly aware that even small errors can lead to catastrophe. This culture is so pervasive that staff at every level is encouraged and even required to share concerns and insight, knowing that leadership and team members alike will defer to their expertise.[3,7,8]

Another common feature of HROs is that they pay close attention to operations.[3] They understand how their systems and processes can affect the entire organization. These types of issues clearly played a role in the example above. HROs focus on predicting problems and understand that their systems may fail in ways that they did not anticipate. Deficiencies are actively pursued as opposed to the common practice of responding only to adverse events. This may be accomplished through regular reporting and rounding to identify issues before problems arise.[5] There is also a reluctance to accept simple explanations when events occur.[3] These organizations always dig deeper to understand all potential sources of failure.[4] Once these deficiencies are identified, HROs have in place and employ powerful process improvement to resolve them.[5]

When problems arise, as they inevitably do, the HRO must be very resilient.[3] An HRO understands that, despite considerable safeguards, a system may fail. They utilize systems of care that catch errors before they can reach patients, yet when failures happen they know how to respond, and use swift problem solving to contain errors and improvise to keep systems functioning.[8] Because of this resilience, HRO health care teams can maintain constant vigilance amidst staffing crises, incessant interruptions, and unexpected changes in patient status.[8]

CREATING AN INFRASTRUCTURE FOR QUALITY

Engaging Leadership

Becoming an HRO requires a true long-term commitment to quality. Having the support of the board of directors and senior leadership is essential to this process.[9,10] The role of leadership is to make safety and quality a high priority focus for their organization. They must frame the agenda, align incentives, and ensure that the overall strategy is aligned with the mission.[5,11] The importance of a fully engaged and supportive leadership cannot be underestimated. Emerging evidence suggests that board's engagement in quality may actually affect organizational performance and patient outcomes.[10] Interviews of hospital board members and CEOs revealed that significant progress is needed in educating hospital leadership about quality improvement (QI) and in recruiting board members with safety expertise.[10]

The Role of Middle Managers

Research on health care innovation implementation has focused on the roles of executives and physicians, but middle managers are largely overlooked.[12] Middle managers function as the intermediary between the executives and the front line. They have the ability to exert upward influence by collating information and elevating issues, as well as downward influence via their interface with the front line. They are the implementers of strategy and are responsible for conveying the company culture to the frontline workers, both through their actions and process development. Their behaviors must consistently support the mission.

Role of Trainees

Trainees are an integral part of many medical services, yet they sometimes do not view themselves as a member of the working team, and therefore not responsible for processes. In actuality, they are important members of the team but require education about their roles and the importance of their participation in established processes. Work flows must be designed to incorporate revolving team members and to ensure that they are properly introduced to the culture of safety. Additional efforts may be required to properly educate trainees about their roles on the team, and it is essential to provide this training. In addition, this is a valuable opportunity to influence behavior early in their careers, which may contribute significantly to a culture of patient safety and the development of HROs.[13]

Responsibility of Frontline Workers

Much of the direct knowledge for successful operations resides here at the front line where the core defining activity for a particular industry takes place.[14] Those working here hold the keys to successful processes. Their knowledge and expertise should be valued, and they must feel empowered to speak up with thoughts and concerns.[14,15]

MANAGING A COMPLEX SYSTEM

Complexity and Normal Accidents

Health care is a high-risk and complex system characterized by multiple component parts that are often tightly coupled. Even trivial failures in two or more system elements may lead to catastrophic outcomes when those failures interact in critical and unanticipated ways. The paradoxical concept of "normal accident" cannot be attributed to poor design, faulty equipment, flawed processes, or operator error as discrete failures but rather is due to the interactive complexity of the system itself. Tightly coupled systems where subcomponents have prompt and significant impact on each other make accidents "normal" or inevitable.

In considering the clinical vignette above, the primary cause of the unnecessary transfusion was not the absent fellow, the unstocked cart, the broken blood gas analyzer, or the defective surgical clamp, all component failures that by themselves might have otherwise been insufficient to produce harm. Instead, the unpredictable and interdependent ways those and several other failures converged and the fact that those failures could not be immediately observed or understood by the operator led to the accidental transfusion.

It is likely that an investigation of the accident above would cite "operator error" as the primary failure. An appropriate read-back technique was not employed by the nurse and lab tech on the phone because of the urgent need for a surgical clamp and the anesthesiology resident did not pursue confirmation of the verbal report prior to administering blood given the feasibility of low hemoglobin in the clinical context. In his work on normal accident theory, Charles Perrow cautions that operator error, cited in 60–80% of accident investigations, is to be expected when operators must respond to anomalous information and unforeseen failures for which no amount of training or standardized operating procedures can prepare them.[16] This is not to suggest organizations should "throw in the towel" and accept accidents as unavoidable and operators unaccountable, but it does highlight the paradoxical demands on organizations in managing risk. On one hand, operators must follow centralized and standardized policies and protocols and avoid taking actions whose consequences have not been analyzed. In contrast, operators must also respond correctly and quickly to all incidents and failures including those that organizations could not imagine and for which operators must think and act independently. It is not reasonable to expect any complex organization to meet both of these criteria without incident. If accidents in complex systems are "normal," then health care organizations must develop strategies to learn from failures and to gain insight into the unplanned and unimaginable.

Ultrasafe versus Resilient Systems

Human factors research uses scientific methods to study why errors occur and how to improve system performance and prevent accidental harm.[17] Human factors is not about eliminating human error or teaching people to modify their behavior, but designing systems that are resilient to unanticipated events. Ultrasafe systems such as civil aviation and nuclear power industries have adopted strategies that have yet to be applied in health care.[18,19] Becoming an ultrasafe industry requires acceptance of certain constraints on activity and a conscious trade-off among safety goals, performance goals, and professional autonomy. Health care must address the same barriers that other industries have faced in striving toward ultrasafety with a few additional industry-specific challenges. The magnitude and impact of human error are unclear in medicine because risks are not homogeneous (i.e., elective vs. emergent conditions) and may be attributed to disease, patient factors, medical decisions, or implementation of those decisions.

Several barriers to reducing unsafe medical care have been identified, chief among them are the need to control maximum production, the use of the equivalent actor principle, and the need for standardization of practices.[20] Increasing economic pressures on health care organizations and providers drive productivity and financial performance goals that may compromise safety and lead to adverse events. When the maximum performance of systems or individuals is unlimited or even encouraged, autonomous decisions are tolerated without regulation or constraints and the risk for adverse events increases. While advances in medicine would not be possible without a willingness to push boundaries or attempt the unthinkable (i.e., organ transplantation or cardiopulmonary bypass), such extraordinary practices are associated with higher levels of risk. Certain sectors of health care such as trauma surgery or labor and delivery are subject to unstable conditions including unpredictable demands, variable patient acuity, and inconsistent team composition, making them inherently less safe. Most sectors of health care, including elective surgery and anesthesia, operate under more stable conditions where achieving ultrasafety will require production limitations, practice standardization, and constraints on provider autonomy. As demonstrated in the vignette above, however, such distinctions may become blurred in a complex health care system where stable and unstable conditions coexist, that is, multiple transplants the prior night strained the system and led to a failure in stocking supply carts for the elective schedule, delayed the OR schedule, overwhelmed intensive care unit (ICU) bed capacity, and created a bottleneck in post-anesthesia care unit (PACU) patient flow. Systemic thinking and planning remain a challenge in health care where teams must anticipate consequences across departments and services.

Another difficult barrier in health care is the concept of the "equivalent actor" in which professionals must abandon their identity as individual craftsmen and accept their equivalence to peers in a highly standardized practice.[20] Anesthesiologists, radiologists, pharmacists, and pilots are examples of professionals that have embraced this concept and perform interchangeably in a highly standardized practice with safety rates that far exceed those who have not yet made that transition.

Unintended Consequences of Quality Initiatives

When a review of a patient safety event leads to a determination that the cause is "human error," it is not uncommon for health care organizations to try and modify the behavior of an individual or group through education or retraining.[21] Unfortunately, this approach has been shown to be ineffective or weak as a safety intervention, and when adopted as the primary solution to eradicate "human error," the organization may fall short of truly achieving reductions in harm.[17] Another common approach to adverse events is to focus on protocols, rules, and checklists.

Safety rules continue to grow rapidly and are essential in a safe system, but the accumulation of guidelines and checklists that are intended to defend against error and constrain human action may make the system overly complex and burdensome. Even when well developed and accepted by end users, checklist repetition has the potential to produce complacency and cognitive drift. If a system is designed with only a limited sphere of safe operation, violations are very likely to occur under real-world conditions.[22,23]

In his work on the subject, Amalberti explains the time course and the manner in which external pressures drive organizations or individuals to violate safety rules and migrate to the boundaries of safety.[24] He advises that while violations are not desirable, they are best understood as adaptations to evolving medical knowledge, staffing, and environment and must be managed at a clinical level, modifying procedures and standards accordingly.

In recent years, much has been published and celebrated about so-called "zero risk" and "never events" in health care.[25,26] Insurance networks have limited reimbursement for several health care–associated conditions on the grounds that they are preventable. This flawed concept ignores the fact that sources of risk in health care are complex and not exclusively attributable to error. Using surgical infections as an example, patients living in chronic care facilities, having higher-risk procedures, requiring more invasive care, or longer length of stay are more likely to develop infection than a low-risk patient undergoing a short "clean" procedure, even when precautions are taken and no "mistakes" are committed. Accepting the notion of zero risk or zero tolerance threatens the very risk management efforts behind voluntary reporting and root cause analyses designed to understand adverse events and improve safety and quality.[27] Carlet et al. suggest the preferred term "zero tolerance to passivity" to distinguish risk reduction from zero risk.

The concern for unintended consequences in the quest for safer health care cannot be overemphasized. Just as clinicians need to learn from their mistakes in their patient care, so too should policy makers. Extrapolation from clinical studies or adoption of unproven, unvalidated measures to develop guidelines and performance indicators can lead to harm. Time to first antibiotic (TFAD) is a measure developed for patients presenting with community-acquired pneumonia, with a target of antibiotic administration within 4 hours from presentation to the hospital. Wachter et al. describe the flaws with the first truly dangerous measure in the era of public quality reporting:

> "In the days before measurement of TFAD, patients with uncertain diagnoses would continue to be evaluated until the diagnosis was clarified. However, the TFAD standard completely transformed the dynamic: Faced with a patient who might have pneumonia, the emergency medicine physician now has a strong incentive (almost always buttressed by social pressure and sometimes by financial incentives) to give antibiotics before 4 hours have passed, even when he or she is still unsure of the diagnosis."[28]

In their cautionary tale, the authors highlight the complexity of improving safety in health care, and urge use of evidence grounded in scientific method, need for engaging end users in measure development, and awareness of potential biases that may corrupt guideline development.

In addition to reviewing the definitions and characteristics of HRO, it is useful to understand the challenges and opportunities of applying this theory to health care. While there are many examples of high-functioning systems in health care, several challenges remain. In comparison to other industries, adoption of recommended standards in medicine is sometimes delayed and inadequate.[29,30] In many instances, there is a lack of clear frameworks with which to measure our progress. Scorecards are not always sufficient.[11] Valid, target-specific data may be lacking,[11] and data acquisition in general suffers from lack of standardization and coordination of databases (even within a single institution). Some of the answers are simply unknown. How can we measure our progress with 30-day postoperative mortality when there is inadequate detail about global perioperative 30-day mortality and no risk-adjusted 30-day mortality data?

In addition to these issues, there are several cultural issues in medicine that may be at odds with HRO theory. Our industry has historically been geared toward physician autonomy. In some instances, this can lead to practices that are not data driven and run counter to standardized process development. The hierarchy in medicine, especially between physicians and nurses, can impede proper coordination required for an HRO.[31] This often leads to communication problems and failure of frontline workers to speak up and participate.

While studying high reliability in other types of industries has proven useful, some argue for caution when extrapolating HRO theory to health care. There is high variability in patients, within teams, and across a single system.[32] Our challenge is to take these ideas and refine concepts that are relevant to health care. Having defined some important concepts, it is useful to consider the path that an organization may take as they strive to improve clinical care and patient safety. The first step is to define the goals. Clearly, one goal should be to eliminate medical errors. These are the most conspicuous aspects of poor patient outcome and can lead to morbidity and mortality.

It is equally important to look at more global outcomes. Medical errors do not always lead to adverse outcomes, and adverse outcomes are not always the result of medical errors; indeed, clear-cut errors cause only a minority of poor outcomes. A true HRO should both prevent errors and minimize preventable adverse outcomes. The second step is to define metrics. What are we trying to accomplish, what should we measure, how are we going to measure it, how will we quantify results, and how will these data be used to improve outcomes? After defining metrics, an organization should then develop tools and protocols aimed at improving outcomes. Unfortunately, for some, this is the end of the operation, when in actuality what follows is the most important and most difficult part of the process, the implementation. This is where all levels of the organization, from leadership to frontline workers, must be engaged. Once processes have been implemented, then proper follow-up, reevaluation, and adjustments are required.

There is much to be learned from high-risk organizational theory as well as other doctrines such as human factors, teamwork philosophy,[31] and normal accident theory.[33] In addition to understanding these ideas, we must work to identify particular concepts that should be applied to health care as well as understanding potential negative consequences of their application. All of these steps as well as addressing cultural or other systemic issues are essential components of achieving high reliability status in health care.

KEY POINTS
- High reliability organizations maintain a strong culture of safety, what has been termed a collective mindfulness.
- High reliability organizations pay close to operations and how these systems can affect outcomes.
- Engaging the entire organization, from senior leadership to frontline workers, is crucial to achieving high reliability status.
- Health care is a complex system whose parts are tightly coupled making it vulnerable to "normal accidents."
- Human factors theory is not about eliminating human error or teaching people to modify their behavior, but designing systems that are resilient to unanticipated events.
- The health care industry must be cognizant of potential unintended consequences of its efforts.
- In addition to understanding organizational theory, the health care must address cultural and other barriers to achieving high reliability status.

ONLINE RESOURCES
1. High Reliability in Healthcare: http://www.jointcommission.org/highreliability. aspx
2. Joint Commission Center for Transforming Healthcare: http://www.centerfortransforminghealthcare.org

REFERENCES

1. Kohn L, Corrigan J, Donaldson M, eds. *To Err Is Human: Building a Safer Health System.* Washington, DC: National Academy Press; 1999.
2. Reason J. Human error: models and management. *BMJ.* 2000;320(7237):768–70.
3. Weick K, Sutcliffe K. *Managing the Unexpected: Assuring High Performance in an Age of Complexity.* 1st ed. San Francisco, CA: Jossey-Bass; 2001.
4. Gamble M. 5 Traits of high reliability organizations: how to hardwire each in your organization. *Becker's Hospital Review.* 2013;29:2013.
5. Chassin MR, Loeb JM. The ongoing quality improvement journey: next stop, high reliability. *Health Aff (Millwood).* 2011;30(4):559–68.
6. May EL. The power of zero: steps toward high reliability healthcare. *Health Exec.* 2013;28(2):16–8, 20, 22 passim.
7. Shabot MM, Monroe D, Inurria J, et al. Memorial Hermann: high reliability from board to bedside. *Jt Comm J Qual Patient Saf.* 2013;39(6):253–7.
8. McKeon LM, Oswaks JD, Cunningham PD. Safeguarding patients: complexity science, high reliability organizations, and implications for team training in healthcare. *Clin Nurse Spec.* 2006;20(6):298–304; quiz 305–296.
9. Punke H. Turning healthcare in to a high reliability industry: memorial Hermann shares 5 steps. *Becker's Hospital Review.* 2013. Accessed 3/18/13.
10. Joshi MS, Hines SC. Getting the board on board: engaging hospital boards in quality and patient safety. *Jt Comm J Qual Patient Saf.* 2006;32(4):179–87.
11. Pronovost PJ, Berenholtz SM, Goeschel CA, et al. Creating high reliability in health care organizations. *Health Serv Res.* 2006;41(4 Pt 2):1599–617.
12. Birken SA, Lee SY, Weiner BJ, et al. Improving the effectiveness of health care innovation implementation: middle managers as change agents. *Med Care Res Rev.* 2013;70(1):29–45.
13. Barnsteiner J. Teaching the culture of safety. *Online J Issues Nurs.* 2011;13(3):5.
14. Matlow A. Front-line ownership: imagine. *Healthc Pap.* 2013;13(1):69–74; discussion 78–82.
15. Frankel AS, Leonard MW, Denham CR. Fair and just culture, team behavior, and leadership engagement: the tools to achieve high reliability. *Health Serv Res.* 2006;41(4 Pt 2):1690–709.
16. Perrow C. *Normal Accidents: Living with High Risk Technologies.* New York: Basic Books; 1984.
17. Scanlon MC, Karsh BT. Value of human factors to medication and patient safety in the intensive care unit. *Crit Care Med.* 2010;38(6 suppl):S90–6.
18. Barach P, Small SD. Reporting and preventing medical mishaps: lessons from non-medical near miss reporting systems. *BMJ.* 2000;320(7237):759–63.
19. Apostolakis G, Barach P. Lessons learned from nuclear power. In: Hatlie M, Tavill K, eds. *Patient Safety: International Textbook.* New York: Aspen; 2003:205–25.
20. Amalberti R, Auroy Y, Berwick D, et al. Five system barriers to achieving ultrasafe health care. *Ann Intern Med.* 2005;142(9):756–64.
21. Dekker S. *The Field Guide to Understanding Human Error.* Burlington, VT: Ashgate Publishing Company; 2006.
22. de Saint Maurice G, Auroy Y, Vincent C, et al. The natural lifespan of a safety policy: violations and system migration in anaesthesia. *Qual Saf Health Care.* 2010;19(4):327–31.
23. Amalberti R, Vincent C, Auroy Y, et al. Violations and migrations in health care: a framework for understanding and management. *Qual Saf Health Care.* 2006;15(suppl 1):i66–71.
24. Amalberti R. The paradoxes of almost totally safe transportation systems. *Saf Sci* 2001;37:109–26.
25. Jarvis WR. The Lowbury Lecture. The United States approach to strategies in the battle against healthcare-associated infections, 2006: transitioning from benchmarking to zero tolerance and clinician accountability. *J Hosp Infect.* 2007;65(suppl 2):3–9.
26. Set a goal of zero central line and VAP infections. Determining what is really preventable. *Hosp Peer Rev.* 2008;33(1):4–5.

27. Carlet J, Fabry J, Amalberti R, et al. The "zero risk" concept for hospital-acquired infections: a risky business! *Clin Infect Dis.* 2009;49(5):747–9.
28. Wachter RM, Flanders SA, Fee C, et al. Public reporting of antibiotic timing in patients with pneumonia: lessons from a flawed performance measure. *Ann Intern Med.* 2008;149(1):29–32.
29. McGlynn EA, Asch SM, Adams J, et al. The quality of health care delivered to adults in the United States. *N Engl J Med.* 2003;348(26):2635–45.
30. Resar RK. Making noncatastrophic health care processes reliable: learning to walk before running in creating high-reliability organizations. *Health Serv Res.* 2006;41(4 Pt 2):1677–89.
31. Baker DP, Day R, Salas E. Teamwork as an essential component of high-reliability organizations. *Health Serv Res.* 2006;41(4 Pt 2):1576–98.
32. Vincent C, Benn J, Hanna GB. High reliability in health care. *BMJ.* 340:c84.
33. Tamuz M, Harrison MI. Improving patient safety in hospitals: contributions of high-reliability theory and normal accident theory. *Health Serv Res.* 2006;41(4 Pt 2):1654–76.

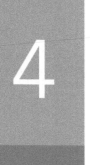

4

Quality Improvement and Patient Safety Tools

Binjon Sriratana and Anshuman Sharma

CLINICAL VIGNETTE

In a large university hospital, the cancellation rate for patients scheduled to undergo elective surgical or diagnostic procedures requiring anesthesia remains more than 1.8%. A preoperative assessment and planning clinic is established to optimize preoperative care and reduce the unwarranted cancellation rate. Using an electronic patient boarding system, waiting times were observed to be increasing. This has resulted in a rise in patient complaints and frustration of nursing staff. The administration wants to decrease the preoperative assessment clinic waiting times (defined as the time from patient's scheduled appointment to MD/advanced practice nurse [APN] encounter) in order to decrease overtime hours and complaints and increase clinic visits.

- What are important components to consider before making a change to the system?
- What tools can the team use to develop and monitor an improvement project?

INTRODUCTION

Current health care delivery is clearly the best and the most complex the world has ever seen. With the help of modern medicine, substantial gains have been made in increasing the life expectancy and in improving the quality of life for millions of patients. Yet, it frequently falls short of its theoretical potential. The Institute of Medicine defines quality as "the degree to which health services for individuals and populations increase the likelihood of desired health outcomes and consistent with current professional knowledge."[1] Quality problems on health care delivery are reflected in the wide variation in the use of medical treatment: underuse of some and overuse of others, and an unacceptable high number of preventable errors. This significant "quality gap" between what is achieved and what can be achieved has been highlighted in medical literature for more than two decades.[1,2] As a result of increasing national attention, patient safety concerns and quality improvement (QI) methods are being integrated in routine medical practices and medical education.

This chapter aims to introduce medical professionals to QI and patient safety tools that are frequently used in health care settings. Most of these tools have been adopted from other high-risk industries. Further references are provided at the end of the chapter for in-depth review.

SCIENCE OF QUALITY IMPROVEMENT

"Every system is perfectly designed to achieve the results it achieves." This fundamental model of health care delivery was conceptualized by Avedis Donabedian MD in 1966.[2] Improvements in individual performances can produce at best a minor, and often nonsustainable, improvement in the output. This shift in focus, from the performance and efforts of an individual health care worker to the system and process-based model of care delivery, is relatively new in modern medicine.

In this chapter, we first describe the basic concepts in the science of QI, followed by commonly used QI tools.

The science of improvement is concerned with how availability of new knowledge of a specific subject matter is applied in routine clinical situations. The fundamental principles of QI are iteration and critical thinking—generating the hypothesis, testing the hypothesis, and, once the hypothesis is confirmed, or negated, executing the cycle again to extend the knowledge further. W. Edward Deming first applied these principles to QI and developed the "System of Profound Knowledge" necessary for making changes that will result in improvement.[3] The word "profound" stresses that deep insightful knowledge of the existing system; an understanding of theories of systems, variance, and human psychology is necessary for making improvement changes.

Appreciating the System

The health care delivery model is a complex, tightly coupled, and dependent system. For example, a detailed preoperative evaluation of a patient requires good communication across the offices of the surgeon, primary care physician, internists, specialist, and anesthesiologist. Depending upon the patient's condition, additional preoperative diagnostic tests may need to be ordered, results of which influence anesthetic plan or may result in the modification, delay, or cancellation of the surgery. Introduction of any change in this complex, highly interdependent, and tightly coupled system has ramifications across many departments. Therefore, it is essential that QI teams develop a deep understanding of the existing system. There are a number of tools that can be used to understand how the current process works. This "mapping" of any process can be achieved by using either of the following tools:

- Flow diagrams: A flow diagram or flowchart is a graphic display of the series of activities that constitutes a process. These charts are extremely helpful in defining the scope of the improvement project, identifying bottlenecks, and understanding relationships between the division and key decision points that affect the final outcome.
- Value stream mapping: Value stream mapping is a variation of flowchart that displays process flow along with the controls for information flow. These types of charts are commonly used in lean improvement projects.
- Causal loop diagram: Causal loop diagram is used to identify and graphically represent dependency between variables and the dynamic nature of the relationship. More complex methods such as dynamic simulation and linkage of processes may be required to develop understanding highly complex processes that cut across many departments or organization.

After developing a thorough understanding of the process system, one must define the boundaries for the QI project. A too ambitious change often results in failure. Additional information is often needed including the opinions of frontline workers.

Understanding Variation

Variance is expected in all processes. For example, time taken to perform a preoperative evaluation in the clinic varies between patients and between health care providers. These differences may stem from differences in the patient's medical history, preoperative tests needed, and their social background. This type of variation is called common cause variation. On the other hand, special cause variation stems from reasons that are not integral to the process. For example, if one of the physicians orders a preoperative echo for every patient over sixty as part of the preoperative testing where as others do not, his visit timings may be high because of this "special cause" variation. Statistical theory developed by Walter A. Shewhart highlights the need to identify the specific cause of variation in any output.[4] Special cause variations are easier to fix but often result in a marginal improvement. On the other hand, to reduce common cause variation, the entire process or system revamp is required. A common mistake made during improvement projects is to assign special cause variance to common cause and thus missing an opportunity to improve the existing system. Control or Shewhart charts are types of run charts (see below) that display quality indicators or summary in a run order (usually over time) and are frequently used to differentiate common cause variation from the special cause variation.

Building Knowledge

Making changes and measuring the results is the basis of all improvement efforts. Lessons learned from measuring effects of the introduction of a small change can form the knowledge required for the next cycle. By repeating these cycles, also known as Plan, Do, Study, Act (PDSA) cycles, one can eventually develop a theory that can reliably predict change. This method of developing new knowledge differs from classic randomized controlled trial (RCT) model of developing new knowledge. The knowledge developed by RCT trials heavy great internal validity but may lack implications for day-to-day clinical care. On the other, knowledge developed by improvement projects is often relevant to a local system.

The Human Side of Change

Change is often difficult, and individuals react differently to the proposed change. Understanding human behavior and human interactions is a necessary skill that is required for successful implementation of any QI project. Human motivations must be considered while selecting members of the improvement team. Team leaders also must understand the need to communicate advantages of the proposed change in a clear manner to all those who will be affected both up- and downstream the process flow. Be sure that the team members have in-depth knowledge of the process, and usually, this knowledge resides with the frontline workers or those who work at the sharp end of spear. Management's role is limited to allocate all the resources necessary for the QI team to accomplish the set goal and facilitate with implementation of the change. For our scenario, an ideal team would include of the anesthesiologist, nursing manager, administrative manager, resident physicians, APNs, and nurses. It may also be necessary to include other individuals to assist the improvement process for data collection, interpretation, and analysis of the data.

TOOLS FOR DEVELOPING A CHANGE: THE MODEL FOR IMPROVEMENT

A common framework for achieving improvement is called the Model for Improvement.[5] This model consists of asking three basic questions and is combined with testing an intervention or a new innovation using a PDSA cycle (see Fig. 4-1). These three questions are:

What Are We Trying to Accomplish?

This question sets the aim or goals for the QI project. Aims or the charter of the project should be in the form of a statement. It must be clear and specific as to what needs to be changed or improved. It should be time specific and measurable. It may

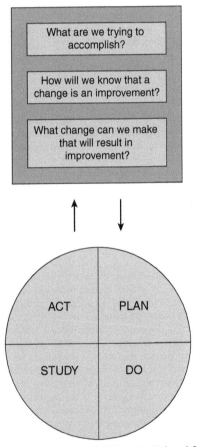

What are we trying to accomplish?

How will we know that a change is an improvement?

What change can we make that will result in improvement?

ACT   PLAN

STUDY   DO

Figure 4-1. The model for improvement and PDSA cycle. (Adapted from Langley GJ, Moen RD, Nolan KM, et al. *The Improvement Guide: A Practical Approach to Enhancing Organizational Performance*, Epub Edition. 2nd ed. San Francisco, CA: John Wiley & Sons Inc; 2009.)

also define the specific population of patients or other systems that will be affected. The following is an example of an effective aim statement for our vignette:

Over the next 6 months we will reduce by 30% the average waiting time, defined as the number of minutes between patient's scheduled appointment and the actual time of encounter with an MD/APN. The aim should specify the system to be improved (the flow of patients), its specific patient population (surgical candidates), its measurable goal (30% decrease in patient waiting time), and specific time frame (within the next 6 months). In addition, the goals have to be realistic. Benchmarking with other successful organizations is one such method that helps the team to avoid utopian goals.

How Will We Know that Change Is an Improvement?

In a complex, tightly coupled system such as a preanesthesia clinic, measurement is a critical part of testing and implementing changes. Measures tell a team whether or not the changes actually yield improvement. A team must develop a set of rigorous, unbiased, quantitative indicators that everyone agrees as an improvement. Donabedian proposed measuring quality of health care by structural, process, and outcome measures.[2] To clarify the perspective of Donabedian, the following are brief descriptions of those measures:

- Structural measures focus on accessibility, availability, and quality of the hospital resources, for example, the number of APNs per 100 patients in a clinic.
- Process measures gauge whether an activity has been accomplished efficiently and reliably. Waiting times in a clinic and frequency of on-time administration of preoperative antibiotic are examples of process measures.
- Outcome measures gauge the impact of treatment on the values of patients, their health, and well-being. Postoperative mortality in 30 days and incidence of severe pain after knee replacement surgery are two such examples of outcome measures. These days, financial and cost measures are commonly being included as outcome measure in most QI projects.
- Balancing measures ensure that improvements made to one system do not sacrifice quality of other measure. In other words, these are related measures that must be maintained or improved but not compromised while implementing the proposed change. For example, surgical cancellation rate could be used as a balancing measure for increased efficiency in the preoperative clinic.

Keep in mind a simple change may not be limited to just one measure. For our vignette, many measures can be considered: minutes of waiting, number of patient complaints, number of patient walkouts (leaving before seeing a doctor), number of overtime hours, number of medical errors (balancing measure), and frequency of surgical cancellations per month due to inadequate preoperative evaluation. These indicators, many of them surrogate for efficient and reliable patient care, are recorded before and after the change is implemented.

What Change Can We Make that Will Result in Improvement?

Change concepts are general notions or approaches found to be useful in developing specific ideas for change that result in improvement. Certain changes are needed to optimize the existing systems and are known as reactive changes. One can say the removing special cause variance is a reactive change. However, if whole new level of performance is required of the system, fundamental changes are needed to revamp the entire system. These changes are aimed to remove or reduce the common cause variance in the system. As mentioned above, making reactive changes to an existing system is easier, but improvement gains are relatively modest. Ideas for developing a fundamental change are readily available and come from the insights of those who have the "profound knowledge" of the system. One simple method is to observe other organizations that have accomplished similar changes. In more complex systems, developing change ideas are complicated and require organized approach. In the last few decades, many tools have been developed to assist with improvement projected related to health care industry. Some of these tools are mentioned below:

• Quality function deployment helps with organizing relationships between process measures and the key factors that affect the performance of these measures. This method provides an efficient way to answer both second and third questions of the model of improvement.
• Pareto Charts: "Pareto principle," commonly called the 80:20 rule, states that relatively few factors are responsible for a majority of the effects. Pareto charts are bar charts that organize various contributing factors according to the magnitude of their effect. This organizing helps identify the "vital few" causes that warrant urgent and most attention.
• Failure mode and effects analysis (FMEA): QI projects will always encounter obstacles, but obstacles can be avoided or manageable if they are planned in advance. The FMEA is one such proactive system that was originally developed by the US military.[6,7] This tool evaluates the processes, identifies the potential failures, and develops methods to prevent potential failures from happening. The Joint Commission has required accredited health care organizations to develop similar risk management strategies.[8] FMEA reviews the steps of the process to identify how and where it might fail (see Fig. 4-2). For our vignette, the preoperative clinic staff can view all of the steps involved in the patient discharge process. One important step to this process is obtaining preoperative labs. Key components to the FMEA are answering these three questions:

1. What could go wrong? (Failure modes) The nurses cannot draw patient blood.
2. Why would the failure happen? (Failure causes) Patient has a difficult venous access. Patient has a port and nurse may not be trained to access the port, provider is inexperienced, or patient refuses.
3. What would be the consequence of each failure? (Failure effects) Delay in clinic discharge and boarding next patient, longer patient waiting time and patient dissatisfaction, and potential delay of surgery.

For each failure mode, a numeric value also known as the Risk Priority Number (RPN) is assigned. This is a subjective value ranging from 1 to 10, meaning "very

Steps in the Process	Failure Mode	Failure Causes	Failure Effects	Likelihood of Occurrence (1–10)	Likelihood of Detection (1–10)	Severity (1–10)	Risk Profile Number (RPN)	Actions to Reduce Occurrence of Failure
1								
2								
3								

Figure 4-2. Failure mode and effect analysis (FMEA) tool. Each step of a process is analyzed to determine the likelihood and severity of failure, and action plans are created to reduce occurrences of failure. Adapted from the Institute for Healthcare Improvement FMEA Tool. (Available on www.IHI.org)

unlikely" to "very likely to occur," respectively. First, use a number to answer the three following questions:

1. How likely will this failure mode occur? (Likelihood of occurrence)
2. How likely will this failure be detected in the failure mode occurs? (Likelihood of detection)
3. What is the severity if this failure were to occur? (Severity)

Next, multiply the three values to calculate the RPN. Compare the RPNs of various failure modes. Those with the lowest number are least likely to occur and/or effect the overall process. However, those with the higher scores create greater burden; therefore, the team should seek actions to reduce the occurrence of failure. The following action plan was developed for a difficult venous access patient: senior nursing staff safely attempts venipuncture on bilateral upper extremities. If not successful, a physician attempts bilateral upper and lower extremities. If still not successful, a physician attempts arterial puncture. Also, consider referring the patient for the placement of preoperative peripherally inserted central catheter (PICC), and make a note in the OR schedule that patient is a difficult access patient.

Health failure mode and effect analysis (HFMEA) is another tool developed by VA's National Center for Patient Safety and is based on FMEA. This method uses hazard analysis by working though the decision tree analysis.[8]

Cause and effect diagram: Also known as fishbone or Ishikawa diagram, it is used to collect, organize, and summarize current knowledge of potential variation. See Figure 4-3. One starts by writing down the problem in a box to the right of an arrow.

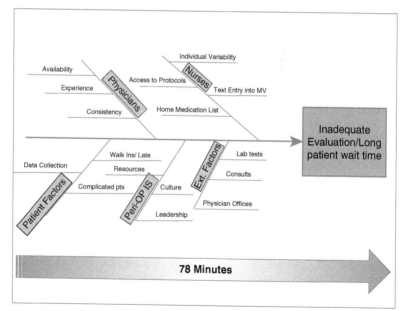

Figure 4-3. Ishikawa or Fishbone diagram: Major factors and variables are shown how they influence the wait time in the clinic.

Identify at least four or more major factors that the team has identified as contributing factors, and add these in the branches of the main arrow. Further subcategories of factors influencing these main factors can be recorded after discussion with the team members. These diagrams can then function as working document that should be updated throughout the project.

Driver diagrams: These are structured logic charts with three or more levels and are commonly used to organize theories and ideas about what changes can be made in order to make an improvement. At minimum, a driver diagram would include a goal, high-level factors, or primary drivers that need to be changed in order to achieve the stated goal and, finally, specific activities that will be needed to make the changes. For more complex projects, number of levels can be expanded.

A meeting was held among the newly assembled team. Feedback from nursing staff was collected using a survey instrument. Ishikawa fishbone diagram was used to identify the major factors that impact patient wait time. It was observed that there was a large variation in how nurses and physicians entered patients' history and physical examination data into electronic medical records. This variance in practice often resulted in inconsistent preoperative workups resulting in higher-than-expected cancellation rate for elective surgeries. A new standardized preoperative form that reduced free text entry was designed and implemented. The team also discovered that the busiest days of the week were Monday afternoons, whereas the number of patients seen on Thursday mornings was consistently low. This coincided to the days with longest and shortest average waiting times of 45 and 25 minutes, respectively. The team proposed a change to staff another resident physician on Mondays.

TESTING THE CHANGE: PLAN, DO, STUDY, ACT CYCLE OR PDSA CYCLE

The PDSA cycles are used to turn the ideas, developed by answering the three above-mentioned questions, into concrete actions. The PDSA cycle is an effective tool that provides detailed steps in testing changes and promotes analytical thinking. The PDSA cycle, initially developed by Deming and later modified by Shewart, has been used by many organizations including health care organization to test and implement change and improve patient care.[4,9] The defining principle of the PDSA cycle is to first test a change in order to provide proof that the proposed change (or a series of changes) will actually result in improvement. This may also help to predict how much improvement can be expected. If a change results in improvement, then it can be implemented on a larger scale. Other option is to extend the tests to gradually include larger samples until you are confident that the change should be more widely adopted. Therefore, it is best to test on a small scale to avoid widespread complications.

As the name suggests, there are four steps in the PDSA cycle:

a. The Planning phase involves answering questions about the change, making predictions about the change, and planning for collecting relevant data. Planning is necessary as it helps team members stay on the same page, prevent hindsight bias, and with designating the responsibilities of team members.
b. During the Do phase, testing the change is begun on a small scale and observations are made in the after-intervention phase. The team also documents other challenges met by the team.

c. During the Study phase, collected data before and after the intervention are compared and other results are studied.
d. During the Act phase, based on the information collected, the team makes a decision about adopting, modifying, or completely abandoning the new change plan. If the plan is modified, another PDSA cycle is initiated.

The PDSA cycle is used sequentially to test changes. Knowledge gained in step "c" and modifications developed in step "d" can be used to develop new cycles. New cycles can also be used to test changes on a larger scale. Once a change is proven to result in improvement, then it should be implemented. As stated before, improvement requires multiple changes. Multiple changes therefore will require multiple tests and PDSA cycles.

After 1 month of introducing new preoperative anesthesia evaluation form and making the changes in the staffing model, significant improvement was noticed in the average time needed to see one patient through the clinic from 78 to 63 minutes. This corresponded with Monday waiting times decreasing from 45 to 39 minutes. The number of overtime hours has decreased by 30%, and the number of complaints has decreased by 40%. Because of the improved patient flow, Thursday clinic times also decreased from 30 to 26 minutes. The team concluded that new preoperative evaluation form and adding a physician on Mondays have resulted in an improvement to the preoperative and assessment clinic. The team also learned from resident physicians that for consistent preoperative testing, guidelines and recommendations from the American Society of Anesthesiology should be posted in the physician offices. Accurate home medication list is another area for improvement identified by the team. Accurate documentation of patient medications is expected to improve preoperative administration of β-blockers and possibly reduce the incidence of postoperative myocardial infarction. The team therefore proposed to make and test these change in a new series of PDSA cycles. The new cycle will need to engage nursing staff from the preoperative surgery area and anesthesiologists that will assist with collection of data regarding postoperative myocardial infarction.

TOOLS FOR MONITORING DATA

There are many tools that provide an easy practical way of tracking and graphically displaying the data collected prior to and after the implementation of the change.

Run Charts

Run charts provide a simple and practical way of tracking and displaying data generated from your changes[10] (see Fig. 4-4). They are essentially line graphs—time intervals are plotted along the x-axis and a measure is plotted along the y-axis. Median and mean values can also be visualized on the chart. For measures and outcomes that happen infrequently, the number of days between two events is a better way to graph the run chart. Annotations can be placed within the chart to show how a change affects the measure and what variables were noted throughout the process. The goal line (at the measured value you aim to achieve) can also be displayed on the chart to better visualize how close the team is to achieving their goal (or aim). Since there are multiple measures used when testing a single change, multiple run charts are developed. Ideally, these charts will prove your changes are yielding improvements. On the other hand, if no improvements are depicted, it can encourage the team that other changes need to be made.

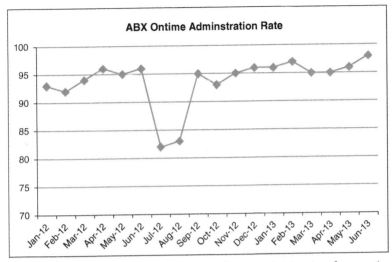

Figure 4-4. Example of a simple run chart. Rate of on-time administration of preoperative antibiotics in patients undergoing total knee replacement surgery. Rates were lowest in July and August of 2012. This may be a case of special cause variation introduced into the system and need further investigation.

Control Charts

A more sophisticated tool is the control chart. As mentioned above, control charts are primarily used as a surveillance tool to monitor the "status quo" of a system. It is used to study how a process changes over time (i.e., how waiting room times have varied over the past couple years). In other words, the primary purpose of the control charts is to display the variance in the existing system and helps in distinguishing between common cause and special cause variations. In commonly displayed control charts, the center line is the mean (or any other measure of central tendency) value of the quality measurement, whereas upper and lower control limits are usually set at 3 standard deviations (σ) above and below the center line, respectively. If the process is in control, or at status quo, 99.7% of all the points will fall between the control limits (upper and lower). If points are found outside the control limits, then it is statistically unlikely due to common cause variation.

There are many types of control charts, and their use depends on the type of data that are being collected and its distribution pattern. For example, p or np charts are used for categorical data, whereas X chart or X bar chart is used for continuous data.[10]

Figure 4-5 is a control chart monitoring our vignettes average waiting times. Note the points lie within the control limits. This means a complete revamp of preoperative clinic is the only method of reducing patient wait time.

ALTERNATIVE APPROACHES TO THE QI PROJECTS

Though PDSA cycles combined with model of improvement are the most commonly used approach to the improvement projects, many other roadmaps are available for use. Some of these approaches are developed for achieving specific aims. For example, lean approach is a systematic approach to identifying and eliminating waste.

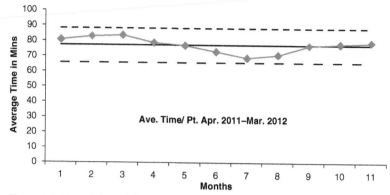

Figure 4-5. Control chart of clinic waiting times over the past 11 months prior to the clinic's improvement project. The upper and lower control limits are shown. Plot demonstrates common cause variation within the control limits. A fundamental change in the system is needed to achieve the stated goal for reducing wait time by 30%.

Six Sigma approach on the other hand assists with reduction in the manufacturing defects. FOCUS-PDCA is another modification of model of improvement where three questions are replaced by Find, Organize, Clarify, Understand, and Select the process improvement. This is followed by the abovementioned PDCA cycle. It is recommended that organization chose one consistent framework for improvement.

SUMMARY

QI is a complex task. However, QI teams are best suited to handle improvement projects only if they develop a good understanding of the process and involve frontline worker in developing the change. A top–down approach usually is met with resistance and produces inconsistent, short-lived benefits if any. Our vignette's improvement team was successful in achieving their goal of decreasing their preoperative clinic waiting times. The team members, in an organized fashion, analyzed the problem using various diagrams and methods of data collection. They made repeated changes, test, and analyzed them using the Model for Improvement and PDSA cycle. They also carefully monitored for improvement using run and control charts. Finally, they were able to identify other improvement ideas that will be tested in the next improvement cycle. Lesson learned from these PDSA cycles may also be used to improve process and patient care in other similar clinics across the hospital.

KEY POINTS

- The three parts of the Model for Improvement are as follows: What are we trying to accomplish? How will we know that change is an improvement? What change can we make that will result in improvement?
- PDSA cycle stands for "Plan, Do, Study, Act."
- Control charts are used to separate common cause variation from special cause variation.

REFERENCES

1. Committee on Quality of Healthcare in America, Institute of Medicine. *Crossing the Quality Chasm: A New Health System for the 21st Century.* Washington, DC: National Academy; 2001.
2. Chassin MR, Kosecoff J, Park RE, et al. Does inappropriate use explain geographic variations in the use of health care services? A study of three procedures. *J Am Med Assoc.* 1987;258:2533–7.
3. Deming WE. *The New Economics.* 2nd ed. Cambridge, MA: Center for Advanced Educational Services, Massachusetts Institute of Technology; 1994.
4. Nolan TW, Provost LP. Understanding variation. *IEEE Eng Manag Rev.* 1996;24:65–74.
5. Langley GJ, Moen RD, Nolan KM, et al. *The Improvement Guide: A Practical Approach to Enhancing Organizational Performance*, Epub Edition. 2nd ed. San Francisco, CA: John Wiley & Sons Inc; 2009.
6. Hughes R. *Patient Safety and Quality: An Evidence-based Handbook for Nurses.* Rockville, MD: Agency for Healthcare Research and Quality, US Dept. of Health and Human Services; 2008.
7. Institute for Healthcare Improvement. http://www.ihi.org/resources/Pages/Tools/FailureModesandEffectsAnalysisTool.aspx. Accessed 11/22/15.
8. Institute for Healthcare Improvement. http://www.ihi.org/resources/Pages/HowtoImprove/default.aspx. Accessed 11/22/15.
9. Donabedian A. *Evaluating the quality of medical care. Milbank Mem Fund Q.* 1966;44:166–206.
10. Wheeler DJ. *Understanding Variation: The Key to Managing Chaos.* 2nd ed. Knoxville, TN: SPC Press; 2000.

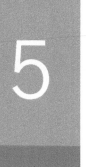

5 Models for Quality
David Vollman, Gokul Kumar, and Michael Stock

CLINICAL VIGNETTE

An 85-year-old man was scheduled to have cataract surgery performed in an outpatient setting. The surgeon had reviewed the patient's preoperative measurements of the eye to select the appropriate lens implant to place after the cataract was removed the night prior to the surgery. On the morning of the surgery, the surgeon became aware that the lens he had selected was out of stock at the surgical facility. He selected a lens that would give a similar refractive outcome for the patient, but it was not his ideal choice. It was later determined that the logistics staff in charge of reordering intraocular lens was bundling lens orders rather than sending in a more timely fashion. In the end, the patient suffered no harm.

- What methodologies can we use to improve systems in health care that ensure patient safety?
- How can we eliminate waste in health care?
- How can Six Sigma and Lean improve quality?

INTRODUCTION

With the increasing cost and growing demand for health care, hospitals, practices, and ancillary services are in need of solutions to both reduce cost and provide higher-quality service with existing resources. Two major models for quality improvement are utilized in health care to identify sustainable solutions: Six Sigma and Lean.

The fundamental goal of Six Sigma is to continuously improve business operations. Originally developed in the 1980s by Motorola, numerous companies started adopting Six Sigma strategies in the 1990s, delivering considerable benefits to operating income. In the 2000s, many authors also suggested Six Sigma applicability to health care.[1] Over the past several years, numerous reports have illustrated the implementation of Six Sigma strategies in multiple health care settings, including some beneficial aspects and some necessary modifications for the health care sector.

Lean is a philosophy accompanied by a varied set of tools that allows an organization to focus on the value it creates for the customer and eliminate wasted resources in its production. The system, which was born and refined in the automobile manufacturing world with Toyota, carries a lot of manufacturing terminology. Its principles and tools, however, can be useful in the design, implementation, and continued execution of all aspects of patient care.

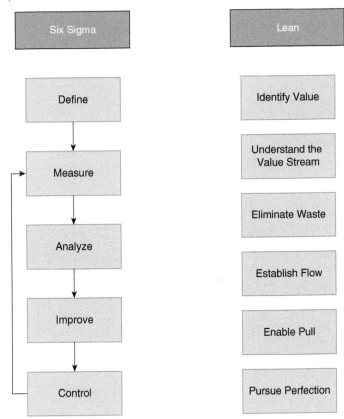

Figure 5-1. Visual representation of Six Sigma and Lean models. (Langley GJ, Moen R, Nolan KM, Nolan TW, eds. *The Improvement Guide: A Practical Approach to Enhancing Organizational Performance.* 2nd ed. San Francisco, CA: Jossey-Bass; 2009.)

This chapter focuses on these two methods of quality improvement by outlining their key concepts and tools to achieve quality improvement and provide some practical applications to the health care industry (see Fig. 5-1).

SIX SIGMA

Methods in Six Sigma

The term sigma, as defined by statisticians, refers to the standard deviation from the mean. In manufacturing and production, a multiple of sigma is used to refer to the amount of defects that are likely to occur in a production process.[2] A widely accepted numerical value is that a Six Sigma process only has 3.4 defects per 1 million opportunities. While the practical application of Six Sigma does not necessitate this statistical occurrence in every process, the use of the term symbolizes the pursuit of significant reduction in the possibility of errors.

The reasoning behind this is straightforward—defects cause an increase in costs. A systematic approach to reducing the occurrence of defects therefore reduces costs overall.

There are two primary project methods used in Six Sigma:

1. DMAIC for established processes (see Fig. 5-1)
   a. Define, Measure, Analyze, Improve, and Control
2. DMADV for new processes
   a. Define, Measure, Analyze, Design, and Verify

A Six Sigma project begins by defining and implementing relevant metrics, which is referred to as the critical to quality (CTQ) characteristics.[3] Then, following the appropriate project methodology above, project leaders guide the execution of a quality improvement project.

Applications of Six Sigma to Health Care

The overall process of Six Sigma is quite applicable to health care, though the nature of the industry and delivery of health care require appropriate adaptations. Generally, four metrics in health care define a system's performance and serve as CTQs for a health care project[4]:

• Service level—for example, wait time, service time, and access to care
• Service cost—for example, cost per unit of service and labor productivity
• Customer satisfaction—patient and family satisfaction and referring physician satisfaction
• Clinical excellence—for example, reduction of infection rates contracted in a hospital and compliance with prescription guidelines

A key concept in translating Six Sigma principles to health care is recognizing that customers are not necessarily patients but can be any person impacted during a particular process. All customers rarely experience the average performance of a metric; instead, they tend to experience the variability.[4] The Six Sigma method attempts to reduce the variability-induced "defect" even if the average performance of a metric is good.

One of the factors that has led to slow adaptation of Six Sigma in health care stems from the perceived discrepancy between an automated manufacturing process and the inherently social interaction of health care, that is, health care is driven by humans.[4] Human variability is often more subtle and variable, leading to difficulty identifying causes of process failures. Multiple reports show that successful implementation of Six Sigma initiative in health care requires a concurrent cultural strategy shift and sound operational strategies to implement change.[4]

DMAIC (Define, Measure, Analyze, Improve, and Control)

For a Six Sigma project following the DMAIC method, once the CTQ is identified, the customer voice needs to be translated into a measurable response variable. For example, a quantifiable clinical excellence variable may be hospital return rate or radiology report time. Next, measurement of the process capability for the appropriate CTQ is performed, yielding a defects per million opportunities (DPMO) number.[4]

In the analyze phase, the Six Sigma team identifies the causal factors likely to have most impact on the previously identified and measured response variable. Then, these factors are categorized as controllable or uncontrollable depending on their contribution to the response variable.[4] Even if a response rate has an acceptable average, if the variability leads to a high DPMO, factors must be identified that lead to this greater variability, as that is the cause of the deficient metric. Controllable factors allow implementation of strategies to directly control the causal factor. Uncontrollable factors necessitate the design of a new process to withstand the variability.[4]

Following the DMAIC protocol, the next phases are improvement and control. These are felt to be most challenging in health care. Organization structure can inhibit process-oriented thinking, and without the necessary oversight and infrastructure, the impetus for change can be limited.[4] The control phase necessitates behavioral changes and translation of project successes in isolated settings to other applicable venues, as the multitude of units and disciplines within health care must function as a cohesive unit.

DMADV (Define, Measure, Analyze, Design, and Verify)

As illustrated above, the DMAIC approach in Six Sigma aims to improve processes that are prone to error due to inherent variability. However, health care institutions also require large changes that cannot come about simply through improvement of existing systems. In these cases, new processes need to be designed altogether. The threshold occurs as optimization is achieved in existing systems, but benefits from those changes plateau. At approximately 4.8 sigma, companies can hit a wall and change is required to achieve further gains.[5] In health care, this wall is felt to occur at earlier levels due to the multitude of old systems and structures in place.[4]

This process is represented by the acronym DMADV (Define, Measure, Analyze, Design, and Verify). A design process in this context includes iteratively breaking down system design requirement into subsystem requirements, in order to properly design a process the first time.[4] For example, staffing needs, reward systems, communication requirements, and information technology needs would be iteratively specified and designed during the process.

Determining Readiness for DMADV

One of the crucial requirements for DMADV projects is to first identify if an organization is ready for these large-scale projects. Institutions with unstable operations and service delivery processes first need to stabilize and optimize these processes through dedicated DMAIC projects. Once this optimization occurs, organizations will always reach the aforementioned "wall."[4] Customer expectations increase and existing legacy systems limit further improvements.

Then, to proceed with DMADV design projects, the following factors need to be considered:

- What is the effectiveness of the current process?
- Is the goal to decrease variability alone or does the entire mean result of a process need to change?
- What are the barriers to change of the current system, including information technology (IT) requirements?
- What upcoming changes are being planned already, such as expansion of facilities, new therapies, and new governmental requirements?

If the above settings seem to necessitate a new design process, a DMADV process can be pursued.[4]

The DMADV Process

The defining and measurement phases of the DMADV process parallel those of the DMAIC process. However, the goal is to predict the performance of the new product or service.[4]

An important tool that can facilitate this process is referred to as quality function deployment (QFD).[4] In QFD, each response variable is plotted against system requirements, with weight given to each response variable by perceived priority. The ability of those system requirements to facilitate change in each response variable is then identified and prioritized. A Pareto analysis can then be utilized to rank each system requirement by its ability to influence the highest priority response variables. It is important to do this measurement and analysis with a focus on the voice of the customer data.[4] A successful execution of the analysis phase then identifies subsystem requirements that will translate into quantifiable result variable improvements.

The design phase then relies upon this mathematical derivation of subsystem requirements to properly correlate with customer satisfaction based on the QFD. This is referred to as capability forecasting.

The validation phase then measures the actual performance of a subsystem process against the predicted performance, as measured by customer satisfaction.[4] While this system may be more straightforward in manufacturing, the ability to test each subsystem in a health care setting may not be feasible. Inherent in this process is targeted changes in recruitment, staff development, communication, and information technology.[4]

Implementation of Six Sigma

Successful implementation of Six Sigma in a large organization is felt to be contingent on implementation of numerous operational strategies outside of Six Sigma. In addition, the system relies on a unique managerial structure by defining quality management professionals in an organization.[6] Specifically, these include the following:

- Executive leadership—CEO and other top management that can oversee continuous quality improvement
- Champions—Oversee Six Sigma implementation throughout the organization
- Master Black Belts—Devote 100% of time to Six Sigma. Roles include statistical analysis, assisting champions, and overseeing Black Belts.
- Black Belts—Lead a team on a project and mentor Green and Yellow Belts
- Green and Yellow Belts—A trained member who participates fully in the projects, including data management and statistical analysis

While the above roles have evolved with time and organization, the fundamental principle of strict organization and commitment to the Six Sigma initiative is integral to success of the projects within the organization.[7]

LEAN

The Philosophy of Lean

The foundation of all Lean thinking is best summarized by Taiichi Ohno, an industrial engineer considered to be the father of the Toyota Production System[8]:

"The basis of the Toyota Production System is the absolute elimination of waste."

Lean's goal is to identify those aspects of a product or service that provide value to the customer, define the processes that produce this value, and eliminate the rest.

TABLE 5-1	Types of Lean Waste	
Type of Waste	Quick Definition	Health Care Examples
Muda	Waste	*Type 1*: Filling out a medical reconciliation for a patient admitted to the hospital adds no direct value from the patient perspective but is necessary as a patient safety tool *Type 2*: Time spent by staff looking for equipment that is not stored properly or in a sensible location
Muri	Overburden	Having a nurse needing to go to multiple floors to find the proper IV supplies because his or her storeroom is continually out while actively participating in patient care
Mura	Unevenness (variation)	The unpredictability of patients arriving to the emergency department can make staffing challenging

Anything that does not directly contribute to the creation of value should be eliminated.

Before eliminating waste, you must identify "value." In Lean, for an action to be value adding, it must fulfill the following three criteria[8]:

1. The customer is willing to pay for it.
2. The action must transform the form, fit, or function of the product.
3. The action must be done correctly the first time.

If any aspect of an action does not meet these criteria, it is considered waste and should be eliminated.

Lean defines three different types of waste (see Table 5-1).[8] Most prominent is "muda," meaning non–value-adding work. Two types of muda exist. Type I muda is work that does not add value but is necessary at the current time and with the current technology to create value. For example, filling out a medical reconciliation for a patient admitted to the hospital adds no direct value from the patient perspective but is necessary as a patient safety tool. Type II is work that does not add value and is not necessary to create value. This type of muda could be illustrated by time spent by staff looking for equipment that is not stored properly or in a sensible location. The tools of Lean focus on identifying and eliminating type II muda.

Within muda, there are seven original (and several subsequently added) categories.[9] Knowledge of these categories allows you to look at the process from many different perspectives to identify and eliminate waste. The original seven muda can be remembered by the mnemonic TIM WOOD.

Transport—the process of relocating resources
Inventory—having more than is needed for the task at hand
Motion—added movement of resources that does not add value

Waiting—wasted time when people, information, or resources are not readily available

Overproduction—redundant or duplicate work

Overprocessing—the wrong tool or sequence of step being used for the task

Defects—work that contains errors or lacks value

Additional types of muda include unmet customer demands and unused human talent.[10] The two other types of waste, mura and muri, may not be as obvious but can provide insight into creating better processes. Mura, "unevenness," is a waste that might be better defined as "inconsistency." If a process has not been standardized or the people implementing it have not been appropriately trained, the process will inconsistently perform—both with respect to time it takes to complete and quality of the outcome. This "unevenness" of the process directly leads to muda.

Muri, "overburdened," is the waste that occurs when a greater level of performance from a process is asked for than it can handle without taking shortcuts and informally modifying decision criteria. This overburdened state directly leads to inconsistency in results for the process (mura), which directly causes non–value-adding work (muda). As an example, when creating a new process for IV placement, if not all of the nurses are trained in the new process (muri), tracking of IV placement outcomes will show great variance in the results (mura). The variability will appear in real time as the muda of defects (poor IV placements), motion (nurse going to get more supplies for alternative attempts), and waiting (needing to get another nurse to help).

Lean has a number of concepts and tools to help identify value and waste and begin the elimination process. Most central to Lean is the concept of "kaizen," continuous improvement.[8] Kaizen is the process of continuously making incremental improvements in processes, consistently eliminating waste, and striving toward sculpting a "perfect" process. Each member of an organization, from the CEO to the janitor, is expected to contribute to kaizen, seeking out and finding new innovative way to eliminate waste.

Pull Systems in Lean

Another center concept of Lean is creating "Pull" systems,[8,11] also known as "just-in-time." Pull is a Lean strategy inherently structured to eliminate waste, especially the muda of overproduction. In a batch-and-queue manufacturing process, managers will attempt to predict the future demand of a product. In this "PUSH" system, the amount of product expected to meet demand is produced and stored in inventory. As demand occurs, the product is pulled from inventory and delivered to the customer. Due to the inherent difficulties of predicting future demand, even with historical trends, they are likely to miss the true mark. If demand is lower than expected, a great deal of overproduction muda will occur. If demand is higher than expected, unless the manufacturing process has been "leaned" out, they will lose customers to the long wait time.

In a Pull system, no product is produced until signaled from a downstream demand. For example, a customer orders a loaf of bread at a bakery. That downstream demand signals to the baker to make a loaf of bread. To make the bread, the baker uses flour, milk, and eggs, which become a signal to the farmer to mill more flour and milk the cows. It is obvious that a Pull system creates less waste especially in terms of inventory. However, such a process in a time-sensitive industry may create long lead times (the time from order to delivery).

In a perfect Lean process, the lead time is short enough to respond in real time to fluctuations in demand. In reality, a Lean process is not completely inventory-free but rather has a buffer of intermediate materials and resources to continue to run while upstream processes have time to respond to the downstream signaling. The important aspect of a Pull system is that clear signaling (called kanban[11]) to upstream processes occurs in real time and directs them to create the appropriate amount and the appropriate time. For example, in the clinical vignette at the beginning of the chapter, most facilities maintain a small consignment of intraocular lenses (usually 2–3) in the most frequently used powers and then the lenses are replaced in consignment as the lenses are utilized so that the hospital or surgical center does not need to maintain a large inventory of lenses, which can take considerable space. Once a lens is used in surgery, the lens sticker from the case is transmitted to the logistics or ordering department so that consignment levels can be maintained.

Implementing the Lean Mind-Set

Lean can be used for "quick fixes," but the gains will be short-lived. True Lean implementation requires a commitment by all parties or all levels of an organization. The organization as a whole organism should express explicitly the goal of "the absolute elimination of waste." From the architecture to the accounting department to the operating rooms, all stakeholders must direct their thoughts and acts toward this goal.

The Lean mind-set in an organization's culture can be seeded and nurtured through having a number of "kaizen events."[12] While a bit of a misnomer, a kaizen event formalizes and encapsulates all of the steps necessary to bring about change. These events introduce the participants to the philosophy, concepts, and tools of Lean. Also, through having a mix of people at an event—both people with intimate knowledge of the process and those inexperienced—it becomes clear that all need to have a hand in kaizen. In this dynamic, the inexperienced participants are forced to ask a series of "why" questions.[8] (Why do you do it this way? Why does this need to happen?) These questions force the more experienced to clearly explain the reason for why things are done and begin to highlight, with each subsequent why, that there may not be a great reason to perform certain tasks in certain ways.

While the "5 Why" is one tool used in Lean, there are a wide array of tools. Each of these tools has been created pragmatically to help solve a different problem using Lean thinking. One of the major tools used in Lean is value stream mapping[13] (see Fig. 5-2). This tool is widely used to analyze and design the flow of materials, information, and resources to deliver a valued outcome. Once a process is mapped out in detail, it becomes clear where waste is occurring and creates a kaizen opportunity (see Fig. 5-3).

From Manufacturing to Service

As is evident from the terminology of Lean, it developed from manufacturing.[14] With care, these concepts can be transferred to other industries including health care services.[15] When making this transition, it is important to translate some of the definitions so as not to leave out important aspects of service. Most notably, identifying value-added aspects in a patient care experience can be far more difficult than the value-added components of a static product. While efficiency and speed are king in manufacturing, certain aspects of patient care should be viewed in the same light. As a general rule, the "things" of health care (notes, procedures, tests) should be "leaned"

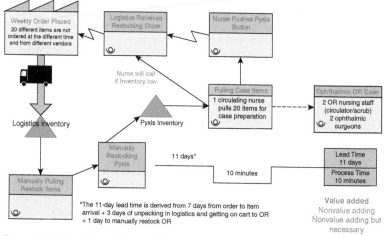

Figure 5-2. Value Stream Current State Map of Ophthalmology OR supply ordering in a hospital-based setting.

out, but in any aspect involving patient interaction, value lies in the direct interaction and human connection. This should not be seen as something to lean out.

Also, in a service industry, certain behaviors can and should be acutely focused on as a source of value or waste. Behaviors such as cheerfulness, courtesy, respect, and well dressed should not be overlooked when planning, implementing, and evaluating processes.

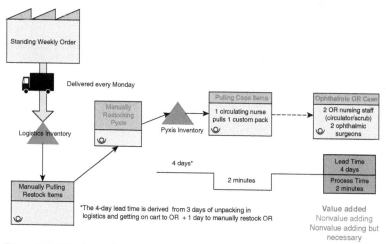

Figure 5-3. Value Stream Future State Map of Ophthalmology OR supply ordering in a hospital-based setting after completing kaizen event analysis.

DIFFICULTIES AND LIMITATIONS OF SIX SIGMA AND LEAN IN HEALTH CARE

One of the biggest obstacles to implementing sustainable Lean or Six Sigma process changes is the required support of upper management. In Six Sigma, both the DMAIC and DMADV processes require appropriate support of leadership in execution of the process and in its implementation. For Lean to be continuous, the mindset must pervade the entire organization.[12,15] Frequently, management believes that for change to occur, it must happen from a top–down approach. However, waste is most easily seen at the level at which it is produced. The frontline worker will recognize the kaizen opportunity long before those not intimately involved in the process. Mentors from upper levels should aid in the process and provide resources to help tackle the identified waste.

The rigid nature of Six Sigma or Lean is felt to focus attention more on methods and tools and not on direct organizational robustness.[16] This emphasis on a model-based approach may hinder practical problem solving by oversimplifying complex interactions, particularly in the multidisciplinary approach to health care.

Another criticism of Six Sigma rests on the observation that sometimes, a "Six Sigma Bureaucracy" can develop within an organization. While the aim of data-focused approaches is to eliminate bureaucratic decision making, the emphasis on the Six Sigma format may instead create a different version of the same problem.[16]

KEY POINTS

- Six Sigma's goal is to eliminate defects, thereby reducing costs.
- DMAIC (Define, Measure, Analyze, Improve, and Control) for established processes.
- DMADV (Define, Measure, Analyze, Design, and Verify) for new processes.
- Lean is the elimination of waste from the process of creating value.
- Kaizen, meaning continuous improvement, is the process through which waste is eliminated.
- Lean uses multiple tools, including value stream mapping, to visualize a process and decide what waste to eliminate.
- Both Six Sigma and Lean require the buy-in of upper management to be properly executed and supported.

ONLINE RESOURCES

1. http://www.innovations.ahrq.gov/content.aspx?id=2148: AHRQ Web site with downloadable Six Sigma and Lean forms.
2. http://www.ihi.org/knowledge/Pages/IHIWhitePapers/GoingLeaninHealthCare.aspx: Downloadable white paper by the IHI ongoing Lean in health care.
3. http://theopenacademy.com/content/introduction-lean-six-sigma-methods: Video lecture series by Professor Earll Murman from MIT on introductory Lean Six Sigma methods.

REFERENCES

1. Snee RD. Six Sigma: the evolution of 100 years of business improvement methodology. *Int J Six Sigma Compet Adv.* 2004;1(1): 4–20.
2. Langley GJ, Moen R, Nolan KM, Nolan TW, eds. *The Improvement Guide: A Practical Approach to Enhancing Organizational Performance.* 2nd ed. San Francisco, CA: Jossey-Bass; 2009.
3. Van den Heuvel J, Does RJMM, Verver JPS. Six Sigma in healthcare: lessons learned from a hospital. *Int J Six Sigma Compet Adv.* 2005;1(4):380–8.
4. Stahl R, Schulz B, Pexton C. Healthcare's horizon: from incremental improvement to design the future. *Six Sigma Forum Mag.* 2003;1(3):17–25.
5. Harry M, Schroeder R. *Six Sigma: The Breakthrough Management Strategy Revolutionizing The World's Top Corporations.* 1st ed. New York, NY: Currency/Doubleday Publishing; 2000.
6. Harry MJ. *The Visions of Six Sigma.* 5th ed. Phoenix, AZ: Tri Star; 1997.
7. Jensen MC. *Foundations of Organisation Strategy.* Cambridge, MA: Harvard University Press; 1998.
8. Ohno T. *Toyota Production System.* Portland, OR: Productivity Press; 1988.
9. Bicheno J, Holweg M. *The Lean Toolbox.* 4th ed. Buckingham, UK: PICSIE Books; 2004.
10. Womack JP, Jones DT. *Lean Thinking: Banish Waste and Create Wealth in Your Corporation.* New York, NY: Free Press; 2003.
11. Japan Management Association. *Kanban: Just-In-Time at Toyota.* Portland, OR: Productivity Press; 1986.
12. Emiliani B. *Better Thinking, Better Results.* Kensington, UK: The Center for Lean Business Management; 2003.
13. Rother M, Shook J. *Learning to See: Value-Stream Mapping to Create Value and Eliminate Muda.* Brookline, MA: Lean Enterprise Institute; 2003.
14. Womack JP, Jones DT, Roos D. *The Machine That Changed the World.* New York, NY: Free Press; 1990.
15. Dean ML. *Lean Healthcare Deployment and Sustainability.* New York, NY: McGraw-Hill Education; 2013.
16. Jarrar Y, Neely A. *Six Sigma—Friend or Foe? Center for Business Performance, Cranfield School of Medicine.* http://yasarjarrar.com/wp-content/uploads/2012/07/Six-Sigma-Friend-or-Foe_paper.pdf

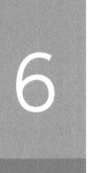

6 Accountability and Reporting

Jonas Marschall and Emily Fondahn

CLINICAL VIGNETTE

A 67-year-old woman with coronary artery disease and diabetes mellitus who was recently diagnosed with endometrial carcinoma is admitted for removal of her uterus, ovaries, and lymph nodes by a resident gynecologist. Her home medications include aspirin, which she has taken up to the day of admission. The patient's family practitioner was aware of the upcoming surgery but has not paused aspirin 7–10 days before surgery as indicated. The resident gynecologist forgets to report this fact to the attending gynecologist who is scheduled to operate on the patient. Aspirin use is not part of the routine questions upon admission for elective surgery. The attending gynecologist does not look at the chart before meeting the patient. The anesthesiologist notices aspirin on the medication list but believes the attending gynecologist is aware of the patient's medications. The next day, the surgery is notable for excessive bleeding and takes 30 minutes longer than usual because of the amount of cauterization required. The attending gynecologist is acutely aware that the tissue damage that resulted will increase the patient's risk of developing a wound infection. After the surgery, he yells at the resident gynecologist and blames him for not stopping aspirin: "You should have told me and I would have cancelled the surgery!" The resident gynecologist is devastated for not having caught this and excuses himself. The patient subsequently develops a postoperative wound infection.

- Is the resident gynecologist responsible, accountable, or to be blamed?
- Who is to enforce accountability?
- Is this an event that should be reported?
- Has this event been used as an opportunity to improve the system?

INTRODUCTION

Few readers of this manual will first skip to the chapter on accountability and reporting, yet this is one of the most important topics in patient safety because it provides the framework for setting standards and enforcing patient safety measures. Hospital staff involved in patient safety and quality should know a few key concepts to understand the legal implications of their work. Here are some definitions:

- *Accountability*: An obligation or willingness to accept responsibility or to account for one's actions, which is closely related to culpability and liability.

- *Public reporting*: The obligation to disclose data that are relevant for patient safety to the public, for example, postoperative infection rates, severe medication errors, or mortality rates of hospitalized patients.
- *Quality indicator*: A measure of medical processes or outcomes that can be used to determine the quality of health care and serve as a basis for improvement initiatives.
- *Regulatory agency*: A government agency that has supervisory capacity over a specific field of human activity.

ACCOUNTABILITY

History

The concept of accountability has long been present in medicine. The opening declaration of the American Medical Association's (AMA) first code of ethics states that for a physician, "there is no tribunal, other than his own conscience, to adjudge penalties for carelessness or neglect" (AMA, 1847, Art. I 1). However, the focus has shifted from the individual physician's own conscience to the health care system as a whole. The individualist concept of accountability has guided health care until recently. Prior to the 19th century, reputation and character largely impacted a physician's practice, especially given the lack of medical therapeutics. In the beginning of the 20th century, with scientific advances, a strong emphasis was placed on medical reform by individuals such as Flexner who proposed reform and standardization of medical education and Codman who advocated for surgical and hospital standards.[1] Following World War I, the image of the autonomous physician who is the "captain of the ship" emerges.

In the 1970s and 1980s, concerns about rising costs of health care lead to the first "report card" being released by the Health Care Financing Administration, which contained hospital-specific data on Medicare mortality rates. Quality measures have become one common method for reporting accountability.[2] In 1998, the ORYX initiative was started by the Joint Commission (JC), which was the first national program to require reporting of hospitals on performance measures.[3] Starting in 2002, accredited hospitals were required to report data on core measures, and this information was made public in 2004.[4] Since then, the number of quality measures endorsed and reported by agencies has skyrocketed. For example, the National Quality Forum (NQF) now endorses over 600 quality measures.

Systems Thinking and Accountability

The patient safety movement is based on the assumption that errors occur when a poorly designed systems allow individuals to make harmful but potentially preventable errors. By redesigning the system, such errors are thought to be no longer possible or at least less likely to occur. Bar coding and computerized physician order entry are examples for systems design. However, if an error does occur, then someone has to assume responsibility for it, work toward further improvement, and provide the victim of the error with a supportive counterpart (who discloses the error and explains to the patient what measures will be taken next). The entity that is *accountable* can either be an individual health care professional or an entire organization, which are linked to each other in the "systems approach." Systems thinking was developed from feedback circles and has, as one of the premises, the "connectivity of elements."[5] As a consequence, errors can be considered as reminders that a system requires further modification to work better.

Individual and Organizational Accountability

Can we pursue a work environment where blame has no place but at the same time expect health care workers to accept responsibility for their actions and take ownership of them? How easy is it in our current health care system to commit an error and "get away with it"? Can we appropriately act upon dangerous behaviors and even more so if they turn out to be repetitive? These are questions that take us in direction of the term accountability. Despite its popularity, accountability is difficult to characterize but most commonly understood as a normative concept, or alternatively, can be used to explain a mechanism by which a system learns.[6] By assuming accountability, each individual is expected to be aware of his/her actions and to understand that poor actions require a response in order to prevent negative outcomes. For an individual health care worker, this response may be a one-time behavioral adjustment. But for the system, there could be a missed learning opportunity if the individual keeps the event to himself/herself. Other health care workers could potentially repeat the same error. Under ideal circumstances, therefore, a hospital's response will be a systems change so that the error in question is more difficult to commit in the future. In their article on "Striking a Balance," Etchells and colleagues argue for a shared responsibility that should emerge between the individual and the system in which the individual acts.[7]

Things get thorny, however, when an individual health care worker will not learn from near misses and errors and becomes a potential danger for patients. A "no-blame" approach might not work in this case. This leads us to the concept of a "Just Culture" outlined by David Marx,[8] which balances an atmosphere of trust that encourages reporting of patient safety issues with clearly stated limits of tolerance beyond which a health care worker will be reminded, counseled, coached, or disciplined. Instead of blamelessness, there should be a sense of obligation to follow best practices and maintain alertness for personal gaps in knowledge and/or performance and system weaknesses. And, instead of punishment that does not necessarily solve the underlying problem, people should only see disciplinary action if other methods fail. There are different suggestions for how an institution should respond to the spectrum of unsafe acts.[7-9] While many errors (and partly a so-called disruptive behavior) can be managed by a behavioral intervention, substance abuse and intentional harm are examples that are thought to always require disciplinary action.

Components of Accountability

At the individual level, accountability is the concept that an individual is responsible for a set of activities and explaining or answering for their actions.[6] At the system level, there is a complex, reciprocating matrix of accountability, which reflects all the diverse components. The model of a single physician being accountable to a single patient has been replaced by multifaceted relationships among multiple different parties in the health care system. Multiple different entities can either be accountable or hold others accountable, such as individual patients, physicians, nurses and other clinical staff, hospitals, the government, and other regulatory agencies. Gamm states that "accountability of health services organizations is defined as taking into account and responding to political, commercial, community and clinical/patient interests and expectations. Accountability is the process by which health leaders pursue the objectives of efficiency, quality, and access to meet the interests and expectations of these significant publics."[10]

How to Foster a Sense of Accountability

A number of ideas have been developed to help create a new safety culture in health care. Their common goal is to empower health care workers. One way is to teach young professionals to "speak up" and question behaviors and practices of coworkers that appear unsafe.[11] This is much more difficult when one is supposed to speak up about one's own errors. However, if health care workers choose to not report their own errors, a large opportunity to improve systems is missed.[12] The Agency for Healthcare Research and Quality (AHRQ) along with the Department of Defense (DoD) has developed a tool box to enhance patient safety beyond communication, which has as its core competencies the following:

1. Leadership
2. Situation monitoring
3. Mutual support
4. Communication[13]

These items suggest that monitoring colleagues could be part of the accountability concept. Another, more difficult approach is to make it a legal requirement to report patient safety incidents, as Denmark's patient safety act did, while at the same time protecting health care workers from sanctions.[14] Before employees can even articulate safety concerns, however, they should be encouraged to be mindful, which is comprised of the following:

1. A constant concern about the possibility of failure
2. Deference to expertise regardless of rank or status
3. Ability to adapt when the unexpected occurs
4. Ability to concentrate on a task while having a sense of the big picture
5. Ability to alter and flatten the hierarchy to fit a specific situation[15]

How to Enforce Accountability

Accountability as a concept that builds upon mature and mindful health care workers may not lend itself to be imposed on an institution. Yet, Wachter and Pronovost proposed strong auditing strategies in order to ensure safe practices but at the same time avoid punitive actions for practices where the benefit for patient safety has not been clearly demonstrated.[16] If there is fear of punishment or blame, the health care provider may not feel encouraged to disclose incidents. Among the suggested auditing strategies are video surveillance, computerized triggers, and secret monitoring of compliance. However, it remains unclear to what degree this enforcement should occur from outside auditors or else if policing should be done by the professional societies themselves.[17] Regulators (such as the JC) or insurers (such as Medicare) will likely mandate accreditation criteria more and more if physicians do not find a balanced way of creating a new safety culture while setting clear lines about what is inadequate behavior in their colleagues and do the corresponding self-policing.

REGULATORY AGENCIES, NATIONAL ORGANIZATIONS, AND THEIR REQUIREMENTS

Regulatory Agencies

Regulatory agencies oversee the different components of the health care system, from individual providers to entire hospitals. The vast amount of different regulatory agencies and their roles can be quite confusing. The stakeholders include federal agencies, state agencies, and private regulators (Table 6-1). The origins of this disjointed system can be traced to the longstanding tension between the federal, state, and local government plus the integration of private organizations. One example of the regulatory maze is the path an individual physician must take to practice. As Field explains, the

TABLE 6-1	Regulatory Agencies		
Federal Agencies	Department of Health and Human Services	DHHS	Implements most of the federal health care regulatory infrastructure through component agencies
Components of DHHS	Agency for Healthcare Research and Quality	AHRQ	Funds research of health services
	Centers for Disease Control and Prevention	CDC	Compiles and disseminates national health care data, investigates disease outbreaks, researches public health threats
	Centers for Medicare and Medicaid Services	CMS	Administers the Medicare program and the federal portion of the Medicaid program and States Children's Health Insurance Program
	Department of Justice	DOJ	Enforces antitrust laws and prohibition on payments for referrals
	Department of Labor	DOL	Administers Employee Retirement Income Security Act of 1974, which applies to employee health benefit arrangements
	National Science Foundation	NSF	Funds basic science research
	Veterans Administration	VA	Operates hospitals and other health care services of veterans, conducts and funds research on health services
State Agencies	Departments of Health		Investigate public health threats, house licensure boards in some states, administer health planning and certificate-of-need programs in some states, regulate clinical operations of managed care organizations
	Boards of Medicine		License and discipline physicians
	Boards (other health professions)		License and discipline allied health professionals
	Departments of Welfare		Administer Medicaid programs in many states
	Departments of Insurance		Regulate the sale and underwriting of private health insurance, including managed care arrangements, except when preempted by ERISA

TABLE 6-1	Regulatory Agencies (*Continued*)		
Local Agencies	Departments of Health		Investigate public health threats, inspect restaurants and other public facilities
Private Organizations	Accreditation Council on Graduate Medical Education	ACGME	Accredits medical residency programs
	American Board of Medical Specialties	ABMS	Coordinates activities of medical specialty societies
	Association of Schools of Allied Health Profession	ASAHP	Coordinates the certification of training programs for allied health professionals
	Educational Commission for Foreign Medical Graduates	ECFMG	Certifies graduates of foreign medical schools to enter ACGME-accredited medical residencies and fellowships
	Federation of State Medical Boards	FSMB	Coordinates some activities of state physician licensure agencies, including maintenance of records of physicians who have been disciplined
	Joint Commission on Accreditation of Healthcare Organizations	JCAHO or JC	Accredits hospitals and other kinds of health care facilities
	Liaison Committee on Medical Education	LCME	Accredits medical schools
	Medical specialty societies		Certify physicians as qualified to practice in medical specialties
	National Board of Medical Examiners	NBME	Develops and administers the examination for medical licensure that is used by all states
	National Committee of Quality Assurance	NCQA	Accredits managed care plans and related organizations

(Adapted from: Field RI. *Health Care Regulation in America: Complexity, Confrontation and Compromise.* New York, NY: Oxford University Press; 2007. By permission of Oxford University Press, USA; www.oup.com)

doctor must "attend a medical school that has received accreditation by a private body, take a national examination administered by another nongovernmental organization, obtain licensure from a state medical boards, complete a hospital residency that is funded and governed by the federal Medicare program, achieve certification from a private specialty board, obtain privileges at a hospital that may operate as either a private or public entity…and receive payment to actually earn a living from Medicare."[18]

Safety and Quality Reporting

There are a number of stakeholder agencies involved in patient safety and quality reporting. All of these have the objective to improve patient safety, by assisting with the measurement and description of events, the design of interventions, the reporting of measures and outcomes, or the proposal of norms. Among them are the JC, the NQF, the AHRQ, the Accreditation Council on Graduate Medical Education (ACGME), the Institute for Healthcare Improvement (IHI), the Centers for Medicare and Medicaid Services (CMS), and the Institute of Medicine (IOM).

Among those entities, the JC has defined National Patient Safety Goals that are updated annually. Details can be found under: http://www.jointcommission.org/assets/1/6/HAP_NPSG_Chapter_2014.pdf. The 2014 goals for hospitals are the following:

NPSG 01.01.01	Use at least 2 patient identifiers when providing care, treatment, and services
NPSG 01.03.01	Eliminate transfusion errors related to patient misidentification
NPSG 02.03.01	Report critical results of tests and diagnostic procedures on a timely basis
NPSG 03.04.01	Label all medications, medication containers, and other solutions on and off the sterile field in perioperative and other procedural settings
NPSG 03.05.01	Reduce the likelihood of patient harm associated with the use of anticoagulant therapy
NPSG 03.06.01	Maintain and communicate accurate patient medication information
NPSG 06.01.01	Improve the safety of clinical alarm systems
NPSG 07.01.01	Comply with either the current Centers for Disease Control and Prevention (CDC) hand hygiene guidelines or the current World Health Organization (WHO) hand hygiene guidelines
NPSG 07.03.01	Implement evidence-based practices to prevent health care–associated infections due to multidrug-resistant organisms in acute care hospitals
NPSG 07.04.01	Implement evidence-based practices to prevent central line–associated bloodstream infections
NPSG 07.05.01	Implement evidence-based practices for preventing surgical site infections

NPSG 07.06.01	Implement evidence-based practices to prevent indwelling catheter-associated urinary tract infections (CAUTI)
NPSG 15.01.01	Identify patients at risk for suicide
UP 01.01.01	Conduct a preprocedure verification process
UP 01.02.01	Mark the procedure site
UP 01.03.01	A time out is performed before the procedure

The **NQF** has compiled a list of Serious Reportable Events (SREs) last updated in 2011 (http://www.qualityforum.org/Topics/SREs/Serious_Reportable_Events.aspx). These SREs are grouped in the following categories: surgical or invasive procedure events, product of device events, patient protection events, care management events, environmental events, radiologic events, and potential criminal events.

The **AHRQ** identified patient safety indicators (PSIs), last updated in 2015 (http://www.qualityindicators.ahrq.gov/Modules/PSI_TechSpec.aspx). These PSIs cover postoperative complications, retained surgical items, death in surgical patients or in patients with low risk for mortality, birth traumas, transfusion reactions, pressure ulcers, and central line–associated bloodstream infections.

Reporting

Health care institutions in many countries have set up *internal* reporting systems for events that jeopardize patients' safety. Known as "incident reporting systems," these systems are supposed to detect unsafe events and make them analyzable. Their goal is to enable quality improvement initiatives. On the other hand, there is a trend toward *public* reporting of patient safety issues as a quality indicator for hospitals; this corresponds to the rise of public reporting of hospital-acquired infections, which is now mandated in the majority of the US (http://www.ncsl.org/documents/health/haireport.pdf). Here, we will discuss intra- and extrainstitutional reporting separately.

Intrainstitutional Reporting

Incident reports (IR) are a form of passive surveillance in that they depend on voluntary reporting by health care workers and do not rely on standardized and objective criteria.[19] Therefore, they mostly produce large amounts of data that require additional classification and labor-intensive analysis. It is unclear what impact incident reporting has on patient safety, in part because incident reporting systems have been understudied.[20,21] Aside from the labor intensity of IR systems, one of their major problems is that they may suffer from both under- and overreporting and therefore cannot produce reliable incident rates.[22] Other requirements of a functional reporting system have been elicited and include the following: (1) supportive environment that protects confidentiality, (2) participation of all types of health care workers, (3) feedback that should be given in a timely manner, and (4) a structured approach for responding to problems and designing interventions.[23] One should add "user-friendliness" and "maximum dissemination within the institution" as further requirements. Current IR systems, however, may not be fully used as learning opportunity for the respective institution. And reporting without corresponding improvement initiatives may be relatively useless. Experts recommend investigating only a small number of incidents but to do so thoroughly as valuable information is often contained in the narrative of the incident.[24]

Public Reporting

As discussed above, there are a number of stakeholders in the field of patient safety and quality improvement, but no single national regulator. Therefore, adverse event reporting to outside the institution is mostly regulated by the individual states (http://oig.hhs.gov/oei/reports/oei-06-07-00471.pdf). Approaches range from requiring broad reporting of medical errors to focusing on the NQF's "Serious Reportable Events." The State of Minnesota is an example for employing these Serious Reportable Events as marker events (http://www.health.state.mn.us/patientsafety/ae/09aheeval.pdf). An example for an organization that has developed a reporting system is the Institute for Safe Medication Practices (ISMP), which operates a database on medication errors (https://www.ismp.org/orderforms/reporterrortoismp.asp).

In summary, the best approach to public reporting of patient safety events remains unknown. The goal should be to extract the maximum amount of information from a select number of well-defined events and use them both for outside reporting and for the institution's learning.

LAWS AND POLICIES

Laws may change, and it is not the purpose of this chapter to review all relevant legislation with regard to patient safety. Of note, no entity *mandates* metrics and measurement of patient safety in the US. Relevant laws include:

- The **Patient Safety Act** of 2005 is a milestone in patient safety legislation (http://archive.ahrq.gov/news/newsroom/press-releases/2008/psoact.html). Its goal is to improve patient safety by encouraging voluntary and confidential reporting of events that adversely affect patients.
- **Medicare's "no-pay" list of conditions** for which US hospitals do not receive reimbursement since October 2008: stage III and IV pressure ulcers; fall or trauma resulting in serious injury; vascular catheter-associated infection; CAUTI; foreign object retained after surgery; certain surgical site infections; air embolism; blood incompatibility; certain manifestations of poor blood sugar control; certain deep vein thromboses; or pulmonary embolisms.

KEY POINTS

- Accountability exists at the individual and system level.
- Multiple regulatory agencies exist in health care at the national, state, and local level and private agencies.
- Hospitals are being evaluated by multiple different agencies based upon their safety and quality indicators.

ONLINE RESOURCES

1. Joint Commission National Patient Safety Goals: http://www.jointcommission.org/assets/1/6/HAP_NPSG_Chapter_2014.pdf
2. National Quality Forum Serious Reportable Events: http://www.qualityforum.org/Topics/SREs/Serious_Reportable_Events.aspx
3. Agency for Healthcare Research and Quality Patient Safety Indicators: http://www.qualityindicators.ahrq.gov/Modules/PSI_TechSpec.aspx
4. NASA's patient safety reporting system (PSRS), which is based on their experience with the Aviation Safety Reporting System: http://www.psrs.arc.nasa.gov/

REFERENCES

1. Sharpe VA. Behind closed doors: accountability and responsibility in patient care. *J Med Philos.* 2000;25(1):28–47. Epub March 25, 2000.
2. Chassin MR, Loeb JM, Schmaltz SP, et al. Accountability measures—using measurement to promote quality improvement. *N Eng J Med.* 2010;363(7):683–8.
3. Lee K, Loeb J, Nadzam D, et al. Special report: an overview of the joint commission's ORYX initiative and proposed statistical methods. *Health Serv Outcomes Res Methodol.* 2000;1(1):63–73.
4. Williams SC, Schmaltz SP, Morton DJ, et al. Quality of care in US hospitals as reflected by standardized measures, 2002–2004. *N Eng J Med.* 2005;353(3):255–64.
5. Waterson P. A critical review of the systems approach within patient safety research. *Ergonomics.* 2009;52(10):1185–95. Epub September 30, 2009.
6. Emanuel EJ, Emanuel LL. What is accountability in health care? *Ann Intern Med.* 1996;124(2):229–39.
7. Etchells E, Lester R, Morgan B, et al. Striking a balance: who is accountable for patient safety? *Healthc Q.* 2005;8 Spec No:146–50. Epub December 13, 2005.
8. Marx D. *Patient Safety and the "Just Culture": A Primer for Health Care Executives.* New York, NY: Columbia University; 2001. http://www.safer.healthcare.ucla.edu/safer/archive/ahrq/FinalPrimerDoc.pdf
9. Leonard MW, Frankel A. The path to safe and reliable healthcare. *Patient Educ Couns.* 2010;80(3):288–92. Epub August 7, 2010.
10. Gamm LD. Dimensions of accountability for not-for-profit hospitals and health systems. *Health Care Manage Rev.* 1996;21(2):74–86. Epub January 1, 1996.
11. O'Connor P, Byrne D, O'Dea A, et al. "Excuse me:" teaching interns to speak up. *Jt Comm J Qual Patient Saf.* 2013;39(9):426–31. Epub October 24, 2013.
12. Moller JL. Leadership, accountability, and patient safety. *J Obstet Gynecol Neonatal Nurs* 2013;42(5):506–7. Epub December 9, 2013.
13. King HB, Battles J, Baker DP, et al. TeamSTEPPS: team strategies and tools to enhance performance and patient safety. In: Henriksen K, Battles JB, Keyes MA, Grady ML, eds. *Advances in Patient Safety: New Directions and Alternative Approaches. Vol 3: Performance and Tools.* Rockville, MD: Agency for Healthcare Research and Quality (US); 2008. http://www.ncbi.nlm.nih.gov/books/NBK43686/
14. Svansoe VL. Patient safety without the blame game. *BMJ.* 2013;347:f4615. Epub 2013/07/26.
15. Boysen PG, II. Just culture: a foundation for balanced accountability and patient safety. *Ochsner J.* 2013;13(3):400–6. Epub September 21, 2013.
16. Wachter RM, Pronovost PJ. Balancing "no blame" with accountability in patient safety. *N Engl J Med.* 2009;361(14):1401–6. Epub October 3, 2009.
17. Wachter RM. Personal accountability in healthcare: searching for the right balance. *BMJ Qual Saf.* 2013;22(2):176–80. Epub September 4, 2012.
18. Field RI. Why is health care regulation so complex? *Pharm Ther.* 2008;33(10):607–8.
19. Tamuz M, Thomas EJ, Franchois KE. Defining and classifying medical error: lessons for patient safety reporting systems. *Qual Saf Health Care.* 2004;13(1):13–20. Epub February 6, 2004.
20. Anderson JE, Kodate N, Walters R, et al. Can incident reporting improve safety? Healthcare practitioners' views of the effectiveness of incident reporting. *Int J Qual Health Care.* 2013;25(2):141–50. Epub January 22, 2013.
21. Pronovost PJ, Thompson DA, Holzmueller CG, et al. Toward learning from patient safety reporting systems. *J Crit Care.* 2006;21(4):305–15. Epub December 19, 2006.
22. Roehr B. US hospital incident reporting systems do not capture most adverse events. *BMJ.* 2012;344:e386. Epub January 17, 2012.
23. Farley DO, Haviland A, Champagne S, et al. Adverse-event-reporting practices by US hospitals: results of a national survey. *Qual Saf Health Care.* 2008;17(6):416–23. Epub December 10, 2008.
24. Vincent C. Incident reporting and patient safety. *BMJ.* 2007;334(7584):51. Epub January 16, 2007.

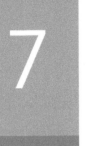

7

Healthcare Information Technology

Feliciano B. Yu Jr.

CLINICAL VIGNETTE

Bianca is a 15-year-old girl with a history of asthma who presented to the emergency department (ED) at a local community hospital with difficulty breathing. She had been using her inhaler for the past 2 days without relief. At the ED, she was noted to have tight breath sounds and obvious increased work of breathing. She was given a nebulizer treatment of a bronchodilator and a dose of oral steroids. Clinicians at the ED reviewed her previous medical history using the electronic medical record (EMR). The EMR also provided the clinicians access to the current best practice guidelines for asthma. Her condition did not improve, and she was admitted to the hospital for further management. After 2 days in the hospital, her condition improved and she was ready to be sent home. Within the EMR, the doctors used the electronic prescribing system to print out a refill of her metered-dose inhaler (MDI), prescriptions for a 5-day course of oral steroids, and a steroid MDI to help prevent future flare-ups. She was also advised to follow up with her primary care physician within a week to assess her response to the therapy.

- How can healthcare information technology facilitate the improvement of care delivered for patients like Bianca?
- What is the role of healthcare information technology in quality and patient safety efforts?

INTRODUCTION

In 21st-century medicine, healthcare information technology (HIT) is an integral aspect of care delivery and is fast becoming ubiquitous in the modern clinical setting. HIT is a collection of computer hardware and software systems that operates within a care delivery ecosystem. When implemented properly, HIT can help improve the quality and safety of care delivery as well as facilitate process improvement and medical research. When designed improperly, it leads to inefficiency, waste, and risks to patient safety. The successful use of HIT depends upon a larger cultural context and organizational framework, where the technology and communication systems are consciously designed and optimized harmoniously to provide an efficient end-user workflow, to improve decision making, and to support a learning health care delivery system. Timely health care data support a "learning" environment by providing all health care stakeholders (providers, patients, families, decision makers) the necessary information and knowledge for making better decisions, improving care, and facilitating population health and research.[1]

Background

The 2001 Institute of Medicine (IOM) publication "Crossing the Quality Chasm: A New Health System for the 21st Century" described the gaps in the quality of care delivered in the US health care system. The report identified the adoption of HIT as an essential component for addressing the gaps in quality and safety. Specifically, modern health care informatics and technology infrastructure need to support timely access to clinical information, evidence-based clinical decision support (CDS), quality measurement, health care research, and education.[2] In 2003, the IOM published the "Patient Safety: Achieving a New Standard for Care" describing a model for a national health information infrastructure based on data standards governing the capture, storage, and transmission of health care information across disparate organizations and computer systems.[3] In order to address the gaps in quality and patient safety, the HIT framework should present clinical information at the point of medical decision making so that care providers can avoid, detect, and address risks to patient safety and quality, even before the adverse event has occurred.[4] In 2004, the George W. Bush administration established the Office of the National Coordinator for Health Information Technology (ONCHIT) within the Department of Health and Human Services to guide the nation's journey toward adopting a national HIT infrastructure and providing Americans access to more robust EHR by the year 2014.

"Meaningful Use" of HIT

Under the Barack Obama administration, the 2009 American Recovery and Reinvestment Act (ARRA) included legislation that promoted the adoption of EHR and other HIT standards that will support health information exchanges (HIE) and interoperability while maintaining the security and privacy of health care information. Through ARRA's Health Information Technology for Economic and Clinical Health (HITECH) Act,[5] financial incentive programs were implemented to rapidly develop the national HIT framework to support a robust and interconnected care delivery system.[6] This program included support for states to adopt HIEs, for providers to adopt certified EHRs, and for communities to educate/train the new HIT workforce. Specifically dubbed as the Meaningful Use EHR incentive program, the effort is executed in successive phases or "stages," designed to incrementally improve the overall function and capabilities of the HIT systems.[7] As of September 2015, over 548,000 providers (hospitals and medical professionals) in the US have signed up to participate in the incentive program and together have received over $31 billion in direct financial support.[8] It is estimated that about 40% of doctor's offices (2012 data) and 85% of US hospitals (March 2013) have adopted EHR technologies that support the goals of the federal HIT framework.[9,10] The Meaningful Use effort is expected to end by 2016 for Medicare and 2021 for Medicaid incentive program.[11] This substantial national investment is an important milestone to consider as we ponder upon the use of HIT in the improvement of quality and patient safety in the US health care system.

HIT and Clinical Practice

The EMR has transformed the way care is delivered in the clinical settings. When compared to paper-based medical records, well-designed EMR systems have been shown to enhance the quality and convenience of care, improve the patient's ability to participate in their care, improve efficiency of medical practice, decrease cost of care, enhance coordination of services, and improve process and outcomes of care. Table 7-1 provides examples of the EMR benefits.

TABLE 7-1	Examples of EMR Benefits
Clinical	
Legible clinical notes	Resolves issues with poor handwriting
Accessible medical records	Patient records can be searched quickly. Minimize efforts in searching for medical records
Simultaneous access to medical record	A number of users can access the patient's record at the same time
Timely laboratory results review	Given connectivity (interface) to laboratory systems or machines, the results are readily available in the EMR
Timely radiology results review	Given connectivity (interface) to radiology/imaging systems or machines, the results are readily available in the EMR
Medication clinical decision support	When equipped with a drug database, the EMR can include a number of CDS rules such as drug dosing, dose range, or drug-to-drug checking. Assists with the medication ordering process
Allergy clinical decision support	When equipped with an allergy module, the EMR can check for allergies, intolerances, and sensitivities against a number of medications, foods, and environmental triggers
e-Prescribing	EMR systems can generate electronic prescriptions and transmit to a local pharmacy through standard electronic communication protocols
Manage problem lists	Ability to maintain a current set of problems pertinent to the patient
Manage physiologic and growth parameters	Ability to record vital signs, growth charts, and other milestones relevant to care and also track these data over time
Improve preventive care services	With proper documentation and use of decision support, clinicians can identify patients who need health care screenings and preventive services such as lab tests, mammograms, immunizations, etc.
Better handoff process	With improved documentation and reports, clinicians can provide a legible patient record during transitions of care, which can eliminate redundant tests through improved communication

TABLE 7-1	Examples of EMR Benefits (*Continued*)	

Financial

Savings on transcription services	EMR documentation minimizes need for transcription: it also reduces need to transport paper medical records
Minimize need for physical storage of paper records	Paper charts storage is no longer needed
Reduce staff needed to maintain paper records	Eliminates need for personnel to manage paper records
Improved billing process	Improved documentation leading to appropriate charge capture and subsequent billing process. Improved documentation leads to a more accurate coding of diagnoses, evaluation, and management

Other

Eligible for incentives	Provider will be eligible for incentive programs such as the Meaningful Use or Leap Frog
Maintain competitiveness	More recent health care workers are seeking workplaces with EMRs
Security for medical records	Ability to provide a more secure environment for patient's records; ability to implement disaster recovery strategies

Overall, the current evidence on the use of HIT in clinical practice tips toward the favorable side.[12] Given the current rate of HIT adoption, we have barely scratched the surface of what it can do to impact care delivery. Adoption of HIT is merely the *first step* in the journey in transforming the way medicine is being practiced today. A cultural transformation following HIT adoption must include human-centered engineering and design of information systems, safe implementation of clinical computer software and algorithms, highly evolved sociotechnical framework for systems implementation, and more robust supporting policies for the effective use of HIT in the clinical settings.[13]

The Electronic Medical Record and the Electronic Health Record

The electronic medical record or EMR is often interchanged with the electronic health record or EHR. For the purpose of this book, the EMR is defined as the digital collection of the patient's medical information (notes, medication, results, physiologic measurements, etc.) that is confined within a scope of practice, whereas the EHR is a compilation of a patient's health care information that spans across organizations (Table 7-2). The EMR is equivalent to a patient's paper chart in a given medical office. The EMR is usually supported by a set of computer hardware and software that are designed for very specific clinical workflow and information requirements.

TABLE 7-2	Difference between Electronic Medical Records and Electronic Health Records

Electronic Medical Records	Electronic Health Records
A record of clinical services for patient encounters contained in a single health care institution	A collection of clinical information from other health care institutions where the patient has been seen
Owned by the health care institution, usually a hospital or doctor's office	Owned by the patient (as in a PHR) or other health care stakeholders such as community or regional health care organizations
Systems are usually purchased through commercial EMR vendors and implemented in hospitals, health systems, or care provider clinics	The system is implemented by commercial vendors and implemented by community, state, or regional stakeholders such as Regional Health Information Organizations (RHIOs)
May have patient access to some results information through a portal	Provides interactive patient access as well as the ability for the patient to append information
Does *not* contain other health care institutions' encounter information	Contains patient encounter information from other health care institutions through HIE or other standard information sharing mechanisms
The legal electronic medical record for a particular health care institution	
Allows for managing other tasks such as scheduling and billing as well as link to other systems such as laboratory and pharmacy systems	
Is a digital version of paper chart in the physician's office or the hospital	

The EMR system is usually owned by the health care provider. Key operational benefits of the EMR include legibility of documentation (and spell check!), accessibility of the patient records, decreased storage space requirements for paper charts, electronic prescribing, and CDS. However, the EMR does not contain all the possible health information pertinent to the patient's care outside its designated scope of practice. For example, the EMR of a doctor's clinic or a hospital may only contain a portion of the patient's entire medical information and may not contain information stored in other institutions' EMR systems.

In contrast, EHRs contain a wealth of patient information that spans across organizations and other health care entities. It can even include health care information derived from the patient such as the personal health record (PHR). Figure 7-1 shows the relationship between EMRs and the EHR. In other words, EHRs store the aggregate digitized health care information about the patient, connecting patient

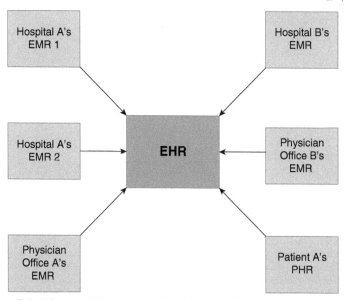

Figure 7-1. Relationship between electronic medical records and electronic health records. Legend: EMR, electronic medical record; EHR, electronic health record; PHR, personal health record.

information across disparate data sources and EMRs. The EHR can scope a region, state, or even a nation. The clinical workflow, information and functional requirements, and governance structures required to maintain EHRs are quite complex. More importantly, EHRs can only be established when interoperability as well as business alignment exists across the participating EMRs and organizations.[14] The Meaningful Use incentive program aims to increase the adoption of EMRs among providers and support the development of HIE standards so that EMRs can connect to each other seamlessly, thus moving the country closer to an ideal national EHR. When implemented properly, EHRs can help improve quality of care, decrease certain medical errors, enhance the organization's bottom line, reduce health care costs, facilitate population health, and contribute to scientific research.[15]

Computerized Provider Order Entry

In the clinical settings, a key functionality of the EMR is to facilitate computerized provider order entry (CPOE). CPOE enables doctors, nurses, and other clinicians to enter orders electronically, as one would use in a paper chart. These electronic orders are routed automatically to other departments, such as a laboratory information system for lab orders or a pharmacy information system for medication orders. As one can imagine, CPOE requires an organization to link, or interface, the EMR to a number of supporting clinical information systems. The degree of incompatibility among these linked systems dictates the complexity (and cost) of the process. The benefits of a properly implemented CPOE include fast connections to supporting systems (labs, pharmacy), avoidance of transcription errors, quick integration of orders into the EMR, and prompting of clinical alerts like allergies, drug–drug interactions, and drug dosing.[16]

HIT AND CLINICAL DECISION SUPPORT SYSTEMS

Strong evidence in the literature shows that Clinical Decision Support Systems (CDSS) improve care delivery processes.[17] CDSS are electronic systems with special computerized algorithms (known as clinical decision support [CDS] rules), designed to assist with medical decision making based on or triggered by certain clinical variables of interest. They can include allergy alerts, reminder pop-ups for medication doses or interactions, automated calculations or notifications, and special electronic views of pertinent patient information. The CDS rules can be simple as in an allergy alert or as complex as following a clinical pathway or guideline.

Supporting Clinicians

The goal of CDSS is to improve medical knowledge and aid human cognition at the point of decision making. For example, CDSS can be integrated into the EMR workflow so that clinicians can be alerted of the clinical services (i.e., preventive, screening) that would be applicable to the patient's visit. When ordering medications via the EMR, CDS rules can be deployed to alert the clinician of specific information in the patient's record such as worsening renal function (i.e., increasing creatinine) or other potential drug reactions. CDSS can also be used to provide the clinician with well-accepted practice recommendations that are tailored to the patient's condition, such as preferred or alternative treatment guidelines based on current medical evidence.[18] One thing to note is that the success of the CDSS in changing clinician behavior depends on how easily the clinician can interact with the system. CDS rules that impede both physical and cognitive workflow tend to be ineffective in changing clinician practice. In fact, indiscriminate firing of alerts from the EMR can induce "alert fatigue" among clinicians, and they can sometimes lead to adverse patient outcomes.[19] EMR-based alerts and reminders can sometimes contribute to information overload and desensitizing the clinician to the importance of the decision support.[20,21]

Supporting Patients

While CDSS has shown to improve clinician performance, the direct effect on patient outcomes is less understood.[17,22] CDSS impacts clinical outcomes by influencing clinician behavior to adhere to best practices, such as promoting preventive services or avoiding complications, by using analytics and informatics to aggregate large datasets for process measurement and surveillance efforts, and by minimizing adverse drug events.[23] However, the direct patient effect is dependent upon the culture of the clinicians using the system as well as those building and implementing the CDSS.[24] Implementing health IT does not guarantee better outcomes. In fact, there are undesirable patient safety consequences of poorly designed computer systems (see *e-iatrogenesis* below).[25]

HIT AND ADVERSE HIT EVENTS (E-IATROGENESIS)

Care delivery is becoming more dependent on computers when rendering care. Thus, it is very important that the sum of all of the hardware and software functions is aligned to maximize the positive effects of health care. However, the science of implementing health IT into the clinical settings is still at its infancy. Coined as "e-iatrogenesis," these new types of errors are a result of the human and computer interaction in the clinical settings.[25] EMR systems constantly introduce change in clinician workflow (both physical and cognitive). If the change is too much burden for end users, then maladaptive behaviors ensue causing work-arounds. Applying human factors and human-centric systems design are critical to the success of EMR workflow adaptation in the clinical settings. More importantly, there are errors that are derived directly from the design of the EMR itself. Poor representation of data, confusing user interface, miscalculations, lack of system navigation feedback, data omissions, poor training and communication, barriers to access, and system performance issues are among the HIT factors that causes end-user problems and subsequent adverse patient safety events.[26] The HIT industry must evolve quickly to design systems that are intuitive and facilitate human cognition and workflow. Encouraging further research on how electronic systems impact patient safety is critical to the success of HIT. In 2011, the IOM publication "Health IT and Patient Safety: Building Safer Systems for Better Care" proposed mechanisms where HIT vendors and users can report HIT-related adverse events and exchange this information across industry to encourage the development of systems that are safe to use in the clinical settings.[27]

HIT AND QUALITY MEASUREMENT

One cannot manage improvement efforts without a good measurement system. Improving the quality of care requires meaningful and actionable data about clinical processes and outcomes. Computer systems have an innate ability to store large amounts of data. The data about clinical processes and outcomes of care are increasingly captured and stored in electronic databases with the advent of health care information systems in the clinical settings. Clinical data derived from EMR systems (i.e., patients, diagnoses, procedures, care providers, etc.) often contain the variables of interest required in studying specific patient populations. In addition, data from EMRs can be linked longitudinally to assess effectiveness of care as well as for epidemiologic research.[28] Clinical data can be used to augment administrative and financial data to understand variations of care and outcomes and to monitor the progress during improvement efforts.

Informatics Implications

At this time, most EMR systems are not specifically designed to support quality measurement and improvement efforts. They are primarily designed to support specific clinical workflow (such as a physician's office, or hospital processes), to document care management and transactions, to schedule patient interventions, and to support billing or reimbursement. The advent of the 2009 Meaningful Use effort incentivizes providers to adopt EMRs that can also be "meaningfully" used in process improvement efforts.[29]

One of the major milestones that EMRs must overcome is to make the clinical information "computable," meaning that clinical information needs to be processed by computer systems, in addition to being readable by humans. Clinical data must be "codified" so it can be processed by computers more efficiently, preferably using standardized and controlled vocabularies.[30] Standard datasets use the same concepts to encode data all throughout the system's database. For example, the patient's "sex" may be represented uniformly as "M" for male and "F" for female or perhaps "1" for male and "2" for female. Regardless of which encoding system one is using, conceptual representation of data must be consistent so it can also be used for cross-sectional and longitudinal analysis and research. In addition, encoded data can be readily used to trigger CDS rules. Today, there are a number of health care terminologies (i.e., LOINC, SNOMED, ICD9, RxNorm) that represent medical concepts like diagnosis, procedures, laboratory tests, medications, etc. This is an important step in ensuring that clinical data can be represented accurately across disparate clinical information systems.

Analytics Implications

Although data standardization is vital to information processing and interoperability, the data necessary for quality improvement must be captured in the EMR system. Often, data that are needed for quality measurement (such as specific clinical interventions, findings, adverse events, etc.) are unstructured, hence not readily "computable." In the EMR, these types of data may be embedded in narrative texts, scanned documents, or dictated notes, posing a challenge to computer-based analysis. Special computer technologies such as optical character recognition (OCR) or natural language processing (NLP) systems can be utilized to "mine" the narrative clinical data; however, the institution must have the right resources (people, software, $$) to leverage these tools.[31] In some cases, data required for quality improvement may not be available in the EMR; hence, efforts must be in place to build and capture these data points within the EMR so that they can be stored as discrete data in the data repository and used in the measurement process. For example, in order to measure the process and outcomes of venous thromboembolism (VTE) care in the inpatient settings, it may be necessary to document the specific data elements (e.g., contraindications for VTE prophylaxis) required to generate the quality measures. More importantly, the information systems stakeholders supporting the implementation of the EMRs must be able to sustain the development of the data capture, data storage, data retrieval, and data mining capabilities of the organization. The skill sets necessary to maintain the analytics process are different from those tasked to implement and maintain the EMRs. The tools involved in deploying analytics are also different from the clinical applications. In addition, the costs required to support the data capture and retrieval are not trivial and can be quite daunting.

HIT WORK FORCE TRANSFORMATION

As of November 2015, only 4.1% of 5454 US hospitals and 7.79% of 35,364 ambulatory offices have achieved the highest level of EMR infrastructure to support clinical analytics, HIE, and continuity of care documentation (also known as HIMSS U.S. EMR Adoption Model Stage 7).[32] Fortunately, an overwhelming number of providers are either implementing EMR or rapidly evolving to have more robust HIT systems. It is projected that by 2019, about 90% of physicians and 70% of hospitals in the US would have adopted robust EMR systems.[33]

Informaticists

With health care institutions adopting EMRs, there is an increased need for a new breed of people with clinical backgrounds to be key contributors to implementing health care information systems. Clinical informatics is a new medical discipline aimed to advance the science, practice, and implementation of HIT into health care. Clinical informaticists come with medical, nursing, or pharmacy skills and IT skills to serve as conduits between IT and the clinical domain.[34-36] Effective implementation of EMRs requires an amalgamation of clinical, managerial, and IT skills. To fill this current void in the workforce, the American Board of Medical Specialties launched the inaugural board certification for the medical subspecialty of clinical informatics in October 2013.

IT Culture

Bridging the gap between the medical and technical cultures is a necessary step for the optimal utilization of IT. As health care services become more dependent on technology, any small change to the system can have a large impact for clinicians and patients.

A software upgrade of the EHR can lead to significant changes in clinical workflow. For example, changing to computer-based medication reconciliation can have huge impacts on the workflow for physicians, nurses, and pharmacists. Stakeholders need to be considered as IT is adapted in the workplace. Health care systems need effective and efficient ways to inform clinicians about upgrades and changes to the EMR. In addition, clinicians need to be able to reach out to the IT department for support, questions, and EMR work flow improvement ideas. Medicine is in a continual flux of new information and new workflows. IT systems (and therefore IT support!) need to respond to these fluctuations while continually striving to improve the quality of care delivered. Health IT must lean forward to becoming more clinical than technical, impacting health more than wealth, and supporting clinical workflow more than cash flow.

CONCLUSION

The health care community is at a critical inflection point for utilization of HIT. The use of computers in the clinical setting has grown exponentially, yet full exploitation of the EMR is still in its infancy. As health care transitions to the information age, there is great promise for improving the safety and quality of care by improving workflow, supporting process measurements, facilitating decision making through CDS and analytics, and creating the platform for HIE for care coordination and population health. Moving forward, the HIT industry must first overcome some of the constraints to fulfill these goals. Foremost, functional requirements and interoperability standards must be adopted so the clinical systems can "talk" to each other in ways that support the care delivery process and ensuring patient privacy and security. Next, the user interface design must evolve to support the human–computer interaction so that clinicians find the systems intuitive and easy to use. Having the ability to customize the EMR systems to accommodate local customs and practices can improve its adoption and enhance its ability to support care delivery. Additionally, the EMR systems should have the capability and flexibility to be used for quality improvement measurements, patient safety, and research. Finally, the barriers (i.e., cost, resources) for acquiring and maintaining HIT systems must be lowered so adoption is increased. Incentive program such as the Meaningful Use effort is a good starting point that can help minimize inequities of resource challenged care providers in adopting HIT. As we look at how IT has profoundly transformed other industries, we have only begun to realize the impact of HIT on the health care community.

KEY POINTS

- The EMR is the digital collection of a patient's medical information, whereas the EHR contains information from multiple EMRs and the PHR.
- Clinical decision support systems assist with medical decision making and are effective in improving clinical performance when properly implemented.
- E-iatrogenesis means errors due to human and computer interaction in the clinical setting.
- The Meaningful Use effort provides incentives to capture clinical data for quality improvement measurements.
- Clinical informatics is an emerging field that will help bridge the gap between clinicians and IT.

REFERENCES

1. National Research Council. *Best Care at Lower Cost: The Path to Continuously Learning Health Care in America*. Washington, DC: The National Academies Press; 2013.
2. Corrigan JM, Donaldson MS, Kohn LT, eds. *Crossing the Quality Chasm: A New Health System for the 21st Century*. Washington, DC: National Academy Press; 2001.
3. Aspden P, Corrigan J, Wolcott J, et al., eds. *Patient Safety: Achieving a New Standard for Care*. Washington, DC: National Academies Press; 2004.
4. Institute of Medicine. IOM report: patient safety—achieving a new standard for care. *Acad Emerg Med*. 2005;12(10):1011–2.
5. *The American Recovery and Reinvestment Act of 2009*. http://www.healthit.gov/sites/default/files/hitech_act_excerpt_from_arra.pdf. Accessed 12/11/13.
6. Centers for Medicare and Medicaid Services. *Medicare and Medicaid EHR Incentive Program Basics*. https://www.cms.gov/Regulations-and-Guidance/Legislation/EHRIncentivePrograms/Basics.html. Accessed 12/11/13.
7. Centers for Medicare and Medicaid Services. *Meaningful Use*. https://www.cms.gov/Regulations-and-Guidance/Legislation/EHRIncentivePrograms/Meaningful_Use.html. Accessed 12/11/13.
8. Centers for Medicare and Medicaid Services. *Data and Programs Reports*. https://www.cms.gov/Regulations-and-Guidance/Legislation/EHRIncentivePrograms/DataAndReports.html. Accessed 11/18/15.
9. Robert Wood Johnson Foundation. Health information technology in the Unites States: better information systems for better care; 2013. http://www.rwjf.org/content/dam/farm/reports/reports/2013/rwjf406758/subassets/rwjf406758_1. Accessed 12/11/13.
10. Office of the National Coordinator (ONC) for Health Information Technology. *ONC Data Brief, No. 9*. 2013. http://www.healthit.gov/sites/default/files/oncdatabrief9final.pdf. Accessed 12/11/13.
11. Centers for Medicare and Medicaid Services. *Electronic Health Record (EHR) Incentive Program FAQs*. https://www.cms.gov/Regulations-and-Guidance/Legislation/EHRIncentivePrograms/downloads/FAQsRemediatedandRevised.pdf. Accessed 12/11/13.
12. Buntin MB, Burke MF, Hoaglin MC, et al. The benefits of health information technology: a review of the recent literature shows predominantly positive results. *Health Aff (Millwood)*. 2011;30(3):464–71.
13. Institute of Medicine. *Health IT and Patient Safety: Building Safer Systems for Better Care*. Washington, DC: The National Academies Press; 2012.
14. Garets D, Davis M. *Electronic Medical Records vs. Electronic Health Records: Yes, There is a difference. HIMSS Analytics White Paper*. 2006. http://www.himssanalytics.org/docs/wp_emr_ehr.pdf. Accessed 12/11/13.
15. Menachemi N, Collum TH. Benefits and drawbacks of electronic health record systems. *Risk Manag Healthc Policy*. 2011;4:47–55.
16. Aarts J, Koppel R. Implementation of computerized physician order entry in seven countries. *Health Aff (Millwood)*. 2009;28(2):404–14.
17. Lobach D, Sanders GD, Bright TJ, et al. Enabling health care decision making through clinical decision support and knowledge management. *Evid Rep Technol Assess (Full Rep)*. 2012;(203):1–784.
18. Kawamoto K, Houlihan CA, Balas EA, et al. Improving clinical practice using clinical decision support systems: a systematic review of trials to identify features critical to success. *BMJ*. 2005;330(7494):765.
19. Carspecken CW, Sharek PJ, Longhurst C, et al. A clinical case of electronic health record drug alert fatigue: consequences for patient outcome. *Pediatrics*. 2013;131(6):e1970–3.
20. Singh H, Spitzmueller C, Petersen NJ, et al. Information overload and missed test results in electronic health record-based settings. *JAMA Intern Med*. 2013;173(8):702–4.
21. Farley HL, Baumlin KM, Hamedani AG, et al. Quality and safety implications of emergency department information systems. *Ann Emerg Med*. 2013;62(4):399–407.

22. Garg AX, Adhikari NK, McDonald H, et al. Effects of computerized clinical decision support systems on practitioner performance and patient outcomes: a systematic review. *JAMA.* 2005;293(10):1223–38.

23. Chaudhry B, Wang J, Wu S, et al. Systematic review: impact of health information technology on quality, efficiency, and costs of medical care. *Ann Intern Med.* 2006;144(10):742–52.

24. Ash JS, Sittig DF, Dykstra R, et al. The unintended consequences of computerized provider order entry: findings from a mixed methods exploration. *Int J Med Inform.* 2009;78(Suppl 1):S69–76.

25. Weiner JP, Kfuri T, Chan K, et al. "e-Iatrogenesis": the most critical unintended consequence of CPOE and other HIT. *J Am Med Inform Assoc.* 2007;14(3):387–8.

26. Campbell EM, Sittig DF, Ash JS, et al. Types of unintended consequences related to computerized provider order entry. *J Am Med Inform Assoc.* 2006;13(5):547–56.

27. National Research Council. *Health IT and Patient Safety: Building Safer Systems for Better Care.* Washington, DC: The National Academies Press; 2012.

28. Aronow DB, Coltin KL. Information technology applications in quality assurance and quality improvement, Part I. *Jt Comm J Qual Improv.* 1993;19(9):403–15.

29. Silow-Carroll S, Edwards JN, Rodin D. *Using Electronic Health Records to Improve Quality and Efficiency: The Experiences of Leading Hospitals. The Commonwealth Fund.* 2012. http://www.commonwealthfund.org/~/media/Files/Publications/Issue%20Brief/2012/Jul/1608_SilowCarroll_using_EHRs_improve_quality.pdf. Accessed 12/11/13.

30. Cimino JJ. Data storage and knowledge representation for clinical workstations. *Int J Biomed Comput.* 1994;34(1-4):185–94.

31. Aronow DB, Coltin KL. Information technology applications in quality assurance and quality improvement, Part II. *Jt Comm J Qual Improv.* 1993;19(10):465–78.

32. *HIMSS Analytics Ambulatory EMR Adoption Model.* http://www.himssanalytics.org/emram/AEMRAM.aspx. Accessed 11/19/15.

33. Steinbrook R. Health care and the American Recovery and Reinvestment Act. *N Engl J Med.* 2009;360(11):1057–60.

34. Lawrence D. Clinical tech trends. Trend: clinical informaticists. *Healthc Inform.* 2010;27(2):34, 36.

35. Leviss J, Kremsdorf R, Mohaideen MF. The CMIO—a new leader for health systems. *J Am Med Inform Assoc.* 2006;13(5):573–8.

36. Detmer DE, Munger BS, Lehmann CU. Clinical informatics board certification: history, current status, and predicted impact on the clinical informatics workforce. *Appl Clin Inform.* 2010;1(1):11–8.

Preventable Harm

Thomas Ciesielski, Emily Fondahn, and
Keith F. Woeltje

CLINICAL VIGNETTE

Patient JV is a 79-year-old woman with mild dementia, diabetes, and hypertension who was admitted to the hospital with acute renal failure. In her evaluation, she was determined to have an unsteady gait. She was deemed to be a high fall risk in her nursing assessment. The nurses placed a bed alarm to alert staff every time she got out of bed, and she was instructed to only get up with assistance. On her fourth night in the hospital, she attempted to get out of bed on her own to use the bathroom. She had an unwitnessed fall and broke her right arm.

- What types of preventable harm happen to patients while in the hospital?
- What strategies can hospitals implement to reduce the risk of preventable harm to their patients?

PREVENTABLE HARM

As the introduction to this manual stated, a founding tenet of medicine is "first, do no harm" to our patients. With the complexity of care increasing and the population generally aging, our most vulnerable patients are at risk for being harmed while in the health care environment. The harms can cause significant morbidity and mortality to patients as well as significantly increase the cost of care. Preventable harm can be defined as "a harm with an identifiable and modifiable cause."[1] Centers for Medicare and Medicaid Services (CMS) has defined hospital-acquired conditions to be reasonably preventable based on the application of published, evidence-based guidelines. However, unpublished data suggest that, for example, many patients have appropriate prophylaxis ordered at the time of a venous thromboembolism (VTE) occurring, suggesting that additional work is necessary to determine which events are truly preventable and to ensure that more effective prophylaxis is developed.

Hospitals can now be penalized for some conditions that are acquired in the hospital—these are preventable harms. Beginning in 2008, the CMS stopped paying hospitals for a subset of conditions that were not present on admission by not allowing the conditions to elevate a patient into a higher paying diagnosis-related group (DRG) category. This list now includes multiple categories, including falls, deep vein thrombosis (DVT)/pulmonary embolism (PE) (following some orthopedic procedures), and stage III/VI pressure ulcers (PUs).[2] CMS initiated a hospital-acquired condition reduction program in 2014, which directly penalizes the bottoms quartile of hospitals based upon three quality measures (Patient Safety Indicator [PSI] 90 composite, central line–associated bloodstream infection, and catheter-associated urinary tract infection).[3] This chapter discusses the scope of many of the preventable harms and identifies major risk factors for the harms and ways to minimize acquiring these conditions.

VENOUS THROMBOEMBOLISM

Introduction

VTE, including DVT and PE, is a well-established risk factor in postoperative patients and certain medical conditions including myocardial infarction (MI) and stroke.[4] A DVT or PE following a total knee replacement or hip replacement is considered a hospital-acquired condition by CMS. A recent review estimated the risk of a hospital-acquired VTE at about 2% of admissions; however, young ambulatory patients were excluded.[4] PE is a significant cause of mortality in the hospital—an estimated 5–10% of all inhospital patient deaths are attributed to PE.[5,6] The US health care system spends between $4.5 and $14.2 billion annually on preventable hospital-acquired VTEs.[7]

Definition

VTE refers to a DVT or a PE. A DVT is the formation of one or more blood clots (thrombus) in one of the body's large veins, most commonly the lower leg or calf.[8] The clot can cause complete or partial blockage of circulation. Some patients develop pain, swelling, discoloration, or redness of the skin, but many patients with a DVT will be asymptomatic. Many patients have no long-term consequences from a DVT, but they can cause significant pain, leg swelling, skin breakdown, and painful ulcers. More significantly, DVTs can lead to significant morbidity and death from a PE.[8]

A PE is the presence of one or more blood clots in the blood vessels of the lungs. A PE can be caused if a portion of the blood clot in the leg breaks loose and travels through the bloodstream to the heart and then to the lungs. Symptoms include shortness of breath, chest pain (especially when taking a deep breath), fast heart rate, coughing up blood, or passing out from low blood pressure.[9] Death can occur if the lungs blood vessels are completely blocked by the clot.

Risk Factors

Most hospitalized patients have at least one risk factor for a DVT.[10] Inherited risk factors include an inherited thrombophilia, such as factor V Leiden gene mutation, prothrombin gene mutation, or a protein C or protein S deficiency.[11] Acquired risk factors include recent major surgery, presence of a central venous catheter, trauma, immobilization, malignancy, pregnancy, use of oral contraceptives or hormonal agents, myeloproliferative disorders, antiphospholipid syndrome, obesity, congestive heart failure, and a history of a prior thrombotic event.[12–14] Virchow triad proposes that VTEs are often due to the following three factors:

1. Alterations in blood flow (stasis) such as prolonged bed rest or immobilization
2. Vascular endothelial injury such as surgery or trauma
3. Hypercoaguable state:
   a. Inherited, which creates a genetic tendency to form VTEs
   b. Acquired such as malignancy, pregnancy, or use of estrogen

Often, patients will have a combination of risk factors for VTE. Even after discharge, these risks persist.

Prevention

VTE Prophylaxis Guidelines

The American College of Chest Physicians published guidelines in *Chest* for VTE prevention in orthopedic surgery patients, nonorthopedic surgery patients, and nonsurgical (medical) patients in 2009 from an exhaustive review of the evidence (Table 8-1).

Ensuring VTE Prophylaxis

Applying appropriate prophylaxis can decrease VTE in hospitalized patients only if administered. Only 30–50% of eligible patients receive VTE prophylaxis.[17] Passive strategies, including guideline dissemination resulted in poor adherence to prophylaxis. Higher prophylaxis rates were seen at centers using proactive strategies, such as computer-based clinical decision support, documentation aids, audit and feedback, and active monitoring. Implementation and dissemination of VTE guidelines can include education, alerts, or a multifaceted approach.

- A tertiary care teaching hospital increased their VTE prophylaxis rate from 63% to 96% using provider education, reminders, and decision support tools as well as monthly audits and feedback over a 4-year period.[18] Unfortunately, similar interventions used in the **S**trategies to **EN**hance venous **Th**romboembolism proph**Y**laxis in hospitalized medical patients (SENTRY) trial did not increase VTE prophylaxis rates across 6 hospitals.[19] A short, three-item checklist encouraging VTE risk assessment and appropriate prophylaxis nonsignificantly increased patients undergoing risk assessment ($p = 0.06$) but did significantly increase inpatients being appropriately prescribed VTE prophylaxis ($p = 0.006$).[20]
- A recent Cochrane Review evaluated results from 54 studies and found that alerts, including computer alerts and stickers on patient charts increased VTE prophylaxis rates by 13% and a multifaceted (education and alerts) approach further increased VTE prophylaxis rates.[21]

TABLE 8-1	*Chest* Guidelines for VTE Preventions
Group	**Recommendation**
Acutely ill medical patients at increased risk of thrombosis	Low molecular weight heparin (LMWH), low-dose unfractionated heparin (LDUH) bid or tid, or fondaparinux.[10]
Acutely ill medical patients at low risk of thrombosis	Recommend against the use of pharmacoprophylaxis or mechanical prophylaxis.[10]
Nonorthopedic surgery patients	For specific type of surgery and patient risk, please consult the 2009 antithrombotic guidelines for VTE prevention in nonorthopedic surgery patients published in *Chest* for recommendation.[15]
Orthopedic surgery patients	For specific type of surgery/joint, please consult the 2009 antithrombotic guidelines for VTE prevention in orthopedic surgery patients published in *Chest* for recommendation.[16]

While education can help convince providers for the need for change, a forcing function may also be necessary to ensure consistent performance.[22] One option is making VTE risk assessment and prophylaxis selection required on every patient and to integrate the orders into the provider's work flow. For example, use of a forcing order set increased VTE prophylaxis rates from 35–55% to 70–85%.[17]

FALLS

Introduction

Falls are a significant issue facing hospitalized patients, affecting up to 12% of all admissions at a rehabilitation hospital; when aged adjusted, falls occur in 18–20% of admissions.[23] At a large academic institution, there is an estimated fall rate of 3.38 falls per 1000 patient days.[24] Some form of injury occurs in approximately 26% of inpatient falls with moderate or major injury occurring in 2.4% of all the falls.[25] Inpatient falls are more likely to occur in evening/night, be unassisted, occur from a loss of balance, and be related to toileting.[24] Costs associated with falling are significant due to an increased length of stay, regardless of degree of harm.[26] Patients that fall and sustain serious injury incur significantly higher costs (>$13,000) than patients who do not experience a fall.[27]

Definition

A fall can be defined as an unplanned descent to the floor with or without injury to the patient.[28] Injuries can include fractures, lacerations, or internal bleeding. The National Database of Nursing Quality Indictors categorizes the types of injury as[28]:

- None—patient did not sustain an injury secondary to the fall
- Minor—those injuries requiring a simple intervention
- Moderate—injuries requiring sutures of splints
- Major—injuries that require surgery, casting, or further examination (e.g., for a neurologic injury)
- Deaths—result from injuries sustained from the fall

Risk Factors

Multiple risk factors exist for patient falls and each patient will have a unique combination of risk factors. Just by being in the hospital, every patient is at risk for a fall. Risk for falling can be broken down into patient factors, environmental factors, and high-risk medications.

Patient risk factors:

- Age ≥75 (crude odds ratio [cOR] 2.6 [95% CI 1.2–5.60])[29]
- Impaired mental status (sedated or unconscious) (cOR 3.8 [95% CI 1.2–11.9])[29]
- History of falls (adjusted odds ratio [aOR] 2.73 [95% CI 1.79–4.16])[30]
- Use of assistive device (aOR 3.17 [95% CI 1.47–6.80]) or person (aOR 2.08 [95% CI 1.31–3.31]) for ambulation[30]
- BMI ≤ 18.5 (aOR 2.35 [95% CI 1.17–4.74]) or ≥30 (aOR 1.58 [95% CI 1.01–2.48])[30]
- Dizziness (aOR 2.12 [95% CI 1.05–4.28])[30]
- Incontinence (aOR 1.53 [95% CI 1.00–2.33])[30]

Environmental risk factors:

- Positioning of the bathroom, flooring, wet floors, lighting, and furniture are all likely contributing factors.[31]
- Geriatric Psychiatry floor (cOR 3.7 [95% CI 1.8–7.4]).[29]

High-risk medications:

- Hydantoin anticonvulsants (3.25 [95% CI 1.33–7.95])[30]
- Haloperidol (aOR 2.80 [95% CI 1.16–6.77])[30]
- Tricyclic anticonvulsants (aOR 2.43 [95% CI 1.21–4.90])[30]
- Benzodiazepines (aOR 2.19 [95% CI 1.46–3.29])[30]
- Insulin (aOR 1.46 [95% CI 1.01–2.13])[30]
- Selective serotonin reuptake inhibitor (OR 1.04 [95% CI 1.04–2.97])[32]
- An opiate (OR 1.59 [95% CI 1.4–2.20])[32]
- A nonantihypertensive diuretic agent (OR 1.53 [95% CI 1.03–2.26])[32]

Multiple tools have been developed to quickly and consistently assess a patient's risk of falling. Assessment of risk factors is an important step in fall prevention to help identify key risk factors, target preventive interventions to the correct patient, facilitate care planning, and facilitate communication between health care workers.[33] Tools that have been studied include the Maine Medical Center Falls Risk Assessment/Interventions (MMC), the New York-Presbyterian Fall and Injury Risk Assessment Tool (NY), St. Thomas Risk Assessment Tool in Falling Elderly Inpatients (STRATIFY), Morse Fall Scale (MFS), and the Hendrich II Fall Risk Model Sensitivity (HFRM) and the Johns Hopkins Fall Risk Assessment Tool. These tools use different combinations of known risk factors (Table 8-2) and have been compared in an acute care setting.[34] There is currently no consensus about which tool is the best to use in the acute care setting, and institutions should adopt a tool that meets their needs.

TABLE 8-2	Fall Risk Assessment					
Category	MMC	NY	Morse	Hendrich	Stratify	Johns Hopkins
≥2 Medical diagnoses			X			
Age	X					X
Agitation					X	
Ambulatory aid			X			
Confined to bed or chair	X					
Day number of hospital stay	X					
Depression				X		

TABLE 8-2 Fall Risk Assessment (*Continued*)

Category	MMC	NY	Morse	Hendrich	Stratify	Johns Hopkins
Dizziness or vertigo				X		
Elimination	X			X		X
Equipment that tethers patient						X
IV therapy/ heparin lock			X			
Frequency of toileting					X	
Gender		X		X		
Get up and go test				X		
History of falling	X	X	X		X	X
Mental status/ cognition	X	X	X	X		X
Impaired gait or mobility	X	X	X		X	X
Visual impairment	X				X	
Medications	X	X		X		X
Antiepileptic				X		X
Benzodiazepine				X		
Sedative	X	X				X
Cardiovascular agent	X					
Anesthesia	X					
Pain medication	X					X
Nine or more medications	X					
Antihypertensive						X
Diuretic						X
Hypnotic						X
Laxative						X
Psychotropic						X

TABLE 8-3	Sensitivity and Specificity of Fall Risk Assessments					
	MMC	NY	Morse	Hendrich II	Stratify	Johns Hopkins
Sensitivity (%)	64.9	78.9	55–77.2	64.9–70	55	100
Specificity (%)	65.8	58.4	72.8–91.2	61.5–69	75.3	47.3–65.9[a]

[a]Based upon scoring cutoff.

Importantly, these tools should be used to aid clinical decision making, not replace it. These tools only predict fall risk rather than prevent falls. Individual patients may have unique risk factors for falls that are not captured in these tools, and the sensitivity and specificity can vary based upon the patient population (Table 8-3).[34–36]

Prevention

- While there have been many interventions that have attempted to decrease falls in the hospital, there are few proven techniques. Calcium/vitamin D (cholecalciferol) supplementation in elderly patients in a long-stay geriatrics unit awaiting placement led to a 49% reduction in falls (Poisson regression estimate: –0.68, 95% CI 14–71% $p = 0.01$).[37]
- Patient education—preprinted care plan with targeted interventions decreased the risk of falling on acute care and community care facility wards, RR 0.79 (95% CI 0.65–0.95).[38]
- Exercise—exercise alone is likely insufficient to reduce falls. A meta-analysis of 13 randomized trials found no reduction in rate of falls in patients assigned to supervised exercise versus usual care (RR 1.03, 95% CI 0.81–1.31).[39]
- Medication review—medication review and adjustment of medication regimen to manage polypharmacy and psychotropic medications may be beneficial. A large randomized control trial demonstrated that a pharmacist review of the medication list in a nursing home lead to decreased falls (RR 0.62, 95% CI 0.53–0.72).[40]
- Hip protectors may be helpful in patients with a high risk of falls. However, there is no evidence to support universal hip protectors and compliance is often poor.[41]
- Bed alarms—the use of bed alarms to prevent falls has not been well established, even though these devices are widely used. One problem with alarms is the common "false-positive" signals that can be irritating to staff and patients.

Given the wide variety of patient, environment, and medication risk factors, there is no one-size-fits-all solution to fall prevention. A number of other strategies, such as toileting interventions and footwear, have been implemented by hospitals. These strategies do not have great evidence supporting their use, but do make common sense. Basic safety measures include fall prevention education, keeping a pathway in the room clear, wearing nonskid footwear, having the call light within reach, having personal items within reach, keeping the bed low with brakes on, orientation to the room and hourly rounding, and having adequate light present. Essentially, the information gained from the fall risk assessment needs to be paired with appropriate interventions for each patient (Fig. 8-1).

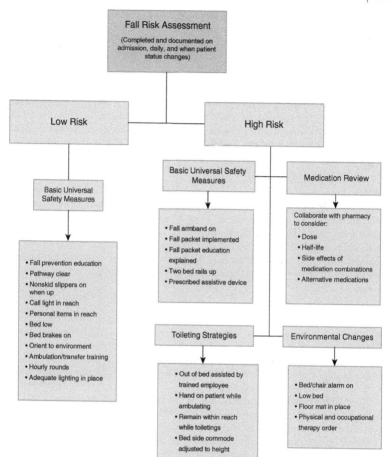

Figure 8-1. Fall risk assessment and interventions. (Adapted from Wolf L, Costantinou E, Limbaugh C, et al. Fall prevention for inpatient oncology using lean and rapid improvement event techniques. *HERD Health Environ Res Des.* 2013;7(1):85–101.[42])

Physical Restraints

A physical restraint is defined as "any physical or mechanical device, material or equipment attached or adjacent to the patient's body that the individual cannot remove easily. This device restricts the freedom of movement or normal access to the patient's own body."[43] Restraints have been applied to patients for issues including fall reduction and agitation. However, use of restraints has not been shown to prevent falls, and in reality, patients with orders for restraints were more likely to fall than patients without such orders, OR 6.3 (95% CI 1.8–22.3), though there was poor correlation between orders for restraints and restraint use at the time of the inpatient falls.[44] Restraints can be used for patients with significant behavioral issues or concern for self-harm; however, a recent systematic review found that use of restraints is associated with a number of bad outcomes, including[45]:

- Failure to be discharged to home (pooled OR 12.42 [95% CI 16–21.52])
- Death during the hospitalization (pooled OR 11.24 [95% CI 6.07–20.83])
- Nosocomial infection (pooled OR 3.46 [95% CI 1.93–6.22])
- Fall during hospitalization (pooled OR 6.79 [95% CI 3.44–13.39])

The authors of a recent systematic review examining the use of physical restraints put forth the following conclusion "…restraints should only be used as a last resort, minimal level of restraint be used, for the minimal duration and that the restrained person should be closely monitored."[45] This recommendation aligns with CMS, which states that "Restraint or seclusion may only be imposed to ensure the immediate physical safety of the patient, a staff member, or others and must be discontinued at the earliest possible time."[46]

Chemical Restraints

Chemical restraints are pharmaceuticals that are given to agitated patients to control behavior. Common medications include antipsychotic agents (e.g., haloperidol) and benzodiazepines (e.g., lorazepam), given either independently or in combination. These medications have significant side effects, including death. There is a further increased risk for adverse events when the two are administered concomitantly to older patients.[43] No current guidelines exist for the proper use of chemical restraints, and care should likely be taken to use chemical restraints sparingly.

PRESSURE ULCERS

PUs are an unfortunate condition that develops from unrelieved pressure to the soft tissue over a bony prominence. Common locations are the hip/buttocks or the heel. PUs range from a slight reddening of the skin to full-thickness loss of tissue and exposed bone.[47] Infections are the most common complication of PUs and can range from a localized infection around the ulcer to osteomyelitis (infection of the bone).[47] A PU can develop within 2 to 6 hours.[48]

A recent study estimates the incidence of a Medicare patient developing a new PU during a hospital stay at about 4.5%.[49] Certain populations are at much higher risk for PUs and more severe complications; one series documented that 17% of patients with PU due to spinal cord injury or stroke developed osteomyelitis.[50] Patients that develop PUs have a higher inhospital mortality, length of stay, and readmission rate.[49] With appropriate systems in place, the risk of developing PUs can be reduced.

Definition

The National Pressure Ulcer Advisory Panel (NPUAP) has a commonly used staging system (Table 8-4).[51] The ulcer should be evaluated for size, depth, presence of sinus tracks, necrotic tissue, exudates, and presence of granulation tissue. The external appearance can underestimate the extent of injury because patients can have the "tip-of-the-iceberg" phenomenon with the largest portion of the wound located deep and less skin involvement.[52] Pictures of the ulcers can be helpful to document changes over time, but the technique for photography should be consistent and include an identification sign with patient identification, date, and wound location.[48]

Hospitals are being penalized if a stage III/IV PU develops during the hospital stay. Documenting of the stages of skin breakdown that are present upon admission to the hospital is exceedingly important.

TABLE 8-4	NPUAP Pressure Ulcer Staging System
Ulcer Category/Stage	Description
Category/stage I	Nonblanchable erythema, skin intact, usually over a bony prominence
Category/stage II	Partial thickness loss of dermis, shallow open ulcer, pink wound bed
Category/stage III	Full-thickness skin loss, fat may be visible, but bones, tendons, or muscle not visible
Category/stage IV	Full-thickness tissue loss with exposed muscle, bone, or tendon
US additional categories	
Unstageable/unclassified	Full-thickness skin or tissue loss with unknown depth—obscured by slough or eschar
Suspected deep tissue injury—depth unknown	Purple/maroon localized area of intact skin or blood-filled blister

Risk Factors

The most important risk factors for developing a PU include immobility, malnutrition, reduced perfusion, and sensory loss. Over 100 risk factors have been identified for PU development (Table 8-5).[47,48] Sores can progress due to the presence of infection, inflammation, and edema.[53]

Furthermore, there are scoring systems available to evaluate an individual patient's risk of developing a PU, including the Braden Scale, the Norton Scale, and the Waterlow Scale—however, there is no current high-quality evidence demonstrating that use of any of the scales decreases the incidence of PUs.[54] The NPUAP recommends the following for a risk assessment[55]:

- Conduct a structured risk assessment as soon as possible (but within a maximum of eight hours after admission) to identify individuals at risk of developing PUs.
- Repeat the risk assessment as often as required by the individuals' acuity.
- Undertake a reassessment if there is any significant change in the individual's condition.
- Include a comprehensive skin assessment as part of every risk assessment to evaluate any alterations to intact skin.
- Document all risk assessments.
- Develop and implement a risk-based prevention plan for individuals identified as being at risk of developing PUs.

Prevention

Management of underlying contributing factors remains the most important aspect of prevention.[56] There are certainly many products available for PU reduction; the following strategies provide the best evidenced at preventing PUs:

TABLE 8-5	Risk Factors for the Development of PUs[47]	
Patient Factors		**Environmental Factors**
• Age (>65) • Limited mobility (stroke, spinal cord injury, postsurgical, etc.) • Poor nutrition • Diabetes • Depression/psychosis • Dementia	• Peripheral vascular disease • Steroids/immunodeficiency • CHF • Malignancy • ESRD • COPD	• Pressure from hard surfaces • Moisture (e.g., bowel or bladder incontinence) • Friction • Shear stress

• Foam mattresses, low-pressure mattresses, and overlays likely reduce the risk of developing PUs compared to "standard" hospital mattresses.[57]
• Optimal nutrition is important for wound healing and should be assessed and corrected for patients with deficiencies.[48] However, there is little evidence to support nutritional supplements in patients without specific deficiencies.[56]
• The NPUAP recommends preventive skin care including avoiding positioning an individual on an area of erythema if possible, keeping skin clean and dry, avoiding vigorously rubbing or massaging the skin at risk of ulcers, protecting skin from excessive moisture, developing an individualized continence management plan, and considering a skin moisturizer to hydrate dry skin.[55]
• Frequent repositioning (e.g., at least every 2 hours) is recommended to reduce duration and magnitude of pressure over vulnerable areas of the body; however, this strategy may not be possible in all patients due to their underlying medical condition. Heels should be free of pressure and knees should be in a slightly flexed position (5–10 degrees).[55]
• Quality improvement projects that track and monitor PUs have been implemented in single hospitals and health systems and have led to a decrease in severe PUs and PUs in general.[58,59]

CONCLUSION

The common theme with the preventable harms presented here is that it is necessary to assess each patient's risks to identify the most at risk population to be able to employ the appropriate prophylaxis or intervention most efficiently. There are interventions that mitigate the harms presented here and strategies need to be employed to introduce these interventions—it may take a quality improvement initiative to be able to effectively add these systems.

KEY POINTS

• Preventable harm is harm to patients that could be potentially avoided.
• Despite prevention guidelines, dissemination and implementation of strategies to avoid harm are needed in hospitals.

ONLINE RESOURCES

1. ACCP Antithrombotic Guidelines: http://www.chestnet.org/Guidelines-and-Resources/Guidelines-and-Consensus-Statements/Antithrombotic-Guidelines-9th-Ed
2. AHRQ Preventing Falls in Hospital Toolkit: http://www.ahrq.gov/professionals/systems/hospital/fallpxtoolkit/fallpxtoolkit.pdf
3. National Pressure Ulcer Advisory Panel: http://www.npuap.org/

REFERENCES

1. Nabhan M, et al. What is preventable harm in healthcare? A systematic review of definitions. *BMC Health Serv Res.* 2012;12:128.
2. Hospital-Acquired Conditions (Present on Admission Indicator). 2014 [cited October 9, 2014]. http://www.cms.gov/Medicare/Medicare-Fee-for-Service-Payment/HospitalAcqCond/index.html
3. Hospital-Acquired Condition (HAC) Reduction Program. QualityNet. March 25, 2015; https://www.qualitynet.org/dcs/ContentServer?c=Page&pagename=QnetPublic%2FPage%2FQnetTier2&cid=1228774189166
4. Dunn AS, Brenner A, Halm EA. The magnitude of an iatrogenic disorder: a systematic review of the incidence of venous thromboembolism for general medical inpatients. *Thromb Haemost.* 2006;95(5):758–62.
5. Sandler DA, Martin JF. Autopsy proven pulmonary embolism in hospital patients: are we detecting enough deep vein thrombosis? *J R Soc Med.* 1989;82(4):203–5.
6. Alikhan R, et al. Fatal pulmonary embolism in hospitalised patients: a necropsy review. *J Clin Pathol.* 2004;57(12):1254–7.
7. Mahan CE, et al. Thromboprophylaxis patterns, risk factors, and outcomes of care in the medically ill patient population. *Thromb Res.* 2013;132(5):520–6.
8. Kearon C. Natural history of venous thromboembolism. *Circulation.* 2003;107(23 suppl 1):I-22–30.
9. Piazza G, Goldhaber SZ. Acute pulmonary embolism. Part I: Epidemiology and diagnosis. *Circulation.* 2006;114(2):e28–32.
10. Kahn SR, et al. Prevention of vte in nonsurgical patients: antithrombotic therapy and prevention of thrombosis, 9th ed: american college of chest physicians evidence-based clinical practice guidelines. *Chest.* 2012;141(2_suppl):e195S–226.
11. Martinelli I. Risk factors in venous thromboembolism. *Thromb Haemost.* 2001;86(1):395–403.
12. Heit JA, et al. Relative impact of risk factors for deep vein thrombosis and pulmonary embolism: a population-based study. *Arch Intern Med.* 2002;162(11):1245–8.
13. Goldhaber SZ, Tapson VF. A prospective registry of 5,451 patients with ultrasound-confirmed deep vein thrombosis. *Am J Cardiol.* 2004;93(2):259–62.
14. Huerta C, et al. Risk factors and short-term mortality of venous thromboembolism diagnosed in the primary care setting in the United Kingdom. *Arch Intern Med.* 2007;167(9):935–43.
15. Gould MK, et al. *Prevention of VTE in nonorthopedic surgical patients: antithrombotic therapy and prevention of thrombosis, 9th ed: American College of Chest Physicians evidence-based clinical practice guidelines. Chest* 2012;141(2_suppl):e227S–77.
16. Falck-Ytter Y, et al. *Prevention of VTE in orthopedic surgery patients: antithrombotic therapy and prevention of thrombosis, 9th ed: American College of Chest Physicians evidence-based clinical practice guidelines. Chest* 2012;141(2_suppl):e278S–325.
17. Maynard G, Stein VF. Designing and implementing effective venous thromboembolism prevention protocols: lessons from collaborative efforts. *J Thromb Thrombolysis.* 2010;29(2):159–66.
18. Bullock-Palmer RP, Weiss S, Hyman C. Innovative approaches to increase deep vein thrombosis prophylaxis rate resulting in a decrease in hospital-acquired deep vein thrombosis at a tertiary-care teaching hospital. *J Hosp Med.* 2008;3(2):148–55.
19. Pai M, et al. Strategies to enhance venous thromboprophylaxis in hospitalized medical patients (SENTRY): a pilot cluster randomized trial. *Implement Sci.* 2013;8:1.

20. Colborne NR, et al. Using a venous thromboembolism checklist significantly improves VTE prevention: a junior doctor led intervention. *Int J Clin Pract.* 2013;67(2):157–60.

21. Kahn SR, et al. Interventions for implementation of thromboprophylaxis in hospitalized medical and surgical patients at risk for venous thromboembolism. *Cochrane Database Syst Rev.* 2013;(7):Cd008201.

22. Streiff MB, et al. Lessons from the Johns Hopkins multi-disciplinary venous thromboembolism (VTE) prevention collaborative. *BMJ.* 2012;344:e3935.

23. Vlahov D, Myers AH, al-Ibrahim MS. Epidemiology of falls among patients in a rehabilitation hospital. *Arch Phys Med Rehabil.* 1990;71(1):8–12.

24. Hitcho EB, et al. Characteristics and circumstances of falls in a hospital setting: a prospective analysis. *J Gen Intern Med.* 2004;19(7):732–9.

25. Krauss MJ, et al. Circumstances of patient falls and injuries in 9 hospitals in a midwestern healthcare system. *Infect Control Hosp Epidemiol.* 2007;28(5):544–50.

26. DunneTJ, Gaboury I, Ashe MC. Falls in hospital increase length of stay regardless of degree of harm. *J Eval Clin Pract.* 2014;20(4):396–400.

27. Wong CA, et al. The cost of serious fall-related injuries at three Midwestern hospitals. *Jt Comm J Qual Patient Saf.* 2011;7(2):81–7.

28. Montalvo I. *The National Database of Nursing Quality Indicators® (NDNQI®).* American Nurses Association. [cited November 4, 2014]; http://www.nursingworld.org/mainmenu-categories/anamarketplace/anaperiodicals/ojin/tableofcontents/volume122007/no3sept07/nursingqualityindicators.aspx

29. Fischer ID, Krauss MJ, Dunagan WC, et al. Patterns and predictors of inpatient falls and fall-related injuries in a large academic hospital. *Infect Control Hosp Epidemiol.* 2005;26(10):822–7.

30. O'Neil CA, et al. Medications and patient characteristics associated with falling in the hospital. *J Patient Saf.* 2015. http://journals.lww.com/journalpatientsafety/Abstract/publishahead/Medications_and_Patient_Characteristics_Associated.99688.aspx

31. Ferris M. Protecting hospitalized elders from falling. *Topics Adv Pract Nurs eJ.* 2009;9(1):8p. http://web.b.ebscohost.com/ehost/detail/detail?vid=4&sid=57727d8d-6462-40da-85a4-b003db5cb3d1%40sessionmgr112&hid=116&bdata=JnNpdGU9ZWhvc3QtbGl2ZQ%3d%3d#AN=105421926&db=jlh

32. Mion LC, et al. Is it possible to identify risks for injurious falls in hospitalized patients? *Jt Comm J Qual Patient Saf.* 2012;38(9):408–13.

33. Ganz DA, Huang C, Saliba D, et al. *Preventing Falls in Hospitals: A Toolkit for Improving Quality of Care. (Prepared by RAND Corporation, Boston University School of Public Health, and ECRI Institute under Contract No. HHSA290201000017I TO #1.).* Rockville, MD: Agency for Healthcare Research and Quality; 2013.

34. Kim EA, et al. Evaluation of three fall-risk assessment tools in an acute care setting. *J Adv Nurs.* 2007;60(4):427–35.

35. Chapman J, Bachand D, Hyrkas K. Testing the sensitivity, specificity and feasibility of four falls risk assessment tools in a clinical setting. *J Nurs Manag.* 2011;19(1):133–42.

36. Hnizdo S, et al. Validity and reliability of the modified John Hopkins Fall Risk Assessment Tool for elderly patients in home health care. *Geriatr Nurs.* 2013;34(5):423–7.

37. Bischoff HA, et al. Effects of vitamin D and calcium supplementation on falls: a randomized controlled trial. *J Bone Miner Res.* 2003;18(2):343–51.

38. Healey F, et al. Using targeted risk factor reduction to prevent falls in older in-patients: a randomised controlled trial. *Age Ageing.* 2004;33(4):390–5.

39. Cameron ID, et al. Interventions for preventing falls in older people in care facilities and hospitals. *Cochrane Database Syst Rev.* 2012;(12):Cd005465.

40. Zermansky AG, et al. Clinical medication review by a pharmacist of patients on repeat prescriptions in general practice: a randomised controlled trial. *Health Technol Assess.* 2002;6(20):1–86.

41. Gillespie WJ, Gillespie LD, Parker MJ. Hip protectors for preventing hip fractures in older people. *Cochrane Database Syst Rev.* 2010;(10):Cd001255.

42. Wolf L, Costantinou E, Limbaugh C, et al. Fall prevention for inpatient oncology using lean and rapid improvement event techniques. *HERD Health Environ Res Des.* 2013;7(1):85–101.

43. Mott S, Poole J, Kenrick M. Physical and chemical restraints in acute care: their potential impact on the rehabilitation of older people. *Int J Nurs Pract.* 2005;11(3):95–101.
44. Shorr RI, et al. Restraint use, restraint orders, and the risk of falls in hospitalized patients. *J Am Geriatr Soc.* 2002;50(3):526–9.
45. Evans D, Wood J, Lambert L. Patient injury and physical restraint devices: a systematic review. *J Adv Nurs.* 2003;41(3):274–82.
46. CMS. *CMS Manual.* 2008. https://www.cms.gov/Regulations-and-Guidance/Guidance/Transmittals/downloads/R37SOMA.pdf
47. Bluestein D, Javaheri A. Pressure ulcers: prevention, evaluation, and management. *Am Fam Physician.* 2008;78(10):1186–94.
48. Lyder CH. Pressure ulcer prevention and management. *JAMA.* 2003;289(2):223–6.
49. Lyder CH, et al. Hospital-acquired pressure ulcers: results from the national medicare patient safety monitoring system study. *J Am Geriatr Soc.* 2012;60(9):1603–8.
50. Darouiche RO, et al. Osteomyelitis associated with pressure sores. *Arch Intern Med.* 1994;154(7):753–8.
51. Panel NPUA. *NPUAP Pressure Ulcer Stages/Categories.* 2007 [cited October 9, 2014]. http://www.npuap.org/resources/educational-and-clinical-resources/npuap-pressure-ulcer-stagescategories/
52. Bauer J, Phillips LG. MOC-PSSM CME article: pressure sores. *Plast Reconstr Surg.* 2008;121(1 Suppl):1–10.
53. Cushing CA, Phillips LG. Evidence-based medicine: pressure sores. *Plast Reconstr Surg.* 2013;132(6):1720–32.
54. Pancorbo-Hidalgo PL, et al. Risk assessment scales for pressure ulcer prevention: a systematic review. *J Adv Nurs.* 2006;54(1):94–110.
55. Haesler E, ed. *Prevention and Treatment of Pressure Ulcers: Quick Reference Guide.* Perth, Australia: National Pressure Ulcer Advisory Panel, European Pressure Ulcer Advisory Panel and Pan Pacific Pressure Injury Alliance; 2014.
56. Reddy M, et al. Treatment of pressure ulcers: A systematic review. *JAMA.* 2008;300(22):2647–62.
57. McInnes E, et al. Support surfaces for pressure ulcer prevention. *Cochrane Database Syst Rev.* 2011;(4):Cd001735.
58. Zaratkiewicz S, et al. Development and implementation of a hospital-acquired pressure ulcer incidence tracking system and algorithm. *J Healthcare Qual.* 2010;32(6):44–51.
59. Harrison MB, Mackey M, Friedberg E. Pressure ulcer monitoring: a process of evidence-based practice, quality, and research. *Jt Comm J Qual Patient Saf.* 2008;34(6):355–9.

9

Health Care–Associated Infections

Rachael A. Lee and Bernard C. Camins

CLINICAL VIGNETTE

A 65-year-old man presents to the hospital for incision and debridement of his left knee prosthesis. He underwent a left knee arthroplasty just 6 weeks prior. Cultures taken in the operating room eventually were positive for methicillin-resistant *Staphylococcus aureus* (MRSA). The prosthetic device was removed and replaced with an antibiotic-impregnated spacer in anticipation for a planned revision after successful treatment with intravenous antibiotics. While reviewing other cases of orthopedic implant infections, the health care epidemiologist and the infection prevention specialist remembered that 2 months prior to this patient undergoing the primary arthroplasty procedure, another patient had undergone an incision and debridement of a right hip prosthesis for MRSA. The patient's isolate and the previous isolate were sent to a reference laboratory for molecular analysis for comparison. The result of the pulsed-field gel electrophoresis, a technique used for genetic fingerprinting, revealed that the two isolates were identical. Since there was no overlap in the dates of the patients' hospitalization, it is plausible that the earlier MRSA isolate was transmitted to the latter patient through environmental contamination or health care workers' hands.

Questions

- What types of health care–associated infections should concern health care workers?
- How is a surgical site infection defined?
- How can one prevent the incidence of health care–associated infections?
- What strategies can hospitals use to increase hand hygiene compliance?

INTRODUCTION

Health care–associated infections (HAIs) represent a major threat to patient safety, affecting about 1 out of 25 hospitalized patients, leading to substantial morbidity, mortality, and excess health care expenditures.[1] An estimated 440,000 infections occur annually, with costs estimated to be $9.8 billion.[2] The types of HAIs include central line–associated bloodstream infection (CLABSI), catheter-associated urinary tract infection (CAUTI), surgical site infection (SSI), and ventilator-associated pneumonia (VAP). Although CLABSIs were found to be the most costly per episode, over a third of these costs was attributable to SSIs.[2] HAIs associated with MRSA are associated with significant morbidity and mortality, with a substantial proportion of colonized patients subsequently developing an MRSA infection.[2] Studies have shown that interventions can reduce the incidence of HAI and at least 50% are estimated to be preventable.[2]

PREVENTION OF HEALTH CARE–ASSOCIATED INFECTIONS

Hand Hygiene

Since Dr. Ignaz Semmelweis demonstrated that the rate of puerperal (childbed) fever can be drastically reduced through appropriate handwashing in the 1800s, hand hygiene remains the most effective preventive method in the prevention and control of nosocomial infections. Alcohol-based hand hygiene solutions have significantly improved the ability for a health care worker to adhere to hand hygiene policies, but adherence to these policies remains as low as 40%.[3]

Monitoring of adherence to hand hygiene guidelines has become standard in acute care facilities but continues to be a challenge, and no national standards of measurement have been established. Direct observation is considered the gold standard method and provides the most detailed information about hand hygiene compliance by health care personnel.[4] The most commonly accepted framework for measuring hand hygiene opportunities is the World Health Organization's (WHO) Five Moments for Hand Hygiene (see Fig. 9-1):

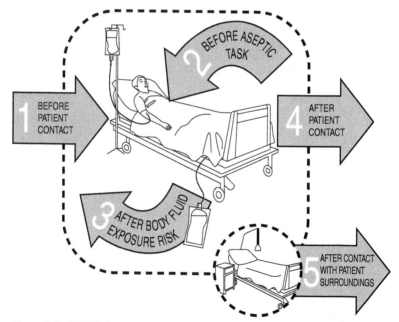

Figure 9-1. WHO's five opportunities for hand hygiene. (Reprinted from World Health Organization: Your 5 Moments for Hand Hygiene, Copyright 2006. http://www.who.int/gpsc/tools/Five_moments/en/. Accessed 5/15/15.)

- Moment 1: before touching the patient, to prevent colonization of the patient with health care–associated microorganisms
- Moment 2: before a clean/aseptic procedure, preventing HAIs that could arise from the patient's endogenous microorganisms or organisms on health care personnel
- Moment 3: after body fluid exposure, reducing the risk of transmission of organisms from a colonized site to a clean site
- Moment 4: after touching the patient, to minimize the risk of transmitting microorganisms to the environment
- Moment 5: after touching the patient surroundings to avoid hand contamination[3]

There are different methods to improve hand hygiene adherence, and each method has strengths and weaknesses:

- Direct observation monitoring of hand hygiene behavior is the gold standard for adherence; it is the only method that can discern all opportunities for hand hygiene within patient care encounters. However, direct observation is labor intensive and subject to the Hawthorne Effect—behavior change based on the awareness of subjects that they are being observed.[3]
- Technology-assisted direct observation includes the use of mobile devices or video-monitoring equipment to document hand hygiene adherence, but video monitoring has limited opportunity for immediate feedback and has potential for impacting patient privacy.[3]
- Product volume or event count measurement can be used as an indirect measurement of hand hygiene adherence. An example is counting all the empty (used) soap containers. This method is not subject to observer bias and may assist in optimal location of soap or foam dispensers but cannot assess adequacy of technique or distinguish between each of the hand hygiene opportunities.[3]
- Intelligent hand hygiene systems are a new technology being developed. Health care personnel will wear a mobile component that can record all hand hygiene opportunities, provide feedback, and respond to personnel behavior. This method is expensive to implement and still cannot distinguish certain types of opportunities within the patient encounter.[3]
- Self-report can raise individuals' awareness of their own practice but is unreliable as health care personnel overestimate their performance.[3]

Several studies have compared the efficacy of hand hygiene products against bacteria. In the majority of studies, alcohol concentrations between 62% and 95% are more effective than antimicrobial soaps.[3] Additionally, alcohol-based regimens have significantly better efficacy in removing several viruses compared with antimicrobial soap.

Hand hygiene technique is important, and the minimal time required by manufacturers of hand hygiene products is generally 15–20 seconds, but recent studies suggest that 15 seconds is insufficient for meeting high-quality hand disinfection standards. In 2009, the WHO published guidance on a standardized multistep technique to promote coverage of all surfaces of the hands, taking approximately 20–30 seconds to complete.[3]

Both hand hygiene and gloves are complementary strategies to prevent transmission of infection within the hospital, but controversy remains about the need for hand hygiene prior to donning nonsterile gloves. The Centers for Disease Control and Prevention (CDC) guidelines emphasize hand hygiene relative to patient contact or contact with patient surroundings, yet the WHO recommends that when an indication for hand hygiene precedes a contact that also requires glove usage, hand hygiene should be performed.[3]

CATHETER-ASSOCIATED URINARY TRACT INFECTIONS

Introduction

CAUTI is one of the most common health care–acquired infections, accounting for 12.9% of health care infections.[5] Recent prevalence surveys report 23.6% of hospitalized patients have a urinary catheter and 70–80% of CAUTIs have been attributable to use of an indwelling urethral catheter.[5–7]

While <3% of patients with bacteriuria develop bacteremia with a urinary isolate, given the high rate of catheter use, CAUTI is one of the most common causes of secondary bacteremia in acute care facilities.[5] Case fatality rate of CAUTIs is approximately 2.3% in US hospitals, with up to 9% morality in bacteremia-associated urinary tract infections and 25–60% in patients with urosepsis.[8]

The annual direct medical cost of CAUTIs is estimated to be $340 to $370 million. As of 2008, the Centers of Medicare and Medicaid Services (CMS) no longer reimburses hospitals for cost related to CAUTI, resulting in renewed effort to prevent and control CAUTIs.[9,10]

Definition

Clinical diagnosis of CAUTI remains challenging, as neither pyuria nor bacteriuria is a reliable indicator of symptomatic UTI.[10] According to the National Healthcare Safety Network (NHSN), CAUTI is defined as a urinary tract infection in which an indwelling catheter was in place for more than two calendar days on the date of the event.[8] Localizing signs and symptoms may not be present or recognized secondary to comorbidity or inability to communicate; the most common presentation is fever and a positive urine culture. Candida species is no longer considered a CAUTI pathogen. While pyuria suggests underlying inflammation, the presence or absence of pyuria is not indicative of CAUTI.[9] This definition lacks specificity given high rates of bacteriuria and will likely lead to overestimation of CAUTI incidence rates.[6]

Risk Factors

Duration of catheterization is a major risk factor for CAUTI and the most important determinant of bacteriuria, with a daily risk of acquisition of 3–7%. Bacteriuria is universal once a catheter remains in place for several weeks.[5,6,8] Bacteriuria develops quickly, and biofilm formation, a complex community of host proteins and organisms that adhere along the catheter surface, can occur.[5,10] Organisms growing within the biofilm are relatively protected from antimicrobials and host defenses.

Catheter trauma and catheter obstruction are well recognized as precipitating events for CAUTI. Other CAUTI risk factors include female sex, severe underlying illness, nonsurgical disease, age >50 years, catheter insertion outside the operating room, diabetes mellitus, and renal function impairment.[9,10] Bacteremia from a urinary source has been linked to neutropenia, renal disease, and male sex.[5]

Prevention

The single most important intervention to prevent CAUTI is avoiding use of an indwelling urinary catheter except in a limited number of accepted indications, including monitoring of urinary output in critically ill patients, perioperative use for selected surgical procedures, and management of urinary retention or obstruction, and to facilitate healing of open pressure ulcers.[5] Unfortunately, 38% of physicians are not aware of urinary catheter use in their patients. Addressing the necessity of the urinary catheter as part of their daily routine may lead to reduction in its use. Additionally, written guidelines for catheter use, insertion, and maintenance should be available at all health care facilities.[6,9]

Catheters should be removed when no longer indicated. Educational reminders have been shown to provide a significant reduction in inappropriate use of urinary catheters by using a nurse-driven multidisciplinary approach to evaluate necessity of urinary catheters.[9] A systematic review of catheter discontinuation strategies for hospitalized patients reported that a stop order reduced duration of catheter use by 1.06 days and decreased rates of CAUTI by 53%.[5]

Catheters should always be inserted under aseptic conditions using sterile equipment with the smallest possible catheter to avoid urethral trauma. Strict adherence to hand hygiene practice is recommended and most outbreaks of urinary pathogens have been linked to inadequate hand hygiene.[10] Both the catheter and collecting system should be replaced if breaks occur in the closed drainage system.[9]

There is limited evidence that antibiotic prophylaxis decreases the rate of bacteriuria; however, it has been shown to select for antimicrobial-resistant organisms.[9] A recent meta-analysis found six trials comparing antibiotic prophylaxis versus no prophylaxis in short-term catheterization (up to 2 weeks) and revealed decreased bacteriuria but no change in the rate of symptomatic CAUTIs.[8]

Introducing a UTI bundle, including avoidance of catheter insertion, maintenance of sterility, product standardization, and early catheter removal, has been shown to decrease catheter utilization from 100% to 73% and CAUTI rate from 5.9 to 2.6 per 1000 catheter days in a neurologic intensive care unit (ICU).[6]

CENTRAL LINE–ASSOCIATED BLOODSTREAM INFECTIONS

Introduction

Central venous catheters (CVC) are ubiquitous in the ICU, with over 15 million CVC days occurring each year.[11] Approximately 250,000 cases of CLABSIs occur yearly, with 30,000–60,000 deaths attributed to infection.[11] CLABSIs are associated with increased length of hospital stay as well as increased cost, varying from $3700 to $39,000 per episode.[12]

Definition

As defined by NHSN, a CLABSI is a laboratory-confirmed bloodstream infection (BSI) where a central line was in place for >2 calendar days from the time the blood culture is drawn.

In order to meet the criteria for laboratory-confirmed BSI, one of the following two situations must be present:

- The patient has a recognized pathogen cultured from one or more blood cultures.
- The patient has at least one sign or symptom of infection, such as fever (>38.0°C), chills, or hypotension, and a positive laboratory result not related to an infection in another site. If the blood culture is positive for a common commensal organism (e.g., coagulase-negative *Staphylococcus*, *Corynebacterium* spp. not *C. diphtheria*, *Bacillus* spp. not *B. anthracis*), two or more blood cultures collected within a calendar day must be positive before this criterion is met.

These criteria include the caveat that the organism cultured from the blood cannot be related to infection at another site, such as a urinary tract infection or intra-abdominal infection cultured with the same bacteria.

Risk Factors

Numerous risk factors have been associated with increased risk of CLABSI (see Table 9-1).[13] Major risk factors include insertion with less than maximum sterile barriers, placement in an old site via guidewire exchange, heavy cutaneous colonization at the catheter hub, and duration of catheter placement >7 days.[13]

Prevention

Use of prevention bundles that focus on catheter insertion has shown to be effective, sustainable, and cost-effective.[12] Their success depends on adherence to each individual measure (see Fig. 9-2).

Education of health care personnel involved in insertion, care, and maintenance of CVCs has been shown to reduce the incidence of CLABSI.[12] Health care professionals who insert a CVC should undergo a credentialing process to ensure competency prior to insertion of a CVC independently; simulation training has been shown to be effective.[12]

Checklists allow institutions to adhere to infection prevention practices at the time of insertion, and health care personnel should ensure that proper aseptic technique is maintained.[12] Checklists should include performing hand hygiene prior to catheter insertion or manipulation.

TABLE 9-1	Risk Factors that Affect Risk for Development of CLABSI
Factors Associated with Increased Risk of CLABSI	**Factors Associated with Decreased Risk of CLABSI**
Prolonged hospitalization before catheterization	Female sex
Prolonged duration of catheterization	Antibiotic administration
Heavy microbial colonization at insertion site or catheter hub	Antibiotic-impregnated catheters
Change of catheter over guidewire	Maximum sterile barriers
Inexperience of operator	Chlorhexidine use prior to insertion
Neutropenia	
Prematurity	
Reduced nurse-to-patient ratio in the ICU	
Total parenteral nutrition	
Substandard catheter care	
Transfusion of blood products	

For Clinicians:

Perform daily audits to assess whether each central line is still needed; remove unnecessary lines promptly

Follow proper insertion practices
- ☐ Perform hand hygiene before insertion
- ☐ Adhere to aseptic technique
- ☐ Use maximal sterile barrier precautions (i.e., mask, cap, gown, sterile gloves, and sterile full body drape)
- ☐ Perform skin antisepsis with >0.5% chlorhexidine with alcohol
- ☐ Choose the best site to minimize infections and mechanical complications (i.e., avoid femoral site in adult patients)

Handle and maintain central lines appropriately
- ☐ Comply with hand hygiene requirements
- ☐ Scrub the access port or hub immediately prior to each use with an appropriate antiseptic (e.g., chlorhexidine, povidone iodine, an iodophor, or 70% alcohol)
- ☐ Access catheters only with sterile devices
- ☐ Replace dressings that are wet, soiled, or dislodged
- ☐ Perform dressing changes under aseptic technique using clean or sterile gloves

For Facilities:

- ☐ Empower staff to stop non-emergent insertion if proper procedures are not followed
- ☐ "Bundle" supplies (e.g., in a kit) to ensure items are readily available for use
- ☐ Provide the checklist above to clinicians, to ensure all insertion practices are followed
- ☐ Ensure efficient access to hand hygiene
- ☐ Monitor and provide prompt feedback for adherence to hand hygiene
- ☐ Provide recurring education sessions on central line insertion, handling and maintenance

Figure 9-2. Checklist for prevention of CLABSI. (Adapted from the 2011 CDC guidelines for prevention of intravascular catheter-associated BSIs. http://www.cdc.gov/HAI/pdfs/bsi/checklist-for-CLABSI.pdf)

The preferred sites of placement for central lines are femoral, subclavian, and internal jugular veins. Previous studies have shown that the femoral site is associated with an increased risk for infection, but a recent meta-analysis showed no difference in the rate of CLABSI between all three sites.[11] Current recommendations recommend avoiding femoral vein catheterization in obese adult patients unless the catheter is placed under planned and controlled conditions.[12] If placing a central line in the internal jugular vein, use of ultrasound guidance is recommended as studies have shown a reduction in the risk of CLABSI and complications.[12]

Full sterile barrier precautions are recommended during insertion, which include mask, cap, sterile gown, and sterile gloves to be worn by all health care personnel involved in the insertion procedure. Full-body sterile drapes should be placed on the patient during insertion. The Seldinger technique for catheter insertion allows for central veins to be cannulated with less risk of pneumothorax and vascular injury. Prospective randomized trials have indicated that exchange of catheter over a guidewire is associated with a twofold increased risk of catheter-related bloodstream infection.[13]

Heavy colonization at the insertion site has been associated with CLABSIs, and reduction of microflora at a potential insertion site is a priority. Chlorhexidine-based antiseptics exhibits prolonged antimicrobial activity on the skin surface after a single application compared to alcohol-only or iodine-based antiseptics.[13] All catheter hubs, needless connectors, and injection ports should be disinfected prior to accessing the catheter with either chlorhexidine–alcohol solution, 70% alcohol, or povidone–iodine. Applying mechanical friction for no <5 seconds reduces contamination.[12]

While the risk of CLABSI is reduced with antiseptic-impregnated catheters and antimicrobial-impregnated catheters, use of these specialized catheters is only recommended in three scenarios: (1) hospital units or patient populations that have CLABSI rates above institutional goals despite compliance with basic CLABSI principles; (2) patients who have limited venous access and a history of recurrent CLABSI; or (3) patients who are at risk of severe sequelae from CLABSI.[12]

VENTILATOR-ASSOCIATED EVENTS

Introduction

The true incidence of VAP is difficult to determine, as surveillance definitions have changed and have poor specificity. Approximately 5–10 health care–associated pneumonias per 1000 hospital admissions occur yearly and 10–20% of ventilated patients will develop VAP, although more recent reports have suggested lower rates of VAP.[14,15] Mortality of VAP is estimated to be 10% but varies depending on patient factors.

Nasally or orally ventilated patients are at risk for a variety of complications including acute respiratory distress syndrome, pneumothorax, pulmonary embolism, lobar atelectasis, and pulmonary edema. These terms have been included in the catch-all phrase ventilator-associated events (VAEs), and approximately 5–10% of mechanically ventilated patients develop VAEs.[14] VAEs extend patient's duration of mechanical ventilation, increase intensive care and hospital length of stay, and increase mortality risk, although excess costs attributable to VAE have not been quantified.[14,16]

Definition

Previously, VAP was defined by clinical, radiographic, and microbiologic criteria, but these signs are neither sensitive nor specific compared to histology.[14] The CDC thus convened in 2011–2012 to develop a new approach to surveillance for mechanically ventilated patients given the limitation of traditional VAP definitions. The CDC thus created a three-tiered definition of VAEs (see Table 9-2).

Risk Factors

The risk of VAP is the highest in the first few days of intubation, with a daily hazard rate of approximately 3% at day 5 of intubation, decreasing to 1% per day by day 15; cumulative risk continues to accrue for the duration of mechanical ventilation.[17]

Prevention

Guidelines for prevention of VAP and other VAEs are divided based on age, but in this chapter, the focus will remain on adults. Avoiding intubation with noninvasive positive pressure ventilation (NIPPV) can be beneficial in patients with hypercarbic or hypoxemic respiratory failure secondary to chronic obstructive pulmonary disease as

TABLE 9-2 Three-tiered Definition for VAE from the CDC

Terminology	Definition
Ventilator-associated condition (VAC)	≥2 days of stable or decreasing daily minimum positive end-expiratory pressure (PEEP) or minimum fraction of inspired oxygen (FiO_2) followed by an increase in daily minimum PEEP ≥3 cm of H_2O or daily minimum FiO_2 ≥0.20 points sustained for ≥2 calendar days
Infection-related ventilator-associated condition (IVAC)	Presence of possible infection concurrent with VAC onset: abnormal temperature (below 36°C or above 38°C) or white blood cell count (≤4000 or ≥12,000 cells/mm³) and 1 or more new antibiotic starts that continue for ≥4 days
Ventilator-associated pneumonia (VAP)	
Possible VAP	Gram stain evidence of purulent pulmonary secretions or a pathogenic pulmonary culture in a patient with IVAC
Probable VAP	Gram stain evidence of purulence plus quantitative or semiquantitative growth of a pathogenic organism beyond specific thresholds

well as cardiogenic congestive heart failure. NIPPV has been shown to decrease VAP risk, shorten duration of mechanical ventilation, decrease length of stay, and lower mortality rates, but if used outside of these special populations, a delay in intubation may lead to increased harm.[14]

While patients are on mechanical ventilation, avoidance of sedatives such as benzodiazepines is recommended. Two randomized control trials have shown that daily sedative interruptions decreased net sedative exposures and reduced the average duration of mechanical ventilation by 2–4 days.[14] Daily spontaneous breathing trials also are associated with extubation 1–2 days earlier compared to usual care.[14]

If possible, minimize pooling of secretions above the endotracheal tube cuff for patients requiring intubation for longer than 48–72 hours. A meta-analysis of 13 randomized controlled trials showed that the use of endotracheal tubes with subglottic drainage reduced VAP rates by 55%, duration of mechanical ventilation by a mean of 1.1 days, and intensive care length of stay by 1.5 days.[14]

Elevating the head of the bed to 30–45 degrees has been evaluated with three randomized controlled trials, and a meta-analysis pooling of these studies did find a significant impact in decreasing VAP rates.[14]

Changing the ventilator circuit is only required if it is visibly soiled or malfunctioning. Changing the circuit on fixed schedules has no impact on VAP rates or patient outcomes.[14]

If high VAP rates are an issue, the following interventions have been shown to decrease duration of mechanical ventilation, length of stay, and mortality although there are insufficient data on their long-term consequences:

- While selective decontamination of the oropharynx with topical antibiotics or of the oropharynx and digestive tract with a combination of oral and parenteral antibiotics has decreased mortality rates by 14% and 17%, respectively, in The Netherlands, this strategy is not adopted in the US given concern for development of antibiotic resistance and *Clostridium difficile* infection (CDI).[14]
- Oral care with chlorhexidine has been studied in 16 randomized controlled trials and 9 meta-analyses and benefits have been shown to be most pronounced in preventing postoperative respiratory tract infections in cardiac surgery patients.[14]
- Four meta-analyses have found lower VAP rates in patients who receive prophylactic probiotics, but no significant impact on mortality has been shown.[14]

Approaches that are generally not recommended include silver-coated endotracheal tubes, kinetic beds, and prone positioning. Stress ulcer prophylaxis lowers the risk of gastrointestinal bleeding, but meta-analyses suggest that there is no impact on pneumonia rates, length of stay, or mortality.[14] Early tracheostomy has been shown to have little impact on VAP rates.[14]

SURGICAL SITE INFECTIONS

Introduction

SSIs occur in 2–5% of patients undergoing inpatient surgery equaling 160,000–300,000 SSIs yearly in the US.[18] SSIs are considered the most common and costly HAI, with 60% considered to be preventable.[18] SSIs add 7–11 additional hospital days to the patient's length of stay and account for $3.5 to $10 billion dollars annually in excess health care expenditures.[18] Furthermore, patients with an SSI have 2–11 times higher risk of death, with 77% of deaths in patients with SSI attributed directly to the infection.[18]

Definition

- SSIs are classified based on depth of infection (see Fig. 9-3).
- Superficial incisional infection involves only the skin and subcutaneous tissues. These infections are most commonly managed in an outpatient setting.
- Deep incisional infections involve the fascia and/or muscular layers and are further broken down by primary or secondary infection. A deep incision primary infection is an SSI identified in a primary incision in a patient who has had an operation with one or more incisions. A deep incision secondary infection is an SSI identified in a secondary incision in a patient with more than one incision.
- Organ/space infections involve any part of the body opened or manipulated during a procedure, excluding skin incision, fascia, or muscle layers.[18] Both deep incisional and organ space infections typically require readmission to the hospital for management.
- For epidemiologic definitions of SSI, see Table 9-3.

Risk Factors

Risk factors can be separated into intrinsic patient-related characteristics and extrinsic procedure-related characteristics.

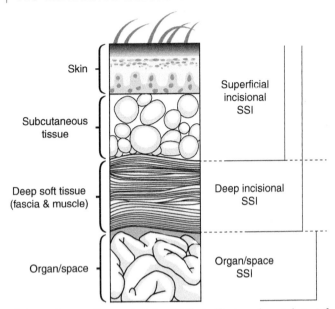

Figure 9-3. A schematic diagram depicting CDC classification of surgical site infections. (Modified from Mangram AJ, Horan TC, Pearson ML, et al. The hospital infection control practices advisory committee. Guideline for the prevention of surgical site infection, 1999. *Infect Control Hosp Epidemiol.* 1999;20:247–80. http://www.cdc.gov/hicpac/pdf/guidelines/ SSI_1999.pdf. Accessed 5/15/15.)

- Age, history of radiation at a surgical site, and previous history of skin infection are all nonmodifiable patient risk factors. Modifiable risk factors include glucose control with a goal of glycosylated hemoglobin A1C levels of lesser than 7%, obesity, smoking cessation, avoidance of immunosuppressive medications in the perioperative period, and hypoalbuminemia.[18]
- Extrinsic procedure-related risk factors include surgical scrub, skin preparation, antimicrobial prophylaxis, avoidance of blood transfusion, minimizing operative time and operating room traffic, and sterilization of surgical equipment according to published guidelines while minimizing immediate-use steam sterilization.[18]

MRSA is a major cause of HAIs, and patients undergoing surgery are at risk of acquiring these infections. Colonization rates of *S. aureus* are approximately 30%.[19] Recently, some hospitals have started screening for *S. aureus* and treating colonized patients prior to surgery as well as selecting the appropriate antistaphylococcal agent in the preoperative setting. A recent meta-analysis of 17 studies concluded that decolonization strategies are effective at preventing SSIs caused by MRSA, MSSA, and other gram-positive pathogens.[18,20] Additionally, bundles that include decontamination, decolonization, and targeted vancomycin prophylaxis have been associated with significantly lower MRSA SSI rates.[21]

TABLE 9-3 NSHN Definitions for SSIs

Superficial SSI

- Infection that occurs within 30 days after any operative procedure
- Involves only skin and subcutaneous tissue of the incision
- The patient has at least one of the following:
  a. Purulent drainage from the superficial incision.
  b. Organisms isolated from an aseptically obtained culture of fluid or tissue from the superficial incision.
  c. Superficial incision that is deliberately opened by a surgeon, attending physician,[1] or other designee and is culture positive or not cultured, and the patient has at least one of the following signs or symptoms: pain or tenderness, localized swelling, redness, or heat. A culture-negative finding does not meet this criterion.
  d. Diagnosis of a superficial incisional SSI by the surgeon or attending physician[a] or other designee.

Deep Incisional SSI

- Infection that occurs within 30 or 90[b] days after the operative procedure
- Involves deep soft tissues of the incision (e.g., fascial and muscle layers)
- The patient has at least one of the following:
  a. Purulent drainage from the deep incision.
  b. A deep incision that spontaneously dehisces or is deliberately opened by a surgeon, attending physician,[a] or other designee and is culture positive or not cultured, and the patient has at least one of the following signs or symptoms: fever (>38°C), localized pain, or tenderness. A culture-negative finding does not meet this criterion.
  c. An abscess or other evidence of infection involving the deep incision that is detected on direct examination, during invasive procedure, or by histopathologic examination or imaging test.

Organ Space SSI

- Infection that occurs within 30 or 90[b] days after the operative procedure
- Infection involves any part of the body, excluding the skin incision, fascia, or muscle layers, that is opened or manipulated during the operative procedure.
- The patient has at least one of the following:
  a. Purulent drainage from a drain that is placed into the organ/space
  b. Organisms isolated from an aseptically obtained culture of fluid or tissue in the organ/space
  c. An abscess or other evidence of infection involving the organ/space that is detected on direct examination, during invasive procedure, or by histopathologic examination or imaging test

[a]Up to 90 days for procedure involving prosthetic devices.
[b]Surgeon(s), infectious disease, other physician on the case, emergency physician, or physician's designee (nurse practitioner or physician's assistant).
(Adapted from NHSN Module. http://www.cdc.gov/nhsn/pdfs/pscmanual/9pscssicurrent.pdf)

Prevention

Guidelines have been published for the prevention of SSIs. The Surgical Infection Prevention (SIP) Project was established by the CMS in 2002 and focused on delivering the most appropriate intravenous antimicrobial prophylaxis at the optimal time, weight-based dose, and proper duration. The Surgical Care Improvement Project (SCIP) was an expansion of SIP created in 2003 that focused on proper hair removal, control of blood glucose postoperatively, and maintenance of normothermia in surgical patients. A comprehensive analysis showed that adherence to SCIP requirements led to an 18% decrease in the odds of developing an SSI.[22] CMS currently requires that hospitals submit data on seven SCIP measures as a part of the Hospital Inpatient Quality Reporting System.[18]

Prophylactic antibiotics, according to evidence-based standards and guidelines, should be administered within 1 hour prior to incision (2 hours for vancomycin and fluoroquinolones) in order to maximize tissue concentrations while the incision is open. These antibiotics should be discontinued within 24 hours after surgery (48 hours for cardiac procedures) as there is no benefit to administering antimicrobial agents after closure of the incision. Prolonged antimicrobial use has shown to confer resistance and increase the risk of CIDs.[18]

Do not remove hair at the operative site unless the presence of hair will interfere with the operation. If hair removal is necessary, clipping with clippers are recommended as opposed to shaving with razors.

Blood glucose levels should be kept below 180 mg/dL in the 18–24 hours after anesthesia end time. More intensive postoperative glucose control has not been shown to reduce the risk of SSI and may only lead to higher risk of adverse outcomes.[18]

Normothermia is imperative during the perioperative period as even mild degrees of hypothermia can increase SSI rates. Hypothermia may directly impair neutrophil function or it may impair it indirectly by triggering subcutaneous vasoconstriction and subsequent tissue hypoxia.[18]

Alcohol-containing preoperative skin preparatory agents are recommended as they are highly bactericidal, but alcohol alone does not have persistent activity; addition of chlorhexidine or povidone–iodine is recommended.

Supplemental oxygen during and immediately following surgical procedures involving mechanical ventilation can be considered as an additional preventive measure. A meta-analysis of 5 studies concluded that perioperative supplemental oxygen led to a relative risk reduction of 25% for SSI.[18]

Education is key to implementing prevention within the hospital. If one surgeon or one area within surgery is noted to have elevation in SSI, providing one-to-one education of evidence-based practices has been shown to decrease SSI rates.[18]

CLOSTRIDIUM DIFFICILE

Introduction

Clostridium difficile is an important transmissible nosocomial pathogen. CDI is the leading cause of infectious diarrhea among hospitalized patients.[23] In a recent survey of US hospitals, gastrointestinal infections were the third most common type of HAI, of which 70.9% were attributed to *C. difficile*.[7] During the past decade, CDI has become more frequent, more severe, and more refractory to treatment. Between the years 2000 and 2009, CDI rates have more than doubled, and recent studies have reported that CDI rates have now surpassed MRSA rates in hospitals.[24,25] CDI increases hospital length of stay by 2.8–5.5 days. Attributable costs have been estimated to be $3006 to $15,397 per episode, and US hospital costs have been estimated to be $1.0 to $4.9 billion per year.[25] The attributable mortality of CDI is estimated to be 5–10%, leading to an estimated 14,000–20,000 deaths each year.[25]

Definition

CDI is defined as a case of clinically significant diarrhea or toxic megacolon without other known etiology that either a stool sample yields a positive result of *C. difficile* toxin, pseudomembranous colitis is seen on endoscopic examination, or pseudomembranous colitis is seen on histopathologic examination (Table 9-4).[25] A positive result of *C. difficile* toxin is the most common method to identify patients with CDI. Patient may be carriers of *C. difficile*, and samples should only be tested when diarrhea is present.[25]

Prevention

Clostridium difficile is a spore-forming bacteria, which poses challenges for hand hygiene and environmental disinfection practices since spores are resistant to the bactericidal effects of alcohol. Although alcohol is not effective at removal of these spores, no clinical study has shown an increase in CDI rates when alcohol-based hand rubs are the predominant hand hygiene product used, nor a decrease in CDI rates if soap and water is the predominant method for hand hygiene.[25] Several controlled studies have found that alcohol-based hand hygiene products to be ineffective at removing *C. difficile* spores from the hands of volunteers. However, a more recent study has found that most alcohol-based hand hygiene products result in a lesser than 1 log reduction

TABLE 9-4 Classification of CDI	
Case Type	Definition
Health care facility–onset, health care facility–associated CDI	CDI symptom onset >3 days after admission to a health care facility
Community-onset, health care facility–associated CDI	CDI symptom onset within the community ≤3 days from admission, <4 weeks after last discharge from a health care facility
Community-associated CDI	CDI symptom onset in the community ≤3 days after admission to hospital, >12 weeks after last discharge from a health care facility
Indeterminate-onset CDI	CDI symptoms >4 weeks but <12 weeks from last discharge from a health care facility
Unknown	Exposure setting cannot be determined because of a lack of available data
Recurrent CDI	An episode of CDI that occurs ≤8 weeks after the onset of a previous episode

in spores despite a 60-second handwash.[25] Contamination of hands is less common when gloves are worn before the patient encounter.

Restriction on antimicrobial use and stewardship are important in the prevention of CDI. Fluoroquinolones have been found to be one of the antimicrobials that are most associated with the development of CDI, but virtually every antibiotic has been associated, including cephalosporins, ampicillin, and clindamycin. Restriction of specific high-risk antimicrobials has been effective in outbreak settings.[25]

Full barrier precautions and hand hygiene prevent indirect transmission by health care professionals. The CDC currently recommends contact precautions to be continued for the duration of illness and up to 48 hours after diarrhea resolves. Patients with CDI can continue to shed spores in the stool and contaminate the environment, but there are no data to support extending contact isolation period beyond 48 hours after resolution of the diarrhea as a measure to decrease CDI incidence.[25] A recent ICU study found admission to a room previously occupied by a patient with CDI to be a risk factor for acquisition, but 90% of patients who developed CDI did not have this risk factor.

When CDI remains higher than the institution's goal, a CDI risk assessment should be performed, and infection prevention with contact precautions and hand hygiene should be intensified. Rooms should be assessed for adequacy of room cleaning. The use of chlorine (at least 500–1000 parts per million in concentration) to disinfect the room may be helpful in reducing CDI rates.

KEY POINTS

- Strict adherence to hand hygiene is essential to decrease the incidence of HAIs.
- Limiting the duration or the complete elimination of use of urinary catheters and CVC decreases the risk of developing CAUTI and CLABSI.
- Encouraging appropriate use of antimicrobials through antimicrobial stewardship programs is essential to prevent the acquisition of CDI in the hospital.
- Use of bundles and checklists can prevent HAIs.
- Surveillance of HAIs by infection prevention teams and proper dissemination of data to staff at all levels leads to a reduction of HAIs within a hospital system.

ONLINE RESOURCES

1. CDC Healthcare-associated Infections: http://www.cdc.gov/hai/
2. IDSA Infection Prevention: http://www.idsociety.org/Infection_Control_Policy/

REFERENCES

1. Yokoe DS, et al. A compendium of strategies to prevent healthcare-associated infections in acute care hospitals: 2014 updates. *Am J Infect Control.* 2014;42(8):820–8.
2. Zimlichman E, et al. Health care-associated infections: a meta-analysis of costs and financial impact on the US health care system. *JAMA Intern Med.* 2013;173(22):2039–46.
3. Ellingson K, et al. Strategies to prevent healthcare-associated infections through hand hygiene. *Infect Control Hosp Epidemiol.* 2014;35(8):937–60.
4. Boyce JM. Update on hand hygiene. *Am J Infect Control.* 2013;41(5 Suppl):S94–6.

5. Nicolle LE. Catheter associated urinary tract infections. *Antimicrob Resistance Infect Control.* 2014;3(23). http://www.aricjournal.com/content/3/1/23

6. Lo E, et al. Strategies to prevent catheter-associated urinary tract infections in acute care hospitals: 2014 update. *Infect Control Hosp Epidemiol.* 2014;35(5):464–79.

7. Magill SS, et al. Multistate point-prevalence survey of health care-associated infections. *N Engl J Med.* 2014;370(13):1198–208.

8. Tenke P, Koves B, Johansen TE. An update on prevention and treatment of catheter-associated urinary tract infections. *Curr Opin Infect Dis.* 2014;27(1):102–7.

9. Tambyah PA, Oon J. Catheter-associated urinary tract infection. *Curr Opin Infect Dis.* 2012;25(4):365–70.

10. Chenoweth C, Saint S. Preventing catheter-associated urinary tract infections in the intensive care unit. *Crit Care Clin.* 2013;29(1):19–32.

11. Marik PE, Flemmer M, Harrison W. The risk of catheter-related bloodstream infection with femoral venous catheters as compared to subclavian and internal jugular venous catheters: a systematic review of the literature and meta-analysis. *Crit Care Med.* 2012;40(8):2479–85.

12. Marschall J, et al. Strategies to prevent central line-associated bloodstream infections in acute care hospitals: 2014 update. *Infect Control Hosp Epidemiol.* 2014;35(7):753–71.

13. Safdar N, Kluger DM, Maki DG. A review of risk factors for catheter-related bloodstream infection caused by percutaneous inserted, noncuffed central venous catheters. *Medicine.* 2002;81(6):466–79.

14. Klompas M, et al. Strategies to prevent ventilator-associated pneumonia in acute care hospitals: 2014 update. *Infect Control Hosp Epidemiol.* 2014;35(8):915–36.

15. Wilke M, Grube R. Update on management options in the treatment of nosocomial and ventilator assisted pneumonia: review of actual guidelines and economic aspects of therapy. *Infect Drug Resist.* 2013;7:1–7.

16. Piazza O, Wang X. A translational approach to ventilator associated pneumonia. *Clin Trans Med.* 2014;3(26). http://www.clintransmed.com/content/3/1/26

17. Bouadma L, Wolff M, Lucet JC. Ventilator-associated pneumonia and its prevention. *Curr Opin Infect Dis.* 2012;25(4):395–404.

18. Anderson DJ, et al. Strategies to prevent surgical site infections in acute care hospitals: 2014 update. *Infect Control Hosp Epidemiol.* 2014;35(6):605–27.

19. Kavanagh KT, et al. The use of surveillance and preventative measures for methicillin-resistant *Staphylococcus aureus* infections in surgical patients. *Antimicrob Resist Infect Control.* 2014;3(18). http://www.ncbi.nlm.nih.gov/pmc/articles/PMC4028005/

20. Schweizer M, et al. Effectiveness of a bundled intervention of decolonization and prophylaxis to decrease Gram positive surgical site infections after cardiac or orthopedic surgery: systematic review and meta-analysis. *BMJ.* 2013;346:f2743.

21. Schweizer ML, Herwaldt LA. Surgical site infections and their prevention. *Curr Opin Infect Dis.* 2012;25(4):378–84.

22. Munday GS, et al. Impact of implementation of the surgical care improvement project and future strategies for improving quality in surgery. *Am J Surg.* 2014;208(5):835–40. doi: 10.1016/j.amjsurg.2014.05.005. Epub Jul 1, 2014.

23. Gabriel L, Beriot-Mathiot A. Hospitalization stay and costs attributable to Clostridium difficile infection: a critical review. *J Hosp Infect.* 2014;88(1):12–21.

24. Miller BA, et al. Comparison of the burdens of hospital-onset, healthcare-facility-associated *Clostridium difficile* infection and of healthcare-associated infection due to methicillin-resistant *Staphylococcus aureus* in community hospitals. *Infect Control Hosp Epidemiol.* 2011;32(4):387–90.

25. Dubberke ER, et al. Strategies to prevent *Clostridium difficile* infections in acute care hospitals: 2014 Update. *Infect Control Hosp Epidemiol.* 2014;35(6):628–45.

Coding and Documentation

Melissa Sum and Robert J. Mahoney

CLINICAL VIGNETTE

A 33-year-old woman with end-stage renal disease presents with swelling and erythema over her dialysis graft site for 5 months. Diagnosed with an infected chronic thrombus, she is admitted for intravenous antibiotics. On admission, she reports an allergy to multiple antibiotics and refuses all medications ending in "-mycin." She is started on cefazolin and metronidazole. After starting this regimen, she notifies staff of a suspected allergic reaction to the metronidazole; the documentation indicates that she appears "well with normal vital signs and no evidence of allergic reaction on exam." Later that day, she is taken to the operating room for debridement and is given intravenous gentamicin, metronidazole, and cefazolin. In recovery, she is noted to be "yelling and scratching" and is given famotidine, diphenhydramine, and hydroxyzine. That evening, the patient complains of feeling unwell and requests prednisone. The request is not documented, nor is a physician evaluation of the patient. The patient receives diphenhydramine and prednisone, "for allergy and itching." The next morning, the patient is found lying across the bed, pulseless. A code blue is called, and cardiopulmonary resuscitation is administered, unsuccessfully. The covering physician reviews the chart and calls the patient's family to inform them of her death.

- Could improved documentation have led to better or safer care?
- Can improved documentation lead to better troubleshooting of unexpected outcomes?

INTRODUCTION

The quality of documentation in medical records has long been subject to improvement. In William Osler's era at the end of the 19th century, house officers worked, slept, and ate at the hospital and were expected to present information to consultants directly. Accordingly, medical record documentation often reflected only superficial aspects of the care provided. Furthermore, Osler and other senior faculty rarely signed chart notes.[1]

With the complexity of modern medical care—encompassing multiple collaborating physicians and complex testing—the medical record now serves a dual role as a critical communication tool and as a repository of clinical information.

Currently, the medical record is the primary means to communicate relevant information about a patient's care to other care providers, to payors, and to allied health professionals. Information from the record is abstracted to determine what services were provided and to provide justification for those services.

The medical record is also a key component of patient safety and serves an important medicolegal function.[2] Medical record documentation is routinely used to assess the severity of illness (SOI) and the likelihood of adverse outcomes.

Given the central role of documentation in capturing and communicating a patient's medical course—and the ease with which multiple providers can now access and contribute to it—high-quality documentation is rapidly becoming synonymous with high-quality care.

PRINCIPLES OF QUALITY DOCUMENTATION

Accuracy

Above all, clinical documentation should reflect the observations and experiences that comprise a given patient encounter as accurately as possible. What is documented during an encounter will likely form the basis for future treatment decisions, making the fidelity of the record essential. When possible, documentation should occur concurrently with the care provided.[3]

Specificity

As we will see in this chapter, a significant amount of information is abstracted from clinical documentation, including indicators of SOI, expected mortality, and the diagnosis and management data used to bill for services. For this reason, the findings and diagnoses in the record should be as specific as possible. Many institutions have hired clinical documentation improvement (CDI) personnel to collaborate with physicians to improve the specificity of the diagnoses provided in their documentation. As the US adopts the tenth edition of the International Classification of Diseases (ICD-10) for coding, the amount of specificity required to properly assign diagnoses for encounters—and, theoretically, the quality of the data extracted from documentation—is expected to increase significantly.[4]

Legibility

Thankfully, the increasing adoption of electronic record systems has reduced the problem of illegible handwritten notes. Nonetheless, many institutions continue to maintain some component of handwritten records. As long as such handwritten notes are a part of the medical record, every effort should be made to make these notes legible.

According to one study of attending and resident physician handwritten records, a considerable portion of the records was illegible.[5] Sixteen percent of the written words were illegible; the complete context could be understood in only 58% of the notes. In addition to medical errors resulting from illegible handwritten medication orders or other documentation, legible records are important to convey to others what has transpired over the course of the day in this era of duty-hour regulations and increasing patient handoffs.

Avoiding Duplicated Documentation ("Copy/Paste")

Many electronic record systems allow providers to copy documentation from other days or other providers into their notes. While this affords convenience, and perhaps more consistent documentation, it can lead to propagation of inaccurate or outdated information.[6] Furthermore, because clinical documentation is abstracted to determine the services provided to a given patient, duplicated documentation can lead to inaccurate—or worse, fraudulent—billing for services.

Out of concern for overpayments provided potentially as a result of duplicated documentation, the U.S. Department of Health and Human Services (HHS) Office of the Inspector General (OIG) announced as part of its work plan for 2013 that it would begin reviewing clinical documentation for evidence of "documentation practices associated with potentially improper payments," including duplicated documentation.[7]

DOCUMENTATION AS A QUALITY COMPONENT

Quality Indicators/Severity of Illness/Risk of Mortality

Since 1992, the Health Care Financing Administration (HCFA)—now the Center for Medicare and Medicaid Services (CMS)—has focused on improving the quality of the medical care in the US.

Instead of relying on clinicians' intuitive criteria to manage patients, peer review organizations (PROs) utilize explicit, nationally uniform criteria to assess patterns of care and outcomes.[8] The PRO program has derived quality indicators (QIs), which measure aspects of health care quality using readily available hospital inpatient administrative data.

The Agency for Healthcare Research and Quality (AHRQ) has developed four sets of QIs:

- Inpatient Quality Indicators (IQIs): These are 32 items reflecting the quality of inpatient care, including inhospital mortality rates for 7 specific medical conditions and 8 surgical procedures, utilization rates for 11 specific procedures, and hospital-level case volume for 6 complex procedures. Each indicator is selected based on evidence that utilization practices or mortality rates vary by institution and may benefit from standardized observation.
- Patient Safety Indicators (PSIs): These are 27 indicators of potentially avoidable complications or other adverse events related to inpatient care.
- Prevention Quality Indicators (PQIs): These are hospital admission rates for 14 conditions wherein admission may reflect shortfalls in outpatient care.
- Pediatric Quality Indicators (PDIs): These are 18 indicators similar to IQIs, PQIs, or PSIs, applied to the pediatric population.

All of the foregoing QIs are derived from hospital documentation at discharge. Originally intended for research and quality improvement activities,[9] they are now publicly available and used to derive pay-for-performance parameters and for grading providers for tiered insurance products.

In addition to deriving QIs, the medical record is also used to determine other important measures. As indicated earlier in this chapter, the diagnoses documented and procedures performed during inpatient encounters are used to determine a key variable, the SOI. The SOI affords reviewers a benchmark for hospital resource use and outcomes by classifying the extent of a given patient's organ system derangement or physiologic decompensation into categories (minor, moderate, major, or extreme). This allows for comparison across hospitals while controlling for the acuity of illness in their patient population.

The risk of mortality (ROM) provides a rough estimate of the likelihood of inpatient survival for a class of patients, again controlled for the degree of illness. Often viewed as a measure of quality, the ROM is used by hospitals and quality organizations across the nation to perform comparison to peer institutions while accounting for the impact of individual risk factors, such as age and SOI. Notably, increasing the consistency and specificity of secondary diagnosis codes has been shown to improve the accuracy of risk-adjusted inpatient mortality rates.[10]

Impact on Quality of Care

While facilitating an accurate assessment of care quality, appropriate documentation could conceivably lead to improved care quality. For example, accurate documentation of the stage of chronic kidney disease could render clinicians more aware of the need for medication dose adjustments to prevent over- or underdosing. A study on wrong-site surgery found that approximately one-third of these sentinel events were attributable to errors that occurred in the weeks prior to surgery, including wrong documentation and inaccurate labeling of radiologic reports.[11] Another study in oncology patients showed that proper documentation of symptoms led to improved symptom management, ultimately improving patients' health-related quality of life.[12]

At the same time, few studies have examined whether improving documentation actually leads to improved quality of care. Authors in one study found a substantial increase in the completion of recommended preventive care such as vaccinations and mammograms after the implementation of an electronic medical record (EMR).[13] Recent studies in the ambulatory setting, however, suggest that outpatient records may not accurately reflect actual provision of quality care components. In one study, investigators assessed 12 quality measures among all eligible adult patients in 2008 at a federally qualified health center using a commercially available health record. They found sensitivities of electronic reporting for each measure ranging from 46% to 98% compared to manual review of what actually was provided. As a result, incentives intended to reward high quality may not necessarily be given to the highest quality provider; rather, these incentives may reward the highest quality documenters.[14]

One of the most important roles for clinical documentation is communication during transitions of care; nowhere is this more evident than at hospital discharge. Communication of a patient's hospital course to the patient's primary care provider is a critical step in the discharge process. Yet, in one systematic review, primary care providers had a discharge summary at only 12–34% of postdischarge visits, and key information was often deemed missing from the discharge summaries.[15] These gaps in communication lead to confusion for the patient and the providers and could be a potential course of adverse events and readmissions.

The fragmentation of inpatient care also means that, increasingly, "cross-cover physicians" get called for patients under the care of another "primary team." Such cross-cover care should be documented whenever a physician is called for a significant event or a change in status. Notes need to include key components of the clinical issue for which the physician was called, relevant subjective and objective data, the physician's assessment and plan, as well as required follow-up. This documented information will be helpful in alerting the primary team that their patient experienced an incident that required a physician's evaluation, will help the primary team (and other teams taking care of the patient) understand the rationale for cross-cover management decisions, and will inform the teams of any follow-up required. A sample template for a cross-cover note is included in Figure 10-1.

Revisiting the clinical vignette at the start of the chapter, it is possible that improved documentation of the patient's symptoms could have led to a recognition

Cross-cover note
Called to see patient for:
Time of patient evaluation:
Symptoms:
Vital signs:
Physical exam and laboratory/imaging data:
Assessment:
Plan (actions taken, orders placed):
Follow-up required:

Figure 10-1. A sample template for a cross-cover note.

of her distress, the need to provide further evaluation, and the opportunity to potentially adjust therapy for a possible allergic reaction—or at least increase the level of monitoring and potentially avoid the adverse outcome.

Litigation

Being involved in medical malpractice is one of the most traumatic experiences any physician can face. More than 42% of physicians have been sued over the course of their careers (American Medical Association survey, 2010, covering years 2007 to 2008). At the same time, fewer than 8% of medical malpractice cases ever reach a jury; at the trial stage, physicians prevail in 80–90% of the cases. According to the Indian Health Service *Risk Management Manual,* "the medical record is the best device we have to protect against malpractice claims."[16]

The characteristics of a defensible medical record include **completeness, objectivity, consistency**, and **accuracy**. Above all else, documentation quality remains the most important factor in the success or failure of most claims.[17] A review showed that documentation in obstetric malpractice cases was more often judged as substandard (13%) rather than acceptable (2%).[18] Since cases often proceed to trial years after the care was provided, an accurate account must exist in the records from the time of the encounter. Documentation should also include informed consent to—or informed refusal of—care deemed medically necessary.

Although informal or "curbside" consultations (in which the consultant may not ever see the patient or review the chart) are a frequent part of medical practice, there is no consensus on proper documentation of such informal consults. In general, such consultations are completely "off the record." Clinicians should avoid documenting the name of the colleague providing the informal consult, or the nature of the recommendations, unless such permission is obtained.[19] Any clinician whose name is entered in the medical record can become entangled in legal proceedings.

When asked to provide such an informal consultation, clinicians should readily suggest formal consultation when appropriate. Finally, when providing informal consultations, it may be advisable to provide academic, generalizable information, rather than patient-specific advice.

DOCUMENTATION AS A TROUBLESHOOTING TOOL

What to Document in Error/Adverse Event

Being able to learn from errors or adverse events is fundamental to prevent them from happening in the future. While a full discussion of error reporting and analysis is provided elsewhere (see Chapters 12 and 13), proper error documentation is an important component of the medical record. In all instances, one should be sure to follow institutional policy.

Completion of medical record documentation should be performed as soon as possible after the error is discovered.[20] Only the facts, not opinion or conjecture, should be recorded in the patient's medical record. Events should be described clearly, as well as any additional treatments given. It is equally important to document the content of any discussions held with the patient and/or family regarding a possible error.

Many institutions have a policy that requires filing an incident report describing the error or adverse event in detail. Here, as in the patient's medical record, it is prudent to avoid conclusions, opinions, conjecture, and assignment of blame in the incident report. While most hospitals maintain these privileged reports for use by their risk management office, these records may be discoverable in some states.

While incident reports are important troubleshooting tools for individual institutions, true safety improvements ultimately require broad reporting. Interestingly, in a study conducted using national surveys, only 21% of physicians, compared to 62% of members of the public, believed that voluntary reporting of serious medical errors to a state agency would reduce future errors.[21]

To return again to the clinical vignette that started the chapter: the patient's repeated complaints and concerns could have alerted staff to a possible adverse reaction to medication. Documentation of a thorough patient assessment, ongoing discussion among staff, and additional treatment/monitoring measures provided could have afforded improved care. Furthermore, comprehensive information about the circumstances surrounding her death could have provided the clinician with crucial information to provide to family members.

KEY POINTS

- All aspects of the medical record must be accurate and legible.
- Documentation is used to assess quality of care.
- Improved documentation may lead to improved quality of care.
- Proper documentation can serve as protection during litigation.
- Documentation of error/adverse events and their disclosure is important.
- Cross-cover services should be documented whenever a patient is evaluated for a significant event or change in status.
- Appropriate documentation can be a valuable troubleshooting tool for physicians.

ONLINE RESOURCES

http://www.qualityindicators.ahrq.gov

REFERENCES

1. Kirkland LR, Bryan CS. Osler's service: a view of the charts. *J Med Biography*. 2007;15(Suppl 1):50–4.
2. Wood DL. Documentation guidelines: evolution, future direction, and compliance. *Am J Med*. 2001;110(4):332–4.
3. Russo R. Documentation and data improvement fundamentals. *2004 IFHRO Congress & AHIMA Convention Proceedings*, Washington, DC. October, 2004.
4. Custodio M, Dixon G, Endicott M, et al. Using CDI programs to improve acute care clinical documentation in preparation for ICD-10-CM/PCS. *J AHIMA*. 2013;84(6):56–61.
5. White KB, Beary JF, III. Illegible handwritten medical records. *N Engl J Med*. 1986;314(6):390–1.
6. Dimick C. Documentation bad habits: shortcuts in electronic records pose risk. *J AHIMA*. 2008;79(6):40–3.
7. Robb D, Owens L. Breaking free of copy/paste: OIG work plan cracks down on risky documentation habit. *J AHIMA*. 2013;84(3):46–7.
8. Jencks SF, Wilensky GR. The health care quality improvement initiative. A new approach to quality assurance in medicare. *JAMA*. 1992;268(7):900–3.
9. Remus D, Fraser, I. *Guidance for Using the AHRQ Quality Indicators for Hospital-level Public Reporting or Payment*. Rockville, MD: Department of Health and Human Services, Agency for Healthcare Research and Quality; 2004. AHRQ Pub. No. 04-0086-EF.
10. Pine M, Jordan HS, Elixhauser A, et al. Modifying ICD-9-CM coding of secondary diagnoses to improve risk-adjustment of inpatient mortality rates. *Med Decis Making*. 2009;29(1):69–81.
11. Kwaan MR, Studdert DM, Zinner MJ, et al. Incidence, patterns, and prevention of wrong-site surgery. *Arch Surg*. 2006;141(4):353–7; discussion 357–8.
12. Williams PD, Graham KM, Storlie DL, et al. Therapy-related symptom checklist use during treatments at a cancer center. *Cancer Nurs*. 2013;36(3):245–54.
13. Gill JM, Ewen E, Nsereko M. Impact of an electronic medical record on quality of care in a primary care office. *Del Med J*. 2001;73(5):187–94.
14. Kern LM, Malhotra S, Barron Y, et al. Accuracy of electronically reported "meaningful use" clinical quality measures: a cross-sectional study. *Ann Intern Med*. 2013;158(2):77–83.
15. Kripalani S, LeFevre F, Phillips CO, et al. Deficits in communication and information transfer between hospital-based and primary care physicians: implications for patient safety and continuity of care. *JAMA*. 2007;297(8):831–41.
16. Heath SW. *Risk Management & Medical Liability: A Manual for Indian Health Service and Tribal Health Care Professionals*. 2nd ed. Rockville, MD: Indian Health Service; 2006.
17. Weintraub MI. Documentation and informed consent. *Neurol Clinics*. 1999;17(2):371–81.
18. Entman SS, Glass CA, Hickson GB, et al. The relationship between malpractice claims history and subsequent obstetric care. *JAMA*. 1994;272(20):1588–91.
19. Curbside Consultations. *Psychiatry (Edgmont)*. 2010;7(5):51–3.
20. Selbst SM, Korin JB. *Preventing Malpractice Lawsuits in Pediatric Emergency Medicine*. Dallas, TX: American College of Emergency Physicians; 1998.
21. Blendon RJ, DesRoches CM, Brodie M, et al. Views of practicing physicians and the public on medical errors. *N Engl J Med*. 2002;347(24):1933–40.

11 Introduction to Patient Safety

Noah Schoenberg, Emily Fondahn, and Michael Lane

CLINICAL VIGNETTE

An outbreak of norovirus has left the nursing staff at the hospital short-handed. Healthy staff members are asked by hospital leadership to cover additional shifts and many shifts are left understaffed. Rob, a new nurse who recently completed his orientation to the unit, feels well and is eager to pitch in and help his colleagues. Rob volunteered to work a double shift even though he was exhausted after coming off of night shift. Joan, a nurse that Rob worked with extensively during his orientation, asked if he could help her out by giving blood pressure medications to her patient, "Jon Smith," since she was busy with an unstable patient. While Rob was obtaining the medication from the Pyxis machine, he was interrupted by Dr. Jones who had a question about the patient in room 2 and the physical therapist who wanted to know if the patient in room 8 was stable to participate in therapy. After the interruptions, Rob removed the medications for Jon Smith. He was unaware that there were two patients with similar names on the floor; one was Jon Smith, the other John Smythe. He entered room 12 and asked the patient to state his name. The patient responded, "John Smythe." Rob thought it was a little strange that the patient pronounced his name differently than Joan had called him but thought this must be the right patient. Although he was taught in school the appropriate steps to verify that he was administering medications to the right patient, the nurses who oriented him to the floor had told him that all of those steps were unnecessary and a waste of time. Rob administered the medication to the patient and returned to taking care of his other patients. Approximately 1 hour later, John Smythe had an episode of syncope while getting out of bed. He was found to be hypotensive. After reviewing the events, it is discovered that the medications for meant Jon Smith where given to John Smythe, causing the hypotension.

- What factors contributed to this error?
- What systems or processes could be put in place to prevent an error like this?

INTRODUCTION

A patient in the hospital should not be harmed due to medical errors while receiving care. However, based upon estimates from the Institute of Medicine report, "To Err is Human," an estimated 44,000–98,000 people are harmed in the hospital each year.[1] Every person can expect to have at least one misdiagnosis during his or her life.[2] These staggering statistics highlight the need to evaluate and reform how health care is delivered. The field of patient safety is a "discipline in the healthcare sector that applies safety science methods towards the goal of achieving a trustworthy system of healthcare delivery…it minimizes the incidence and impact of, and maximizes recovery from, adverse events."[3] Patient safety is a relatively new discipline in health care and focuses on preventing harm to patients. The components of patient safety include a culture of safety to limit blame to individual providers, redesigning systems to create high reliability, promoting transparency and learning from medical errors, and making health care systems accountable to eliminate preventable harm.[3] Approaches to analyzing patient safety include Donabedian "Structure–Process–Outcome" Model, Reason "Swiss Cheese" Model, Rasmussen Model of System's Migration, and error analysis.

PATIENT SAFETY MODELS

Donabedian Structure–Process–Outcome Model

In 1966, Avedis Donabedian published a seminal paper titled "Evaluating the Quality of Medical Care" in which he outlines a formalized approach to patient safety and quality improvement, now known as the Structure–Process–Outcome Model.[4]

- Outcomes include all the effects of health care on patients or populations, such as recovery, restoration of function, and survival. Examining outcomes is the most natural and intuitive means of evaluating quality since the goal of "good" health care is a positive outcome. Any outcome is, by definition, linked to a series of actions, which are dependent on the structure where health care is provided and the processes by which health care is delivered.
- Structure comprises the setting in which health care occurs. The structure consists of the physical infrastructure, the staffing, the material and supplies, and all the various support systems involved in providing health care.[5] The quality of care provided inherently depends upon the structure in which it is provided. A flaw in the structure can propagate, resulting in an error and potentially in a bad outcome. In the above clinical scenario, the structure of the medical unit requires the nurse, Joan, to divide her time among too many patients due to understaffing. The structure creates the backbone for the health care process and outcomes.
- Process encompasses all of the actions and interventions undertaken by the health care providers operating within the above-defined structure. Process includes the decisions, operations, orders, and procedures that lead to a given outcome. The process in which health care is delivered is dependent upon the structure of the health care setting but can also be an independent factor in patient outcomes. For example, the process of medication administration is influenced by the structure of the unit but has specific procedures and protocols. In the previous example, the failure by the nurse, Rob, to confirm that the right medication was given to the right patient would be considered a failure of process. At times, processes can help to balance or correct shortcomings in structure. For example, the Pyxis machine is often located in a busy area on a medical unit, causing nurses to be frequently interrupted while obtaining medications. Establishing a "no interruption zone" around the Pyxis machine could have helped prevented this error by not allowing Rob to be interrupted as he obtained the medications.

Swiss Cheese Model

James Reason proposed the Swiss Cheese Model in his 1990 paper "The Contribution of Latent Human Failures to the Breakdown of Complex Systems."[6] Recent human

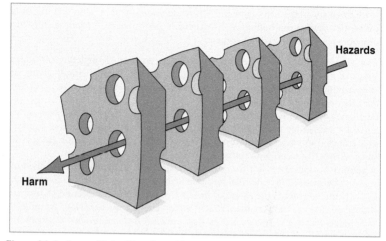

Figure 11-1. Reason "Swiss Cheese" Model. (From Reason J. Human error: models and management. *BMJ*. 2000;320:768–70.)

history has seen the evolution of multiple very complex, high-risk systems, including aviation, nuclear power, and health care, that have developed multiple safeguards to prevent bad outcomes. Medicine, like many complex high-risk systems, is perpetually devising and revising procedural safeguards to attempt to minimize the potential for harm. Overlapping layers of safeguards often catch an error before harm occurs. In the Swiss Cheese Model, multiple failures in safeguards must happen in order for an error to reach a patient. None of the individual failures is sufficient to cause harm; multiple failures must occur along the system safeguards.[6] The model's name arises from the analogy that each barrier to a bad outcome is akin to a slice of Swiss cheese, with the holes in the cheese being analogous to potential errors, circumstances, or events that could overcome that particular barrier. If a sufficient number of holes line up in a series of slices of cheese, a bad outcome could occur (Fig. 11-1).

In the opening vignette, multiple safeguards designed to prevent incorrect medication administration had to fail. The multiple holes in the Swiss cheese included having two patients with very similar names, lack of following the policy for medication administration, understaffing of the unit due to a norovirus outbreak, and multiple interruptions while retrieving the medication. A combination of unusual circumstances, deliberate choices, and unintentional errors led to an adverse event. This example demonstrates that despite the engineering of multiple procedural safeguards designed within a system, the correct alignment of system failures can overcome these barriers, potentially leading to patient harm.

The Human Component of Patient Safety

A key component of any model of patient safety must take into account the human component of a system. A series of high-profile accidents, including the Chernobyl reactor meltdown and the Zeebrugge ferry incident, highlighted the human component of safety. In both these examples, humans deliberately drifted away from standard operating procedure. Rasmussen describes the human tendency to drift toward the minimal acceptable safety margin. Rasmussen states there is "a natural migration of activities toward the boundary of acceptable performance."[7] Many factors may cause humans to cut procedural corners.

- Pressure exists to increase productivity and decrease cost. Completing the appropriate steps of medication administration takes more time than simply giving the medication. The time spent on medication administration means there is less time for other work to be completed.
- As humans frequently perform routine tasks, habit and memory are often substituted for knowledge-based decision making. As individuals become more comfortable completing a task, they have a decrease in analytic thought and increased laxity in adherence to precise procedure.
- A person who does not follow the policy will usually not see patient harm. Individuals may not be aware of the potential for harm because subsequent safeguards catch any errors before they reach the patient. The fact that harm does not occur each time the individual deviates from standard practice may reinforce the behavior.[7] As multiple individuals within a system or process begin to stray from established practices, the entire system slowly becomes increasingly unsafe until an accident or bad outcome occurs that forces a re-evaluation and realignment of the general safety practices.[7] Amalberti et al. have applied Rasmussen's ideas to the tendency to drift toward unsafe practices over time in medicine (Fig. 11-2).[8]
- "Legal zone" is where practices begin and all rules are followed.
- "Illegal–normal zone" is where minor variations in safety practices occur, and adaption is not only tolerated but sometimes encouraged depending upon the circumstance. Migration is due to pressure for greater performance (horizontal axis) and personal gain (vertical axis). Borderline tolerated conditions of use (BTCUs) are violations that

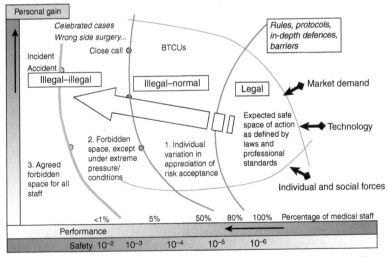

Figure 11-2. The tendency to drift toward unsafe practices over time in medicine. (From Amalberti R, et al. Violations and migrations in health care: a framework for understanding and management. *Qual Saf Health Care.* 2006;15:i66–71.)

are considered to provide the maximum benefit for the minimum and accepted probability of harm. On the medical unit in the clinical vignette, staff believed that not following the protocol for medication administration was accepted and encouraged to increase productivity and the probability of harm to the patient was low.

- "Illegal–illegal zone" where safety practices become extreme and most practices are considered "forbidden" under essentially all circumstances. The boundary between "illegal–normal" and "illegal–illegal" is where close calls occur. The "illegal–illegal" territory is where the majority of accidents and bad outcomes occur.
- A commonly used analogy is how most individuals follow the speed limit. If the speed limit is 30 miles per hour, few people drive in the legal zone of <30 miles per hour under normal circumstances. Most people drive in the illegal–normal speed of 30–40 miles per hour. People driving above 45 miles per hour are considered in the illegal–illegal category.

In the medical field, long work hours, large patient care burdens, and immense financial pressures provide a perfect mix of conditions to promote migration toward minimal acceptable safety practices. This erosion was examined more closely in the field of anesthesia in a 2010 paper looking at anesthesia practices in the operating room (OR).[9] The authors noted that there are two different types of perceived safety regulations: "need-to-follow" and "nice-to-follow." They found that failure to observe "nice-to-follow" rules frequently leads to violations of "need-to-follow" rules, endangering patients and leading to further accidents and bad outcomes.

ERROR DEFINITIONS

Types of Errors

Many different terms are often used to describe a bad outcome. Clarifying these terms is important both to prevent misunderstanding and to facilitate more efficient communication. Using the correct terminology is crucial to communicate the etiology of the error and nature of the outcome. When discussing bad outcomes, one can describe it as an *adverse event*, a *near miss*, or simply as an *error*. These terms are not interchangeable.

- An *adverse event* implies a bad outcome due to medical management that could be, but is not necessarily, the result of a mistake or flaw in the system. If a patient with a known penicillin allergy receives amoxicillin because no one ever asked about her allergies, that would be an adverse event. An adverse event is also if a penicillin-naive patient has an allergic reaction to an amoxicillin; there is no way to foresee and prevent an allergic reaction. The term does not imply causation, merely an undesirable outcome due to interaction with the medical system.
- A bad outcome is an undesirable outcome due to a disease process.[10] A patient with septic shock who dies despite receiving appropriate antibiotics and medical therapy had a bad outcome, not an adverse event.
- An error means an unintended event or a mistake. An error does not necessarily imply outcome. An error can be caught and corrected before reaching the patient, can reach the patient but not cause harm, or can directly lead to a bad outcome for a patient. Regardless of whether or not the patient with the penicillin allergy actually receives the medication, the act of prescribing a medication to a patient with a known allergy is an error. The prevention of errors is a central focus of the field of patient safety and one of the driving forces behind the evolution of new safeguards and precautions.

• A *near miss* is an error without a subsequent adverse event. If the patient with the penicillin allergy is prescribed amoxicillin, but the nurse notices the error prior to giving the medication and alerts the physician, who cancels the order and prescribes a new medication, that is classified as a near miss. Near misses are difficult to track and address and are some of the most frequent errors. In a complex system with multiple redundant safeguards, much of the design of the system is intended to *create* near misses in lieu of adverse events. However, by their very nature, they are less noticeable and thus harder to track. In addition, there is an inherent reluctance by health care workers to report the event, due to either embarrassment by the individual who made the error or concern by the individual who caught the near miss that they might get someone else in trouble. A tendency exists to see near misses as "no big deal" since an adverse event actually occurred. As a result, near misses, though a frequent product of a well-designed series of safeguards, are often underreported and obscure.

Classification of Human Behavior

A critical aspect of evaluating an error or adverse event lies in analyzing the intentions underlying the behavior that lead to the error. Though there is increasing emphasis on a Just Culture in medicine, in which individuals are not held solely responsible for errors, individuals are still responsible for their actions. There are three different categories into which individual actions leading to an error can fall: human error, at-risk behavior, and reckless behavior. The crucial difference between each category is the awareness of the individual regarding the risk inherent in their actions and their choices regarding how to proceed. Evaluating the individual's intentions is a critical step in event analysis to identify system changes to prevent similar errors.

• Reckless behavior, or a deliberate disregard of risk, is the easiest to define and the category most clearly requiring individual consequences. Most commonly, this behavior occurs when someone, despite knowing the risks of their behavior, chooses to ignore safeguards and proceed with their actions, deliberately putting patients and coworkers at risk. This behavior leaves the individual culpable and requires that the individual's choices and behavior be explicitly addressed in rectifying the situation. Designing safeguards against consciously reckless behavior is very difficult.
• At-risk behavior involves a person putting a patient or coworker at risk through unsafe practices, without necessarily realizing the situation is unsafe. This behavior usually occurs due to an effort to save time or improve efficiency, thereby accidently leading to an unsafe situation. A nurse drawing blood to match for a transfusion and not immediately labeling the blood per policy is engaging in at-risk behavior. The distinction between reckless behavior and at-risk behavior revolves around that fact that with reckless behavior, the individual deliberately places another at risk through their actions, but in at-risk behavior, unsafe actions are taken without awareness of the risk involved. The individual remains culpable, however, as they are nonetheless engaging in unsafe behavior. Prevention of at-risk behavior frequently involves training in appropriate safety practices and sufficient oversight to ensure practices and policies are followed.
• Simple human error involves an individual taking action they believe to be safe, which nonetheless can result in a bad outcome. Fatigue, miscalculation, and lack of attention often underlie these types of errors. These errors include an accidental

contamination of a sterile field, mislabeling of a specimen, wrong-side surgery, or even just ordering the wrong dose of a medication. Many of the system safeguards and redundancies focus on attempting to prevent or correct human error. Witnessed blood draws, procedural checklists, and surgical site marking are common safety practices intended to prevent human error. Of note, the category of human error does not include mechanical or technical errors. An intra-venous pump breaking, an incorrect lab result, or a computer glitch would not be counted as human errors given that they are not directly due to human actions. A slip of the hand, a mental miscalculation, and a failure of human memory are inherent dangers in any system that involves a human component and the potential for error implicit in the human presence that drives much of the development of the field of patient safety.

Active Failures and Latent Conditions

In his paper proposing the Swiss cheese model, Reason notes that the majority of failures leading to an adverse event are human in nature and are frequently present long before the actual event occurs. He states that prior to an adverse outcome occurring, two different types of errors can occur: active failures and latent conditions.[6]

- An active failure consists of "those errors and violations having an immediate adverse effect." Active failures are events that usually occur on the "front line" (in the OR, the patient's bedside, etc.) that directly lead to adverse events.
- A latent condition includes "decision or actions, the damaging consequences of which may lie dormant for a long time, only becoming evident which they combine with local triggering factors" to create an adverse event. Latent failures are errors or mistakes that set up conditions for failure.

Most often, an adverse event depends upon both types of events occurring. A surgeon operating on the wrong arm is an active failure. However, this active failure depends upon a latent condition: the hospital not having a policy regarding advance labeling of the appropriate limb. In the majority of highly complex systems with multiple safeguards, the only way the "Swiss Cheese holes" all line up is for a latent condition (or several of them) to prepare a situation that is triggered by an active failure.

CONCLUSION

In the opening vignette, a patient was harmed from a preventable medical error due to receiving the wrong medications. Yet, patients safely receive medications in the hospital every day. So what happened to this particular patient? What can be done about it? Using the ideas and patient safety modeling systems outlined in this chapter, let us look back at the events to decipher what went wrong. The structure of the medical unit and the process of medication administration led to the bad outcome. The policies and procedure were not followed due to the natural tendency to drift toward the minimal safety standards. An active failure by a tired, overworked nurse aligned with the multiple latent conditions allowed the error to reach the patient. The patient safety models presented in this chapter help us analyze and classify this error and begin redesigning systems to eliminate preventable harm to patients.

KEY POINTS

- There are often multiple safeguards in place to prevent errors from reaching patients and causing harm. However, when all the holes in the "Swiss Cheese" align, errors may reach patients.
- Although errors have the potential to cause harm, they are not all due to negligent behavior.
- Both active failures and latent conditions may align to result in patient harm.
- In order to fully understand the factors that contribute to patient harm, one must have a full understanding of human behavior and the systems and processes involved in delivering health care.

ONLINE RESOURCES

1. Institute for Healthcare Improvement: http://www.ihi.org/Topics/PatientSafety/
2. VA National Center for Patient Safety: http://www.patientsafety.va.gov/media/factsheets.asp
3. National Patient Safety Foundation: http://www.npsf.org/?page=professionals
4. Agency for Healthcare Research and Quality: http://www.ahrq.gov/professionals/quality-patient-safety/index.html

REFERENCES

1. Kohn LT, Corrigan JM, Donaldson MS, eds. *To Err Is Human: Building a Safer Health System*. Washington, DC: The National Academies Press; 1999.
2. National Academies of Sciences, Engineering, and Medicine. *Improving Diagnosis in Health Care*. Washington, DC: The National Academies Press; 2015.
3. Emanuel L, Berwick D, Conway J, et al. What exactly is patient safety? In: Battles JB, Henriksen K, Keyes MA, et al., eds. *New Directions and Alternative Approaches*. Rockville, MD: Agency for Healthcare Research and Quality; 2008.
4. Donabedian A. Evaluating the quality of medical care (Reprinted from The Milbank Memorial Fund Quarterly, vol 44, pp 166–203, 1966). *Milbank Q.* 2005;83(4):691–729.
5. Runciman WB, et al. Tracing the foundations of a conceptual framework for a patient safety ontology. *Qual Saf Health Care.* 2010;19(6):1–5.
6. Reason J. The contribution of latent human failures of the breakdown of complex-systems. *Philos Trans Royal Soc London Ser B Biol Sci.* 1990;327(1241):475–84.
7. Rasmussen J. Risk management in a dynamic society: a modelling problem. *Saf Sci.* 1997;27(2–3):183–213.
8. Amalberti R, et al. Violations and migrations in health care: a framework for understanding and management. *Qual Saf Health Care.* 2006;15:i66–71.
9. De Saint Maurice G, et al. The natural lifespan of a safety policy: violations and system migration in anesthesia. *Qual Saf Health Care.* 2010;19(4):327–31.
10. World Alliance for Patient Safety. *WHO Draft Guidelines for Adverse Event Reporting and Learning Systems: From Information to Action*. Geneva, Switzerland: World Health Organization; 2005.

12

Culture of Safety

Richard A. Santos and Myra Rubio

CLINICAL VIGNETTE

Mrs. M, a 56-year-old woman with hypertension, presented to the hospital with a complaint of black, tarry stools. She was found to be anemic and admitted for evaluation of gastrointestinal bleeding. She was transferred to a semiprivate room, hospital bed A, which was closest to the patient room door. Her admitting physician ordered a type and screen and crossmatched 2 units of packed red blood cells. The patient noted that hospital bed B, which was closest to the window with a garden view, was vacant and requested the nurse to transfer her to bed B. The nurse agreed to move the patient from bed A to bed B. That evening, the unit had several new patients that arrived simultaneously, and the nurse for Mrs. M forgot to notify admitting to change her location in the hospital computer order entry system. In addition, the nurse caring for Mrs. M was on her 15th hour of working because she had agreed to work an extra 6-hour shift for double pay. In the meantime, transporters of a new patient with dementia arrived to the floor and assumed that the empty bed A was for the new patient. Overnight, the patient care technician drew blood on the wrong patient in bed A, which was not Mrs. M, but still had Mrs. M's name in the computer. The technician did not follow protocol of checking the patient's identification prior to drawing blood. Later that night, the nurse for Mrs. M realized she had forgotten to notify admitting of the room change and called admitting to correct the room assignment. The nurse for Mrs. M proceeded with the blood transfusion, which was unfortunately crossmatched for the other patient's blood. Mrs. M had a severe transfusion reaction and required subsequent treatment in an intensive care unit.

- How should we address this adverse event in a culture of safety?
- How can the patient safety culture be assessed on this inpatient unit?
- How can information about this event be disseminated to prevent future, similar events from occurring?

INTRODUCTION

Health care leaders today are challenged to develop and support an infrastructure based on a foundation centered on a culture of safety in their acute care settings. In 1983, the fundamentals of safety culture were defined by Uttal as "shared values (what is important) and beliefs (how things work) that interact with an organization's structures and control systems to produce behavioral norms (the way we do things around here)."[1] The safety culture in acute care settings in health care has since been described in this manner as "the norms, practices, values, and beliefs of the people working in a given unit, department, hospital, or hospital system."[2,3] According to James Reason, known for his work on human error, "safety cultures evolve gradually in response to local conditions, past events, the character of the leadership and the mood of the workforce."[4] Positioning these parts strategically in order to establish a safety culture in health care can prove to be challenging. Many have suggested that organizations need to establish attitudes, behaviors, and practices that are engrained as a "new normal" structured in a way to prevent errors.[5]

Developing a safety culture involves acquiring insight on the perceptions of frontline workers and on multifaceted areas such as teamwork, accepted behaviors, job satisfaction, leadership, stress recognition, availability of resources, learning environment, error reporting, feedback, and communication in their work environment.[4] The Agency for Healthcare Research and Quality (AHRQ), the national federal agency with the goal of improving safety and quality through research and practice implementation, has identified four key features in health care patient safety culture. These features include recognition of high-risk activities to obtain reliable operations, presence of blame-free environments in reporting errors or near misses, practicing collaboratively to identify solutions to safety problems, and having leadership commitment to address patient safety concerns.[5] AHRQ has defined the safety culture of an organization as "the product of individual and group values, attitudes, perceptions, competencies, and patterns of behavior that determine the commitment to, and the style and proficiency of, an organization's health and safety management."[6]

A weak safety culture is exemplified by health care workers who do not communicate; fail to use safety policies, procedures, or tools; and refrain from reporting mistakes due to a "blame and shame" phenomenon.[3] Institutions with strong health care safety cultures have highly reliable, engaged, health care workers who communicate effectively, have strong teamwork perceptions, and respond to errors by utilizing reporting systems and root cause analysis, which foster a continuous learning environment from mistakes and near misses.

ESTABLISHING A "JUST CULTURE"

On May 24, 2001, Dr. Lucian Leape, a professor at the Harvard School of Public Health, prepared a statement for the Senate Committee on Health, revealing that "identifying systems failures and correcting them will not occur if workers are punished for making errors. Safe industries create a non-punitive environment, and also pay attention to factors that affect performance, such as hours and work loads, work conditions, and team relationships, an agenda that health care must now address."[7] Developing a safety culture, which learns and improves by openly identifying and examining its own strengths and weaknesses, is a priority in preventing errors in health care. However, the environment in which this occurs must be nonthreatening and nonpunitive but balanced with personal accountability.[8] The culture must also be engaged in a degree of professionalism with codes of conduct that expect mutual respect and integrity and address disruptive and inappropriate behaviors nonconducive to learning or working.[9]

A pioneer in Just Culture, David Marx, a US attorney and engineer, focuses his safety culture model on establishing open reporting and accountability as crucial elements in improving patient outcomes.[10] When medical errors occur, personal accountability constitutes a key role in respecting a Just Culture (see Chapter 11 for more information about classification of human behavior). According to Marx, accountability for errors can be divided into:

1. Human or inadvertent error
2. Errors due to at-risk behavioral choices
3. Errors due to conscious reckless behavior

Human error, in this model, requires careful examination of systems, processes, training, and design. When behavioral choices play a role in errors, managing positive and negative incentives and increasing situational awareness must be examined. However, when conscious, reckless behavior is involved, corrective disciplinary actions must be pursued. Disciplinary models can be based on rules, outcomes, or risks.[10] Some consider a Just Culture to be established when an organization has balanced the fine line of acceptable and unacceptable behaviors, with a cushion of psychological safety in reporting errors to improve systems and decrease patient harm.[11]

TOOLS FOR ASSESSING PATIENT SAFETY CULTURE

Measuring and analyzing the patient safety culture in health care settings plays an important role because it identifies strengths and weaknesses of organizations in regard to patient safety issues. Assessment of a safety culture allows institutions to establish a reference point for baseline data before interventions are started, prioritization of areas for patient safety efforts, and monitoring of trends or changes in patient safety culture after interventions. Several tools have been developed to help organizations measure patient safety culture.

AHRQ SURVEYS ON PATIENT SAFETY CULTURE

In 2004, AHRQ developed a tool known as the Hospital Survey on Patient Safety (HSOPS) Culture, which explored 12 components of safety culture[12]:

1. Communication openness
2. Feedback and communication about error
3. Frequency of events reported
4. Handoffs and transitions
5. Management support for patient safety
6. Nonpunitive response to error
7. Organizational learning—continuous improvement
8. Overall perceptions of patient safety
9. Staffing
10. Supervisor/manager expectations and actions promoting safety
11. Teamwork across units
12. Teamwork within units

In order for hospitals to compare their patient safety culture with other organizations, AHRQ established a database in 2006 from over 382 US hospitals who volunteered and over 108,621 hospital staff data. In 2007, AHRQ first published their results. This was subsequently updated in the HSOPS Culture: 2008 Comparative Database Report, which included over 519 hospitals and 160,176 hospital staff respondent.[13] This database has allowed hospitals to compare their patient safety culture survey results with each other and has enabled the monitoring of trends in patient safety culture over time within and between institutions.

Establishing a patient safety culture is not unique to hospitals and acute care settings. Ambulatory settings and medical offices are also prone to medical errors and preventable adverse events.[14] Creating a safety culture in medical offices has grown widespread interest. In 2009, AHRQ released the Medical Office Survey on Patient Safety Culture.[15] Similar to the HSOPS, the Medical Office Survey on Patient Safety Culture examines 13 areas that include the following:

1. List of patient safety and quality issues
2. Teamwork
3. Information exchange with other settings
4. Work pressure and pace
5. Staff training
6. Office processes and standardization
7. Communication openness
8. Patient care tracking/follow-up
9. Communication about error
10. Leadership support for patient safety
11. Organizational learning
12. Overall perceptions of patient safety and quality
13. Overall ratings on quality and patient safety

In 2010, AHRQ developed a database of their results in patient safety culture in medical offices. Updated in 2012, this database included over 234 US medical offices and over 23,679 medical staff respondents. In addition to hospital and medical office settings, AHRQ has also developed patient safety culture assessment tools tailored for nursing homes and pharmacies supporting the goal of improving the patient safety culture in other health care settings.[16,17]

PATIENT SAFETY CLIMATES AND SAFETY ATTITUDES QUESTIONNAIRES

Within a safety culture, unique patient safety climates exist, comprising of multiple components that are specific to each unit or clinical area. Measurements of attitudes and beliefs relevant to patient safety issues have grown with widespread interest. The Safety Attitudes Questionnaire (SAQ), funded by the Robert Wood Johnson Foundation and AHRQ, was developed in 2006 by Bryan Sexton, Eric Thomas, and Bob Helmreich.[18] Modifications of the SAQ and variations of safety climate surveys are frequently utilized in organizations to provide a snapshot representation of perceptions of safety culture in individual areas. Versions of the SAQ have been adapted for use in operating rooms, inpatient settings, ambulatory outpatient settings, and intensive care units. Modifications of these types of questionnaires often target central themes surrounding patient safety, such as teamwork, stress recognition, communication, resources, discipline, working conditions, job satisfaction, organization, and leadership. Results of these questionnaires are often utilized to display strengths and weaknesses of health care units in specific areas. These areas can then be a focus for future interventions to improve patient safety climates.

CREATING A CULTURE OF SAFETY THROUGH ERROR REPORTING

Implementation and Use of Error Reporting Systems

The Institute of Medicine (IOM) in 1999 called for the implementation of error reporting systems in health care organizations.[19] At that time, eight states had mandatory adverse event reporting systems in place, the earliest being South Carolina in 1976. The Joint Commission on Accreditation of Healthcare Organizations (JCAHO) (now called the Joint Commission) created a sentinel event system in 1996 for voluntary reporting of what the commission defined as sentinel events. The purpose of this system was for member organizations to submit not only the details of the event itself but also the root cause analysis performed and the response undertaken by the health care organization. Other reporting systems in place at that time included the medication errors reporting (MER) program started by the Institute for Safe Medication Programs in 1975, which shared medication error reports with the Food and Drug Administration (FDA) and pharmaceutical companies. These reporting systems were in many ways limited. The state adverse reporting systems and the JCAHO sentinel event system focused mostly on events that led to significant harm or death. Programs like MER looked at medication errors and may not have captured errors in other aspects of health care delivery system. None of these reporting systems attempted to address the more common no harm or near miss events, which, although no patient harm occurred, may actually better highlight the vulnerabilities in the health care delivery system.

The IOM described the dual roles envisioned for error reporting systems: to hold providers accountable for performance and to improve patient safety through learning from errors. Two tiers of error reporting systems were proposed. Mandatory reporting systems were envisioned to hold providers accountable for performance by focusing on errors that lead to serious injuries or death. These systems were to be run by state regulatory programs with the power to investigate specific cases and, if deemed appropriate, levy penalties or fines. The model for these systems was the state mandatory adverse event reporting systems already in place. The goals of such a reporting system were to create a level of protection for patients and, by holding health care organizations accountable for their actions, incentivize health care organizations to invest in patient safety and quality improvement efforts.

The Office of Inspector General (OIG) for Health and Human Services sought to identify states with adverse event reporting systems and how this information was utilized by the states.[20] By 2008, 26 states had hospital adverse reporting systems, although a 27th state has implemented an adverse event reporting system in the interim. In their report, the OIG noted a large disparity in the adverse events each state required to be reported. For example, the types of adverse events requiring reporting varied based upon the level of resultant harm to the patient. All states listed at least one adverse event that leads to death listed as a reportable event. However, only one state (Pennsylvania) required certain near misses as reportable adverse events. Similarly, adverse events associated with medical devices not functioning as intended are reportable in some states if death, disability, or loss of body part occurs but in other states are only reportable if death occurs. Only three states used a standardized list of serious reportable events such as one generated by the National Quality Forum,[21] a nonprofit public service organization that endorses the use of standardized health care performance measures. Although the creation of state mandatory reporting systems in at least half of the states is a marked improvement over the absence of such reporting systems, the disparity by state of what information is collected makes aggregating such data into national trends exceedingly difficult. The IOM recognized this problem, calling for a standardized report format with basic required elements such as how the event was discovered, details of the adverse event itself, contributing factors, any causal analysis, and the recommendations derived from this analysis.[22] Such a standardized report would also require the generation of a standardized taxonomy for adverse events to allow for classification and comparison of similar events. However, such standardization would allow for national trends to be compiled and analyzed.

Voluntary reporting systems were envisioned by the IOM to act as a complement to mandatory reporting systems to drive improvements in patient safety and quality care. Such error reporting systems would attempt to capture all errors, regardless of severity of harm, as well as near misses that were corrected before any harm occurred to the patient. Through the gathering of such information from multiple, frontline reporters, potential trends or persistent vulnerabilities in health care delivery would hopefully become apparent. One potential model cited by the IOM was the Aviation Safety Reporting System operated by National Aeronautics and Space Administration (NASA) for the aviation industry.[23] This system collects incident reports submitted confidentially about aircraft operations, which could affect safety. All incident reports are indexed in a database where the identifier information is kept anonymous and is analyzed by a group of experts. If further expert analysis identifies potential hazards or possible system improvements, this information is disseminated to the aviation industry through bulletins and monthly safety publications. Currently, this model is used in health care by the Veteran's Administration through the Patient Safety Reporting System (PSRS).

Regardless of whether states have adverse event reporting systems, hospitals are required by Federal regulation to maintain a Quality Assessment and Performance Improvement Program as a condition of participation in Medicare.[24] Within this code, hospitals must measure quality indicators, including adverse patient events, and use this data to identify areas for improvement in safety and quality of care. Nearly all hospitals have an internal incident reporting system accessible by all hospital personnel in which adverse events can be reported. However, the capabilities and utilization of these systems vary, with only 79% able to document severity of harm to patient, 58% able to collect patient's medical history, and only 47% allowing for anonymous reporting.[25]

Barriers to Error Reporting

Unfortunately, multiple studies have highlighted the many barriers to error reporting. Perceived barriers to error reporting include lack of knowledge about the reporting system, time involved in reporting an error, fear of reprisal/culture of blame, and the belief that there was no need to report errors that cause no harm to the patient.[26] A study performed in South Australia noted these barriers and also highlighted that lack of feedback from errors that were reported was a major deterrent from further error reporting.[27] The majority of current error reporting is being done by nursing and not by physicians, therapists, or other members of the health care team. In one survey, 96% of the hospitals involved stated that nursing generated most to all of the incident reports with only 2% from physicians in training and 1% from attending physicians.[25] Such barriers, whether real or perceived, lead to substantial underreporting of adverse events, errors, or near misses.

The OIG in a follow-up report further quantified the problem of underreporting of adverse events in error reporting systems.[28] The OIG performed a chart review of 780 Medicare beneficiaries hospitalized in the month of October 2008 and identified 293 adverse events in 189 hospitals with internal error reporting systems. The review found that of these events, only 35 (14%) were actually captured by the hospital's incident reporting system. The most common reasons given for why the vast majority of adverse events were not reported was that hospital staff did not perceive the events as reportable, usually due to lack of perceived error or the belief that the event was an expected side effect of treatment. When the adverse events were then compared to data obtained by state mandatory reporting systems, it was found that 60% of the events occurred in states with mandatory reporting systems, only 12% met state reporting requirements, and that only three total events (1%) of all events were actually reported to the state.[29] All three events were reported in Pennsylvania, which as noted earlier requires reporting of certain events regardless of the severity of patient harm. Therefore, this study concluded that only 1% of adverse events are actually being captured by mandatory state reporting, showing that health care still has a large deficiency in capturing all adverse events, much less no harm events or near misses.

Ideally, error reporting systems would be ubiquitous in all health care settings. A vigorous collection of error reporting would allow organizations to learn from experience. There must be a supportive, nonpunitive environment that encourages the reporting of adverse events, errors, or near misses. Although a Just Culture should reduce the fear of reprisal, anonymous submissions should be allowed to ensure a supportive environment and encourage error reporting. The reporting system must protect confidentiality not only of the patients but also of the reporters. The reporting would come from a range of staff to ensure that all health care providers are invested in the process and that multiple viewpoints are being observed within the health care organization. Finally, there must be prompt feedback, relevant expert analysis, and distribution of lessons learned to encourage further error reporting from frontline providers. Dr. Charles Billings, one of the founders from NASA of the Aviation Safety Reporting System, summarized it thusly when he stated the best error reporting systems are safe (nonpunitive), simple (easy to report), and worthwhile (expert analysis with timely feedback and dissemination).[30]

LEARNING FROM ERRORS

Transparency

As described in the previous section, one must report errors to learn from errors. From the earliest stages of medical training, we are asked to learn from our experiences, which include learning from our mistakes. Through openness in reporting, we can also learn from errors performed by others before we repeat such mistakes in our patients. However, this principle of transparency also requires us to admit fallibility, which is not easy in the setting of medical care. Transparency calls for health care providers to factually report errors, both to error reporting systems as well as to patients. Quality improvement through full analysis of any error benefits from full transparency from the reporter. Although anonymous reporting should be allowed in a supportive environment, that same anonymity does not allow for further context to be obtained from the reporter in the form of follow-up questions. Anonymity also precludes providing feedback to the reporter. Full transparency from the initial reporter about the adverse event, corresponding situation, and the error that occurred is vital in determining the root causes for the adverse event. Transparency through acknowledgement of errors to the patient also fulfills the need to establish trust with the health care consumers.

Transparency also may lie in conflict with liability, another perceived barrier to voluntary reporting of error. Health care providers are often concerned that error reporting could be utilized in discovery in civil liability cases. Full disclosure of errors to patients was perceived as an invitation to further malpractice claims, although such an increase in claims has not been demonstrated at health care organizations that have implemented full disclosure.[31] In the absence of a Just Culture, concerns for sanctions, loss of reputation, and loss of livelihood also stood in the way of full transparency.[32]

In an attempt to address these issues, the US Congress passed the Patient Safety and Quality Improvement Act (PSQIA) in 2005. The PSQIA defined data involved in patient safety programs as patient safety work products, which would be granted legal protections from discovery. The Act also authorized the Agency of Healthcare Research and Quality to create patient safety organizations (PSO), external agencies that would receive and analyze error reporting data from health care organizations. The PSO could then disseminate its findings throughout health care to drive quality improvement, similar to the role played by the Aviation Safety Reporting System. Of note, the legal protections for patient safety work products (PSWP) were specifically for data reported to PSO; data utilized for internal use would not fall under PSQIA but may fall under state rules of peer review.[33]

The establishment of PSO with legally protected patient safety work product may allow for the greater transparency needed for the creation of national databases of error reporting and analysis. Certified PSO could analyze error reporting from multiple health care organizations and potentially identify common system weaknesses present throughout health care. The ability to share PSWP with external organizations without fear of sanction may encourage more comprehensive error reporting. Finally, the ability to widely disseminate the findings from subsequent adverse event analysis would ideally keep health care organizations from repeating such errors before they occur at their facility.

Morbidity and Mortality Conference

Morbidity and mortality (M&M) conferences are one important setting for learning from adverse events. One of the earliest proponents of learning from patient outcomes was Dr. Ernest Codman, who in the early 20th century was a strong proponent of "The End Result System." In this system, all surgical patients upon entry into the operating room would have a card created upon which would be documented the initial diagnosis, operative details, postoperative diagnosis, and immediate complications. The cards would then be revisited annually with updates given to assess the "end result" from each surgery. If the desired end result was not achieved, the case was further analyzed to determine the causes and possible errors that led to the nonoptimal end result.[34] The "End Result System" was one of the first recorded surgical systems to use patient outcomes to further drive physician education and quality improvement.

The most immediate precursor to the modern M&M conference was the Anesthesia Mortality Committee (later renamed the Anesthesia Study Commission) created in 1935 in Philadelphia.[35] This group was made up of area surgeons, anesthesiologists, and internists who solicited reports of any mortalities that occurred in the county resulting from anesthesia. Monthly open meetings were held at which all attending physicians, residents, and interns were invited to attend. The commission chairman would present to the group cases selected for review, and an open discussion would then occur under the guidance of the chairman. After this discussion was held, the commission would vote on whether the mortality was preventable and, if so, what factors were involved that may have contributed to the adverse event. The findings of the commission were recorded by a secretary, and public reports were generated. Also, the physicians present would be encouraged to report back to their home institutions the findings generated at these meetings to further disseminate the findings of the commission.

The morbidity and mortality conference has been a requirement of the Accreditation Council for Graduate Medical Education (ACGME) for accredited training programs since 1983.[36] Recent surveys in internal medicine and surgical residency programs reveal that morbidity and mortality conference is practically ubiquitous in residency training, with the majority of internal medicine programs holding M&M or quality improvement conference at least monthly and almost all surgical programs conducting M&M conference weekly.[37,38] These conferences are almost universally described as similar to the format originally created by the Anesthesia Study Commission: cases are presented to the group for review, an open discussion is held among attending physicians and trainees, and conference attendees attempt to learn from errors and adverse events. Morbidity and mortality conference attendees uniformly rank highly the perceived educational value of the conference, highlighted by one survey of surgical trainees in which 80% of those surveyed stated that they would continue to attend M&M conference even if attendance was no longer mandatory.[38]

However, these surveys also demonstrate potential areas of improvement in the morbidity and mortality conference. One survey of internal medicine M&M conference attendees noted the rationale for case selection is not uniform, with less than half of selected cases actually addressing unexpected morbidity or mortality.[37] Presentation format and discussion practices are neither uniform nor standardized, with many programs allotting <10 minutes for open discussion.[39] The persistent barrier of underreporting has also been shown in case selection, with one study revealing that postdischarge review by a trained nurse–reviewer captured twice as many cases with mortality and over four times as many cases with morbidity than identified and presented at that institution's M&M conference.[40] Finally, despite the call for a supportive, Just Culture, resident physicians still cite more openness and less defensiveness/blame as the top improvement needed in morbidity and mortality conference.[36]

A number of studies have attempted to address these shortcomings. As noted, one method to address underreporting is through a trained nurse–reviewer to evaluate for morbidity and mortality through chart review, computerized hospital diagnosis coding, and follow-up with patients through letters and phone calls.[40] In another study, all surgical patients had a potential complications form placed into the chart on admission. During the course of the hospitalization, any complications that occurred were to be immediately documented on this form. Follow-up was also performed with all patients at 6 weeks to capture complications up to 30 days postdischarge. Through this method, a 10% increase in mortality and 106% increase in morbidities were captured for review.[41]

Regarding uniformity of presentation, one study evaluated the benefit of a standardized format to M&M conference.[42] In this study, M&M presenters were asked to utilize a presentation format adapted from SBAR (Situation, Background, Assessment, Recommendations). Specifically, all case presentations were now broken down by Situation (admitting diagnosis, operative procedure, adverse outcome), Background (patient history, procedural detail, hospital course, recognition and management of complication), Assessment (error analysis, root cause analysis), and Recommendations (areas for improvement, learning points). Pre- and postintervention outcomes measured were user satisfaction, presentation quality, and educational outcomes. All measures improved postintervention, but most interesting was the significant improvement in educational outcomes based upon performance on a multiple-choice test given postconference. In another study of internal medicine M&M conferences, a "systems audit" was created to give the discussant a framework with which to review and analyze each case.[43] The systems audit required (1) all documentation be reviewed, (2) interviews performed with all stakeholders, (3) performance of a root cause analysis using a quality improvement tool, (4) calculation of overcall cost of care and cost of adverse outcomes, (5) identification of systems issues, and (6) proposal of system improvements and prioritization of implementation. Through this audit, resident awareness of systems-based practice increased and multiple system interventions were proposed and implemented within the institution.[43] Studies such as these show the educational value and systems improvement potential of morbidity and mortality conference. These studies also highlight the need for standardized formats and formal guidelines to the required elements of morbidity and mortality conference.

In summary, morbidity and mortality conferences are a vital component to learning from errors, especially in the realm of physician education. A standardized format may ensure that the educational value is maximized. Formal guidelines on the goals of M&M conference should be created. At a minimum, M&M conference should identify adverse events, generate open and blameless discussion of how errors occur, and attempt to identify the root causes for such error. The lessons learned should be subsequently disseminated widely to all health care providers. In short, the ideal M&M would identify that medicine is difficult, acknowledge our accountability in providing quality care, but recognize that errors also allow for further learning and quality improvement.[39]

SPREADING AND SUSTAINING CHANGE

Dissemination

As noted, the hard-earned lessons that can be derived from an error reporting and analysis must subsequently be disseminated to achieve full value from these lessons. For external reporting systems, one potential model is again from the Aviation Safety Reporting System (ASRS) run by NASA. From NASA, monthly safety newsletters are issued in which case reports are discussed and a monthly update on ASRS alerts is reported. Also, alert bulletins are generated as needed to highlight subjects that have arisen through incident report analysis regarding conditions or situations that may compromise safety.[23]

Current medical external error reporting systems attempt to disseminate information in a similar fashion. The PSRS for the Veterans Administration distributes quarterly safety newsletters to disseminate the lessons learned from its incident evaluations. The Joint Commission (TJC) Sentinel Event System issues Sentinel Event Alerts to highlight potential system issues identified through its error reporting database and propose potential improvement measures. As of 2013, 50 Sentinel Event alerts have been generated through this system and are sent to their member organizations. These reports are also available for review (www.jointcomission.org). The Institute for Safe Medication Practices generates a biweekly e-mail newsletter called Medication Safety Alert Acute Care, which is sent to subscribers at hospitals, pharmacies, pharmaceutical companies, and the FDA to report up-to-date information on medication and device errors as well as adverse drug reactions.

Dissemination of knowledge learned from internal, voluntary error reporting is just as vital to ensure a culture of safety. As noted, one deterrent to voluntary error reporting is lack of feedback creating a perception that error reporting is not worthwhile.[27] At a minimum, successful error reporting systems have timely feedback to the reporters to both spur quality improvement as well as encourage future reporting.[30] Hospital-wide newsletters and e-mail may represent an efficient way to disseminate lessons learned from adverse events; however, these media may have lower impact if lost in the flurry of electronic messages generated on a daily basis in a typical hospital setting. One program that has shown promise is the use of executive walk rounds in which senior executives, such as the hospital president or chief nursing officer, held weekly rounds in different areas of the hospital with senior patient safety officers.[44] At each area, the group holds with the present physicians, nurses, and staff informal rounds to obtain information about potential safety issues, such as near misses or system vulnerabilities. Also, the staff is encouraged to discuss possible solutions or describe their own practices to improve patient safety. The goal of this program was to further inculcate a culture of safety by both obtaining information about safety issues as well as reinforcing the importance of safety in the delivery of health care. At least one study suggests that implementation of these rounds can lead to improvements in the safety climate of an institution, with nurses reporting a stronger perception that patient safety is constantly reinforced and that senior leadership is appropriately prioritizing patient safety.[45]

Implementation

The ultimate goal of a safety culture is the implementation of significant changes and quality improvement using the lessons learned from adverse events and errors. As will be discussed in the next chapter, event analysis must be performed on adverse events with an emphasis on determining systems improvements that can strengthen patient safety. Root cause analysis, with a focus on identifying the myriad of contributing underlying causes that lead to adverse events, can allow for the identification and correction of suboptimal processes. Through this process, organizations can encourage continuous improvement in providing the safest, most efficient, and most effective delivery of health care to its patients.

However, organizations must be willing and eager to embrace change to allow process improvements to be sustained. In a series of case reports describing health care organizations implementing wide-scale safety improvements,[46] the common theme for all of these organizations was the need to change the existing culture by raising expectations, rewarding safety improvements, and supporting a learning culture in which reforms are based on data derived from internal and external data. Closing the feedback loop by implementing improvements derived from error reporting and event analysis sends a clear signal to all stakeholders that error reporting is worthwhile and can lead to significant change. Strong follow-up from senior leadership to ensure that action plans generated by root cause analysis are implemented not only ensures accountability but also reinforces to all members of the organization leadership's emphasis on a culture of safety.[47]

In summary, sustaining change can only occur if there is a system-wide commitment to evolve. The organization must be ready to embrace change and recognize that the present state is not satisfactory. There must be strong leadership to clearly and consistently communicate the importance of patient safety and implement process improvements. Feedback must be timely and continuous, encouraging the use of techniques that reduce errors and addressing suboptimal system processes as they are identified. Finally, the commitment to change cannot waver as improvements are made; otherwise, the desired permanent change to culture may not occur.[45,48,49]

KEY POINTS

- Safety culture surveys are necessary to obtain baseline data on the current culture environment prior to any interventions used to improve patient outcomes.
- Establishing a Just Culture requires balancing error reporting, avoiding blame, analyzing systems, holding personal accountability, and having the highest degree of professionalism to prevent errors and near misses.
- Error reporting systems work best in a nonpunitive environment, when reporting is simple and easy to perform, and when clear feedback is provided to reporters.
- Adverse events and error reporting systems require timely, expert analysis of events with appropriate focus on root causes and potential system improvements.
- Morbidity and mortality conference is a powerful yet still underutilized opportunity to promote accountability and quality improvement.
- Hard-earned lessons derived from adverse events and error reporting must be disseminated widely to obtain full value from these lessons.
- Sustained change can only be achieved through strong leadership emphasizing the importance of patient safety.

ONLINE RESOURCES

1. Agency for Healthcare Research and Quality (AHRQ): http://psnet.ahrq.gov/primer.aspx?primerID=5
2. Safety Attitudes Questionnaire (SAQ): https://med.uth.edu/chqs/surveys/safety-attitudes-and-safety-climate-questionnaire/

REFERENCES

1. Uttal B. The corporate culture vultures. *Fortune.* 1983;108(8):66–72.
2. Wachter R, Sexton JBS. Conversation with…J. Bryan Sexton, PhD, MA. http://www.webmm.ahrq.gov/perspective.aspx?perspectiveId=143. Cited July/August 2013.
3. Sexton JBS, Grillo S, Fullwood C, et al. Assessing and improving safety culture. In: Frankel A, Leonard M, Simmonds T, Haraden C, Vega KB, eds. *The Essential Guide for Patient Safety Officers.* Oak Brook, IL: Joint Commission Resources; 2009:11–9.
4. Reason J. Achieving a safe culture: theory and practice. *Work Stress.* 1998;12(3):293–306.
5. Hoff TJ. Establishing a safety culture: thinking small. http://webmm.ahrq.gov/perspective.aspx?perspectiveID=35. Cited December 2006.

6. Patient Safety Primer. http://psnet.ahrq.gov/primer.aspx?primerID=5
7. Prepared Statement of Lucian L. Leape, MD. Harvard School of Public Health Subject— Reporting and Prevention of Medical Errors Before the Senate Committee on Health, Education, Labor and Pensions. http://md-jd.info/leap2001.html. Cited May 2001.
8. Wachter RM. Personal accountability in healthcare: searching for the right balance. *BMJ Qual Saf.* 2013;22(2):176–80.
9. DuPree E, Anderson RM, Brodman M. Professionalism: a necessary ingredient in a culture of safety. *Jt Comm J Qual Patient Saf.* 2011;37(10):447–55.
10. Marx D. Patient safety and the "just culture:" a primer for health care executives medical event reporting system—transfusion medicine (MERS-TM). http://www.safer.healthcare. ucla.edu/safer/archive/ahrq/FinalPrimerDoc.pdf. Cited April 2001.
11. Frankel AS, Leonard MW, Denham CR. Fair and just culture, team behavior, and leadership engagement: the tools to achieve high reliability. *Health Serv Res.* 2006;41(4):1690–709.
12. Westat R, Sorra J, Nieva V. Hospital survey on patient safety culture. AHRQ Publication No. 04–0041. http://www.ahrq.gov/professionals/quality-patient-safety/patientsafetyculture/hospital/resources/hospcult.pdf. Cited September 2004.
13. Hospital Survey on Patient Safety Culture Comparative Database. http://www.ahrq.gov/professionals/quality-patient-safety/patientsafetyculture/index.html
14. Clancy CM. New patient safety culture survey helps medical offices assess awareness. *Am J Med Qual.* 2009;24:441–3.
15. Agency for Healthcare Research and Quality. Medical office survey on patient safety culture. http://www.ahrq.gov/professionals/quality-patient-safety/patientsafetyculture/medical-office/
16. Agency for Healthcare Research and Quality. Nursing home survey on patient safety culture. http://www.ahrq.gov/professionals/quality-patient-safety/patientsafetyculture/nursinghome/index.html
17. Agency for Healthcare Research and Quality. Pharmacy survey on patient safety culture. http://www.ahrq.gov/professionals/quality-patient-safety/patientsafetyculture/pharmacy/index.html
18. Sexton JB, Helmreich RL, Neilands TB, et al. The safety attitudes questionnaire: psychometric properties, benchmarking data, and emerging research. *BMC Health Serv Res.* 2006;6:44.
19. Kohn L, Corrigan J, Donaldson M, eds. *To Err is Human: Building a Safer Health System.* Washington, DC: National Academies Press; 1999.
20. Office Inspector General. *Adverse events in hospitals: state reporting systems.* OEI-06-07-00471, 2008.
21. National Quality Forum. *Serious Reportable Event in Healthcare 2006 Update.* Washington, DC: National Quality Forum; 2007.
22. Aspden P, Corrigan JM, Wolcott J, et al., eds. *Patient Safety: Achieving a New Standard for Care.* Washington, DC: National Academies Press; 2004.
23. National Aeronautics and Space Administration. Aviation Safety Reporting System. ASRS: the case for confidential incident reporting systems. *NASA ASRS Pub. 60.* 2001.
24. Condition of participation: quality assessment and performance improvement program, *42 C.F.R. Sect. 482.21,* 2011.
25. Farley DO, Haviland A, Champagne S, et al. Adverse-event-reporting practices by US hospitals: results of a national survey. *Qual Saf Health Care.* 2007;17:416–23.
26. Uribe CL, Schweikhart SB, Pathak DS, et al. Perceived barriers to medical-error reporting: an exploratory investigation. *J Healthc Manage.* 2002;47(4):263–80.
27. Evans SM, Berry JG, Smith BJ, et al. Attitudes and barriers to incident reporting: a collaborative hospital study. *Qual Saf Health Care.* 2006;15:39–43.
28. Office Inspector General. Hospital incident reporting systems do not capture most patient harm. *OEI-06-09-00091,* 2012.
29. Office Inspector General. Few adverse events in hospitals were reported to state adverse event reporting systems. *OEI-06-09-00092,* 2012.
30. Leape LL. Reporting of adverse events. *N Engl J Med.* 2002;324(20):1633–8.
31. Kraman SS, Hamm G. Risk management: extreme honesty may be the best policy. *Ann Intern Med.* 1999;131(12):963–7.

32. Paterick ZR, Paterick BB, Waterhouse BE, et al. The challenges to transparency in reporting medical errors. *J Patient Saf.* 2009;5(4):205–9.
33. Fassett WE. Patient safety and quality improvement act of 2005. *Ann Phamacother.* 2006; 40:917–24.
34. Kaska SC, Weinstein JM. Historical perspective: Ernest Armor Codman, 1869–1940. *Spine.* 1998;23(5):629–33.
35. Ruth HS. Anesthesia study commissions. *JAMA.* 1945;127(5):514–7.
36. Harbison SP, Reghr G. Faculty and resident opinions regarding the role of morbidity and mortality conference. *Am J Surg.* 1999;177:136–9.
37. Orlander JD, Fincke GF. Morbidity and mortality conference: a survey of academic internal medicine departments. *J Gen Intern Med.* 2003;18:656–8.
38. Gore DC. National survey of surgical morbidity and mortality conferences. *Am J Surg.* 2006;191:708–14.
39. Orlander JD, Barner TW, Fincke GF. The morbidity and mortality conference: the delicate nature of learning from error. *Acad Med.* 2002;77(10):1001–6.
40. Hutter MM, Rowell KS, Devaney LA, et al. Identification of surgical complications and deaths: an assessment of the traditional surgical morbidity and mortality conference compared with American College of Surgeons-National Surgical Quality Improvement Program. *J Am Coll Surg.* 2006;203(5):618–24.
41. McVeigh TP, Waters PS, Murphy R, et al. Increasing reporting of adverse events to improve the educational value of the morbidity and mortality conference. *J Am Coll Surg.* 2013;216(1):50–6.
42. Mitchell EL, Lee DY, Arora S, et al. Improving the quality of the surgical morbidity and mortality conference: a prospective intervention study. *Acad Med.* 2013;88(6):824–30.
43. Szostek JH, Wieland ML, Loertscher LL, et al. A systems approach to morbidity and mortality conference. *Am J Med.* 2013;123(7):663–8.
44. Frankel A, Graydon-Baker E, Neppl C, et al. Patient safety leadership WalkRounds. *Jt Comm J Qual Patient Saf.* 2003;29(1):16–26.
45. Thomas EJ, Sexton JB, Neilands TB, et al. The effect of executive walk rounds on nurse safety climate attitudes: a randomized trial of clinical units. *BMC Health Serv Res.* 2005;5(28):1–9.
46. McCarthy D, Blumenthal D. Stories from the sharp end: case studies in safety improvement. *Milbank Q.* 2006;84(1):165–200.
47. Gandhi TK, Graydon-Baker E, Neppl Huber C, et al. Closing the loop: follow-up and feedback in a patient safety program. *Jt Comm J Qual Patient Saf.* 2005;1(11):614–21.
48. Narine L, Persaud DD. Gaining and maintaining commitment to large-scale change in healthcare organizations. *Health Serv Manage Res.* 2003;16(3):179–87.
49. Weaver SJ, Lubomski LH, Wilson RF, et al. Promoting a culture of safety as a patient safety strategy. *Ann Intern Med.* 2013;158(5):369–74.

13

Event Analysis

Rosalyn Corcoran and Katherine E. Henderson

CLINICAL VIGNETTE

Ms. W is a 67-year-old woman with lung cancer admitted to the hospital for shortness of breath. During the initial intake, she was noted to have a history of falls at home. Standard fall precaution orders were placed. At 9:40 PM, the patient used the call system to request someone assist her to the bathroom. The unit secretary indicted that someone would be in shortly. At 9:43 PM, the patient's nurse entered the room and found the patient on the floor. The patient had a small laceration to the right elbow and complained of right hip pain. A femur x-ray demonstrated an acute right femoral neck fracture. The patient's roommate witnessed the patient fall. According to the patient's roommate, the patient was trying to walk to the bathroom even though there was a bedside commode present.

- Who should be notified about this event?
- What are the next steps that should be taken?
- How would this event be classified?

INTRODUCTION

Medical errors are devastating events for both patients and caregivers. Having a well-thought-out plan for how you and your institution will respond when an error occurs before it actually happens will ensure a more effective response. In this chapter, we cover the basics of event analysis including initial response to an error, classification of events, debriefing, root cause analysis, and crisis management.

WHAT TO DO IF AN ERROR OCCURS

Immediate Actions

- The error should be reported immediately to the patient's attending physician if he/she is not already aware of the situation. Risk management should also be made aware of the error either by entering the details into the institution's event reporting system or, especially if the event has resulted in harm to the patient, by calling risk management directly.
- The facts as known should be disclosed to the patient. The attending of record should perform the disclosure to the patient. Please refer to Chapter 14 for a more detailed explanation of disclosure.

- Any devices involved in the event (e.g., intravenous [IV] pump and tubing, cardiac monitor, etc.) should be taken out of service immediately and sequestered for evaluation.
  - In accordance with the Safe Medical Devices Act of 1990 (SMDA) (Public Law 101–629),[1] all medical devices that may have caused or contributed to a death or serious injury must be reported to the Food and Drug Administration (FDA) and/or to the manufacturers within 10 working days.
  - The FDA may impose civil penalties for failure to comply with this reporting requirement.
  - To further the safety evaluation process, many hospitals encourage the reporting of all failed medical devices, regardless of level of harm.
  - Reportable events of failed medical devices may include the following:
    - Failure of a diagnostic device when there is information to reasonably suggest a probability that misdiagnosis or lack of diagnosis has or could have caused or contributed to a death and serious injury.
    - Event due to user error or failure to service or maintain the device.
    - Failure of a surgically implanted device.
    - Malfunction of a device that supports or sustains life.
    - Device malfunction or failure that necessitates medical or surgical intervention to preclude permanent impairment of a body function or permanent damage to a body structure.
    - Device causes permanent impairment of a body function or damage to a body structure.
- Risk management should perform an evaluation for immediate jeopardy. *Immediate jeopardy* is a situation in which the hospital's noncompliance with one or more requirements of the Centers for Medicare & Medicaid Services (CMS) Conditions of Participation (CoP) has caused, or is likely to cause, serious injury, harm, impairment, or death to a patient (see Table 13-1).[2]

If an immediate jeopardy situation exists, corrective measures must be taken to abate the immediate jeopardy situation and correct deficient practices. If a hospital receives an immediate jeopardy citation, that hospital and any other hospital in its system must undergo a complete inspection within 23 days or risk losing their Medicare and Medicaid funding. Of note, surveyors may place a hospital in immediate jeopardy even if only 1 patient has been harmed or is at risk of harm. Consequences of noncompliance with the CMS CoP can include the following:

- Termination from both the Medicare and State Medicaid program
- Loss of deemed status from its accrediting body—resulting in jurisdiction shift to the state agency
- Loss of public goodwill and trust
- Loss of third-party payor contracts if linked to continued Medicare participation

Event Investigation

- After an error occurs, it is important to establish the facts surrounding the event. This is best done with a *debriefing*. A debriefing is a meeting of all of those directly involved in the care of the patient. It is best done within the first 48–72 hours following the event, before memories begin to fade. The debriefing meeting is a fact-finding mission with the purpose of understanding and identifying vulnerabilities in the care delivery system (the "holes in the Swiss cheese"), which allowed harm to reach the patient. A debriefing is specifically *not* an opportunity to point fingers or

TABLE 13-1 CMS Immediate Jeopardy Triggers

Issue	Triggers
A. Failure to protect from abuse	1. Serious injuries such as head trauma or fractures
	2. Nonconsensual sexual interactions, for example, sexual harassment, sexual coercion, or sexual assault
	3. Unexplained serious injuries that have not been investigated
	4. Staff striking or roughly handling an individual
	5. Staff yelling, swearing, gesturing, or calling an individual derogatory names
	6. Bruises around the breast or genital area, or suspicious injuries, for example, black eyes, rope marks, cigarette burns, unexplained bruising
B. Failure to prevent neglect	1. Lack of timely assessment of individuals after injury
	2. Lack of supervision for individuals with known special needs
	3. Failure to carry out doctor's orders
	4. Repeated occurrences such as falls that place the individual at risk of harm without intervention
	5. Access to chemical and physical hazards by individuals who are at risk
	6. Access to hot water of sufficient temperature to cause tissue injury
	7. Nonfunctioning call system without compensatory measures
	8. Unsupervised smoking by an individual with a known safety risk
	9. Lack of supervision of cognitively impaired individuals with known elopement risk
	10. Failure to adequately monitor individuals with known severe self-injurious behavior
	11. Failure to adequately monitor and intervene for serious medical/surgical conditions
	12. Use of chemical/physical restraints without adequate monitoring
	13. Lack of security to prevent abduction of infants
	14. Improper feeding/positioning of individuals with known aspiration risk
	15. Inadequate supervision to prevent physical altercations

(Continued)

TABLE 13-1 CMS Immediate Jeopardy Triggers (*Continued*)

Issue	Triggers
C. Failure to protect from psychological harm	1. Application of chemical/physical restraints without clinical indications 2. Presence of behaviors by staff, such as threatening or demeaning, resulting in displays of fear, unwillingness to communicate, and recent or sudden changes in behavior by individuals 3. Lack of intervention to prevent individuals from creating an environment of fear
D. Failure to protect from undue adverse medication consequences and/or failure to provide medications as prescribed	1. Administration of medication to an individual with a known history of allergic reaction to that medication 2. Lack of monitoring and identification of potential serious drug interaction, side effects, and adverse reactions 3. Administration of contraindicated medications 4. Pattern of repeated medication errors without intervention 5. Lack of diabetic monitoring resulting or likely to result in serious hypoglycemic or hyperglycemic reaction 6. Lack of timely and appropriate monitoring required for drug titration
E. Failure to provide adequate nutrition and hydration to support and maintain health	1. Food supply inadequate to meet the nutritional needs of the individual 2. Failure to provide adequate nutrition and hydration resulting in malnutrition, for example, severe weight loss, abnormal laboratory values 3. Withholding nutrition and hydration without advance directive 4. Lack of potable water supply
F. Failure to protect from widespread nosocomial infections, for example, failure to practice standard precautions, failure to maintain sterile techniques during invasive procedures, and/or failure to identify and treat nosocomial infections	1. Pervasive improper handling of body fluids or substances from an individual with an infectious disease 2. High number of infections or contagious diseases without appropriate reporting, intervention, and care 3. Pattern of ineffective infection control precautions 4. High number of nosocomial infections caused by cross-contamination from staff and/or equipment/supplies

TABLE 13-1 CMS Immediate Jeopardy Triggers (*Continued*)

Issue	Triggers
G. Failure to correctly identify individuals	1. Blood products given to wrong individual 2. Surgical procedure/treatment performed on wrong individual or wrong body part 3. Administration of medication or treatments to wrong individual 4. Discharge of an infant to the wrong individual
H. Failure to safely administer blood products and safely monitor organ transplantation	1. Wrong blood type transfused 2. Improper storage of blood products 3. High number of serious blood reactions 4. Incorrect cross match and utilization of blood products or transplantation organs 5. Lack of monitoring for reactions during transfusions
I. Failure to provide safety from fire, smoke, and environmental hazards and/or failure to educate staff in handling emergency situations	1. Nonfunctioning or lack of emergency equipment and/or power source 2. Smoking in high-risk areas 3. Incidents such as electrical shock, fires 4. Ungrounded/unsafe electrical equipment 5. Widespread lack of knowledge of emergency procedures by staff 6. Widespread infestation by insects/rodents 7. Lack of functioning ventilation, heating, or cooling system placing individuals at risk 8. Use of nonapproved space heaters, such as kerosene, electrical, in resident or patient areas 9. Improper handling/disposal of hazardous materials, chemicals, and waste 10. Locking exit doors in a manner that does not comply with NFPA 101 11. Obstructed hallways and exits preventing egress 12. Lack of maintenance of fire or life safety systems 13. Unsafe dietary practices resulting in high potential for food-borne illnesses
J. Failure to provide initial medical screening, stabilization of emergency medical conditions, and safe transfer for individuals and women in active labor seeking emergency treatment (Emergency Medical Treatment and Active Labor Act)	1. Individuals turned away from ER without medical screening exam 2. Women with contractions not medically screened for status of labor 3. Absence of ER and OB medical screening records 4. Failure to stabilize emergency medical condition 5. Failure to appropriately transfer an individual with an unstabilized emergency medical condition

(From: *CMS State Operations Manual, Appendix Q – Guidelines for Determining Immediate Jeopardy,* http://www.cms.gov/Regulations-and-Guidance/Guidance/Manuals/downloads/som107ap_q_immedjeopardy.pdf) lay blame. When conducting a debriefing, it is important that leadership does not assume going into the meeting that they already know what happened during the event. Very often, initial assumptions prove to be either incorrect or incomplete. The Joint Commission has published a collection of 12 best practices for debriefings (Of note, these practices can be applied to recurring events such as postprocedure debriefings or to critical incidents such as medical errors)[3]:

- Debriefings must be diagnostic: The team should understand that the debriefing is intended to be a learning opportunity aimed at better understanding the inherent weaknesses in the system in which they work.
- The debrief environment should be a supportive learning environment where all team members feel comfortable contributing to the conversation and sharing observations and opinions. Leadership should appreciate the benefits of debriefing and make time for team members to participate.
- Teamwork behaviors such as coordination, effective communication, shared situation assessment, and leadership should be addressed during the debriefing.
- Debrief leaders/facilitators should be educated in the art and science of leading a debriefing and understand their role and responsibilities as facilitators.
- It is vitally important that team members feel comfortable during the debriefing. The atmosphere should be collegial and nonthreatening. All participants should be given an equal role and have an equal voice regardless of their roles on the patient care team (i.e., attending physicians, residents, nurses, and students should all have an equal voice). Ideally, team members should be comfortably seated at eye level with each other in a quiet space where they can easily hear one another.
- Focus on critical performance issues. There is typically a limited amount of time available to accomplish the debriefing, so it is important that the team focus on bringing out and highlighting all of the elements that contributed to the event.
- Describe specific teamwork interactions and processes that were key elements of the team's performance including issues of leadership, delegation, communication, and problem assessment.
- Support feedback with objective performance indicators.
- Provide outcome feedback later and less frequently than process feedback, as even with successful outcomes an opportunity may exist to improve processes.
- Provide individual and team-oriented feedback but know when each is most appropriate.
- Shorten the delay between task performance and feedback as much as possible.
- Record conclusions made and goals set during the debriefing to facilitate feedback during future debriefings and to track progress over time.

Debriefings should be used with near misses as well as actual events, since the same circumstances surrounding one patient's near miss may lead to harm for the next patient.

CLASSIFICATION OF EVENTS

The Institute of Medicine (IOM) report "To Err is Human" defines medical errors as "the failure of a planned action to be completed as intended or the use of a wrong plan to achieve an aim."[4] In order to respond to errors and work to prevent them, we must first study them and understand why they happened. Several classification systems exist to aid in the study of medical errors.

- **The Joint Commission's sentinel events**
  - The Joint Commission defines a sentinel event as "an unexpected occurrence involving death or serious physical or psychological injury, or the risk thereof."[5]

TABLE 13-2	**The Joint Commission List of Reviewable Sentinel Events**

Events resulting in an unanticipated death or major permanent loss of function not related to the natural course of the patient's illness or underlying condition

Suicide of any patient receiving care, treatment, and services in a staffed round-the-clock setting or within 72 h of discharge

Unanticipated death of a full-term infant

Abduction of any patient receiving care, treatment, and services

Discharge of an infant to the wrong family

Rape, assault (leading to death or permanent loss of function), or homicide of any patient receiving care, treatment, and services

Rape, assault (leading to death or permanent loss of function), or homicide of a staff member, licensed independent practitioner, visitor, or vendor while on site at the health care organization

Hemolytic transfusion reaction involving administration of blood or blood products having major blood group incompatibilities (ABO, Rh, other blood groups)

Invasive procedure, including surgery, on the wrong patient, wrong site, or wrong procedure

Unintended retention of a foreign object in a patient after surgery or other invasive procedures

Severe neonatal hyperbilirubinemia (bilirubin >30 mg/dL)

Prolonged fluoroscopy with cumulative dose >1500 rads to a single field or any delivery of radiotherapy to the wrong body region or >25% above the planned radiotherapy dose

(Adapted from: *The Joint Commission Sentinel Event Policy and Procedures in the Comprehensive Accreditation Manual* for *Hospitals*, http://www.jointcommission.org/assets/1/6/CAMH_2012_Update2_24_SE.pdf)

These events (see Table 13-2) require immediate investigation and response. Of note, the Joint Commission recognizes that not all sentinel events occur due to an error and not all errors result in a sentinel event.

- Response to a reviewable event:
  - Prepare a root cause analysis (see Root Cause Analysis section below) and action plan within 45 calendar days of the event or of becoming aware of the event.
  - Submit the root cause analysis and action plan to the Joint Commission with 45 calendar days of the known occurrence of the event. The Joint Commission will then determine if the root cause analysis and action plan are acceptable.
- **World Health Organization (WHO) taxonomy**

The WHO has published a set of standardized concepts for organizations worldwide to use when reporting and classifying incidents (see Table 13-3). The product, called the International Classification for Patient Safety, is a conceptual framework designed to standardize definitions and terms to facilitate the trending, monitoring, and analysis of events to improve overall patient safety.[6]

TABLE 13-3	WHO Conceptual Framework for the International Classification for Patient Safety
Incident type	Incidents of a common nature grouped because of shared, agreed features (e.g., "clinical process/procedure" or "medication/IV fluid" incident). A patient safety incident can be classified as more than one incident type.
Patient outcomes	Concepts that relate to the impact upon a patient, which are wholly or partially attributable to an incident. They can be classified according to type of harm, degree of harm, and any social and/or economic impact.
Patient characteristics	Categorizes patient demographics, the original reason the patient sought care and the patient's primary diagnosis.
Incident characteristics	Classifies information about the circumstances surrounding the incident such as where and when the incident occurred, who was involved in the incident, and who reported it.
Contributing factors/hazards	Circumstances, actions, or influences felt to have played a part in the origin or development of an incident or to increase the risk of an incident. Usually, more than one contributing factor and/or hazard is involved in a particular patient safety incident.
Organizational outcomes	The direct impact upon an organization, which is wholly or partially attributable to an incident, such as an increased use of resources to care for the patient, media attention, or legal ramifications. Organizational outcomes differ from patient outcomes, which would include clinical or therapeutic consequences.
Detection	An action or circumstance resulting in the discovery of an incident. Detection mechanisms may be informally developed or built into the system as official barriers (e.g., monitor alarms, audits, etc.).
Mitigating factors	Actions or circumstances that prevent or moderate the progression of an incident that could harm the patient. Mitigating factors are designed to minimize the harm to the patient after the error has occurred by triggering damage control mechanisms. Detection and mitigation factors working together represent incident recovery (secondary prevention) and can impede the progression of an incident from reaching and/or harming a patient.

TABLE 13-3	WHO Conceptual Framework for the International Classification for Patient Safety (*Continued*)
Ameliorating actions	Actions taken or circumstances altered to make better or compensate any harm to the patient and the organization after an incident (e.g., disclosure and apology, clinical management of patient harm, team debriefings, etc.). Ameliorating actions are utilized in the rescue phase of incident recovery (tertiary prevention).
Actions taken to reduce risk	These are the steps taken to prevent the reoccurrence of the same or similar patient safety incident and to improve system resilience and may be directed toward the patient, the therapeutic agents, or equipment involved in patient care or the organization itself.

(Adapted from: More than words: Conceptual framework for the international classification for patient safety, version 1.1. *WHO Technical Report*, January 2009.)

- **Eindhoven Classification Model**

  The Eindhoven model[7] was originally designed for the chemical processing industry but has since been adapted for health care. The model classifies factors contributing to errors into three different types: technical (e.g., problems with equipment design/installation, software, forms, etc.), organizational (e.g., organizational culture, policies, or priorities), and human. The model uses a predefined order of operations—which specifies that human error be considered last—to counteract traditional bias toward stopping event analysis at the employee level without considering technical or organizational contributions to the system failure.

- **Harm or severity grading**

  Some scales categorize errors based on the severity of the outcome.

  - **National Coordinating Council for Medication Errors Reporting and Prevention (NCC MERP) Index**

    Although the NCC MERP initially developed their categorization process for medication errors, the index has been widely adopted across health care as a tool to categorize all medical errors. This Index uses an A to I rating scale that spans unsafe conditions without harm to events that result in death (see Table 13-4).[8,9]

ROOT CAUSE ANALYSIS

As the IOM report "To Err is Human" highlighted in 1999, most medical errors are made by bright, well-intentioned people coming to work each day doing the best they can in a very complex environment that, in many ways, sets them up to fail. In many cases, one could swap out all of the people involved in a medical error—the physicians, staff, and even the patients themselves—and, if the same circumstances aligned again, the same results would be achieved. To truly prevent medical errors, we must focus on making changes to the environment in which they occur.

TABLE 13-4	Modified NCC MERP Index for Reporting Medical Errors or Adverse Events
No Actual Event	
A	Unsafe condition
Event, No Harm	
B1	The event did not reach the patient do to chance alone (near miss)
B2	The event did not reach the patient do to active recovery efforts of caregivers (near miss)
C	The event reached the patient but did not cause harm
D	The event reached the patient and required additional monitoring or treatment to prevent harm
Event, Harm	
E	Patient experienced temporary harm and required treatment or intervention
F	Patient experienced temporary harm and required initial or prolonged hospitalization
G	Patient experienced permanent harm
H	Patient experienced permanent harm and required intervention necessary to sustain life (e.g., ICU transfer)
I	Patient died

(Adapted from: Griffin FA, Resar RK. *IHI Global Trigger Tool for Measuring Adverse Events.* 2nd ed. IHI Innovation Series White Paper. Cambridge, MA: Institute for Healthcare Improvement; 2009, Available on www.IHI.org)

The Joint Commission defines a root cause analysis (RCA) as "a process for identifying the factors that underlie variation in performance, including the occurrence or possible occurrence of a sentinel event." The focus of a root cause analysis should be on systems and processes rather than on individual performance, and the product of this analysis is an action plan that identifies strategies to reduce the risk of similar events occurring in the future. Action plans should address responsibility for implementation and oversight, pilot testing (when appropriate), timelines, and measures of effectiveness of the plan. Events that meet criteria for a sentinel event (see Table 13-2) require a root cause analysis and action plan to be submitted to the Joint Commission within 45 days. The Joint Commission will then review the root cause analysis to decide if it is acceptable, thorough, and credible based on the criteria outlined below[5]:

- An *acceptable* root cause analysis has the following characteristics:
  - The analysis focuses primarily on systems and processes, not on individual performance.
  - The analysis progresses from special causes in clinical processes to common causes in organizational processes.
  - The analysis repeatedly digs deeper by repeatedly asking "Why?"
  - The analysis identifies changes that could be made in systems and processes (either through redesign or by development of new systems or processes) that would reduce the risk of such events occurring in the future.
  - The analysis is thorough and credible.

- A *thorough* root cause analysis must include the following:
  - A determination of the human and other factors most directly associated with the sentinel event and the process(es) and systems related to its occurrence
  - An analysis of the underlying systems and processes through a series of "why?" questions to determine where redesign might reduce risk
  - An inquiry into all areas appropriate to the specific type of event (e.g., behavioral assessment, patient identification process, care planning process, continuum of care, staffing levels, orientation/training, competency assessment/credentialing, supervision, communication between staff and with patient/family, availability of information, adequacy of technologic support, equipment maintenance/management, physical environment, security systems/processes, medication management)
  - An identification of risk points and their potential contributions to this type of event
  - A determination of potential improvement in processes or systems that would tend to decrease the likelihood of such events in the future, or a determination, after analysis, that no such improvement opportunities exist
- A *credible* root cause analysis must do the following:
  - Include participation by the leadership of the hospital and by individuals most closely involved in the processes and systems under review.
  - Be internally consistent (not contradict itself or leave obvious questions unanswered).
  - Provide an explanation for all findings of "not applicable" or "no problem."
  - Include consideration of any relevant literature.

In more recent years, the study of human factors engineering has been integrated into the RCA process. The Human Factors and Ergonomics Society defines human factors as "the application of what we know about people, their abilities, characteristics, and limitations to the design of equipment they use, environments in which they function and jobs they perform."[10] Addressing factors that affect performance (e.g., fatigue, stress, task interruptions/distractions, familiarity with task, etc.) during the RCA process will help to ensure that the team has truly highlighted the system and process issues that led to the error. Incorporating human factors engineering design strategies such as forcing functions, checklists, and redundant processes, into the resulting action plan will lead to designing systems that are more resilient to unanticipated events. (See Chapter 16, Human Factors, for a more detailed description of human factors engineering in health care.)

CRISIS MANAGEMENT

As Benjamin Franklin once said, "By failing to prepare, you are preparing to fail." All health care organizations will, at some point, experience a crisis, whether that be a natural disaster, a mass casualty event, or a medical error that allows harm to come to a patient. At such times, the organization will be judged as much by its response to the crisis as it is to the actual event itself. Organizations need to be prepared for, rather than just react to, unexpected crises. Most organizations have a management plan to deal with the unexpected facility or weather crisis, but few have adapted this process to respond to a patient safety event. The Institute for Healthcare Improvement (IHI) has developed a white paper that contains tools to assist organizations to manage

TABLE 13-5 Key Elements of Clinical Crisis Management

Advanced planning	The organization should develop a work plan that prompts specific actions in the first hour, day, week, month, and beyond. Key members of the crisis management team should be identified in advance.
C-suite leadership responsibility and focus	The CEO should have immediate and ongoing visibility during the crisis and sets the tone for the organization's response.
Clear priorities for patients and families, staff, and the organization	Senior leaders should have early and respectful communication with those harmed by the event, understanding this includes the staff member(s) as well as the patient and family.
Communication strategy	Stakeholders should hear frequently and directly from a senior staff member of the organization.
The investigation	A root cause analysis should be used to systematically analyze all contributing factors.
Learning and improving	The results of the root cause analysis of the current crisis should be seen as an opportunity to positively impact all areas of the organization by disseminating "lessons learned."

(Adapted from: Conway JB, Sadler BL, Stewart K. Planning for a clinical crisis. *Healthc Exec.* 2010;25(6):78–81.)

crises and has identified some key elements of effective clinical crisis management (see Table 13-5).[11,12] The IHI white paper highlights the importance of establishing a plan and then implementing the plan when a serious event occurs stating, "The risks of not responding to a serious event in a timely and effective manner include, but are not limited to, loss of trust among patients, sending of mixed messages to employees regarding the organization's commitment to safety and quality, absence of healing, absence of learning and improvement, increased likelihood of regulatory action or lawsuits, and media that are all too willing to play 'gotcha' with an organization that is not prepared to publicly address a serious clinical event."[12]

Based on feedback from readers, the IHI white paper was revised in 2011 to contain a more in-depth focus on four key areas: the apology, reimbursement and compensation, second victims, and creating a "burning platform" for change.[13] The updated version is an excellent reference for health care systems to create a proactive blueprint for crisis management.

ROLE OF RISK MANAGEMENT

Historically, the risk manager's role was to act as a resource to staff as well as to protect the organization *after* something bad had already happened. Partnering with the quality staff was not consistent. Many times the reporting structures were not aligned, resulting in silos of information, ineffective communication, overlapping efforts, and ineffective process improvement efforts. Traditional functions of risk management centered around protecting the organization's financial assets and reputation (e.g., loss prevention, claims management, policy and contract review, worker's compensation, etc.). Quality managers, on the other hand, typically focused on improving patient care and outcomes while not necessarily worrying about financial loss or litigation.[14]

Over the last decade, the roles of risk management and quality improvement have converged to develop a partnership with the goal of advancing patient safety in a coordinated manner. Some key changes that have promoted this new collaboration include[15]:

- Establishment of new organizational models in which risk management, quality improvement, and patient safety functions are all embedded within one department
- Development of new terminology to encompass traditional roles (e.g., "quality risk management" and "clinical effectiveness")
- Change in culture from being reactive to proactive in response to patient safety events
- Joint investigation and analysis of patient safety events
- Need to respond to continually expanding and evolving requirements from external regulatory agencies

Regardless of how the changes are implemented, open communication between risk managers and quality managers is becoming critical. In the current era of patient safety, these roles have begun to overlap. In order to further advance patient safety, risk managers and quality managers must communicate effectively and align their activities.

KEY POINTS

- All medical errors and near misses should be reported into the institution's safety event reporting system.
- Any devices involved in the event should be taken out of service immediately and sequestered for evaluation.
- Debriefings of events should be done as close in time to the event as possible and with the involvement of all those directly involved in the patient's care.
- Root cause analysis should be performed to identify system and process issues, which contributed to the event.
- All health care organizations should have a proactive plan in place to respond to patient safety events.

ONLINE RESOURCES

1. The Joint Commission Web site: http://www.jointcommission.org/
2. Centers for Medicare & Medicaid Services (CMS) Web site: http://www.cms.gov/
3. National Coordinating Council for Medication Error Reporting and Prevention: http://www.nccmerp.org/
4. IHI whitepaper: "Respectful Management of Serious Clinical Adverse Events": http://www.ihi.org/resources/Pages/IHIWhitePapers/RespectfulManagement SeriousClinicalAEsWhitePaper.aspx

REFERENCES

1. Safe Medical Devices Act of 1990. Government Printing Office. http://www.gpo.gov/fdsys/pkg/STATUTE-104/pdf/STATUTE-104-Pg4511.pdf. Accessed 8/25/13.
2. CMS State Operations Manual, Appendix Q—Guidelines for Determining Immediate Jeopardy. http://www.cms.gov/Regulations-and-Guidance/Guidance/Manuals/downloads/som107ap_q_immedjeopardy.pdf. Accessed 9/8/13.
3. Salas E, Klein C, King H, et al. Debriefing medical teams: 12 evidence-based best practices and tips. *Jt Comm J Qual Patient Saf* 2008;34:518–27.
4. Kohn LT, Corrigan JM, Donaldson MS, eds. *To Err is Human: Building a Safer Health System*. Washington, DC: National Academy Press, Institute of Medicine; 1999.
5. *The Joint Commission Sentinel Event Policy and Procedures in the Comprehensive Accreditation Manual for Hospitals*. Available at: http://www.jointcommission.org/assets/1/6/CAMH_2012_Update2_24_SE.pdf. Accessed 9/8/13.
6. More than words: Conceptual framework for the international classification for patient safety, version 1.1. World Health Organization Technical Report. January 2009. http://www.who.int/patientsafety/taxonomy/icps_full_report.pdf. Accessed 9/29/13.
7. Van Vuuren W, Shea CE, Van Der Schaaf TW. *The Development of an Incident Analysis Tool for the Medical Field. ETU Report.* Eindhoven, The Netherlands: Eindhoven Institute of Technology; 1997.
8. National Coordinating Council for Medication Error Reporting and Prevention. http://www.nccmerp.org/. Accessed 10/1/13.
9. Griffin FA, Resar RK. *IHI Global Trigger Tool for Measuring Adverse Events*. 2nd ed. *IHI Innovation Series White Paper*. Cambridge, MA: Institute for Healthcare Improvement; 2009. http://www.IHI.org
10. Human Factors and Ergonomics Society. *Educational Resources*. http://www.hfes.org/Web/EducationalResources/HFEdefinitionsmain.html. Accessed 10/3/13.
11. Conway JB, Sadler BL, Stewart K. Planning for a clinical crisis. *Healthc Exec*. 2010;25(6):78–81.
12. Conway J, Federico F, Stewart K, et al. *Respectful Management of Serious Clinical Adverse Events*. 2nd ed. *IHI Innovation Series white paper*. Cambridge, MA: Institute for Healthcare Improvement; 2011. Available at: http://www.IHI.org
13. Federico F, Conway J. Planning for a clinical crisis: next steps. *Healthc Exec*. 2011;26(6):74–6.
14. *Risk Management, Quality Improvement and Patient Safety*. Vol. 2. ECRI Institute; July 2009. http://www.scribd.com/doc/241454752/Risk-Quality-Patient-Safety#scribd. Accessed 10/3/13.
15. Perry DG, Bokar V. Different roles, same goal: risk and quality management partnering for patient safety. By the ASHRM Monographs Task Force. *J Healthc Risk Manag*. 2007;27:17–25. Available at: http://www.ashrm.org

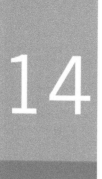

14

Disclosure of Adverse Events and Medical Errors: Supporting the Patient, the Family, and the Provider

Stephen Y. Liang, Mary Taylor, and Amy D. Waterman

CLINICAL VIGNETTE

A 79-year-old man was admitted to the intensive care unit (ICU) with multifocal pneumonia and sepsis. He had been emergently intubated for respiratory failure and placed on mechanical ventilation. The patient had only one peripheral venous catheter in the right hand through which he was receiving intravenous fluids and antibiotics. In the face of refractory hypotension, it was determined that central venous access was needed to administer vasopressors. After more than five failed attempts, a resident physician was finally successful in inserting a right-sided subclavian central venous catheter and a norepinephrine infusion was subsequently started. Thirty minutes later, the patient became acutely hypoxemic and tachycardic. The ventilator registered an increase in airway pressures and a nurse noticed diminished breath sounds on the right side with tracheal deviation to the left. Needle decompression was performed with some improvement in vital signs. A portable chest film confirmed a large right-sided pneumothorax.

INTRODUCTION

Unanticipated adverse events and harmful medical errors are unfortunate yet common occurrences in health care. An **adverse event** is defined as harm caused by medical care (e.g., medication-related anaphylaxis, contrast-induced nephropathy, pneumothorax due to central venous catheter insertion) rather than an underlying disease process. While the outcome is undesirable, an adverse event does not imply error, negligence, or poor care. A **medical error** has occurred when a planned action is not completed as intended or an incorrect action fails to achieve a desired effect (e.g., ordering a medication to which a patient has a documented drug allergy, administering intravenous contrast to a patient in acute renal failure, performing orthopedic surgery on the wrong extremity). Medical errors are generally unintentional but often arise in the setting of incorrect diagnoses, complex processes, inadequately designed systems, insufficient training or clinical experience, and breakdowns in team communication.

The impact of adverse events and medical errors on our patients and their families ranges from temporary harm to death, and costs can be financial, emotional, and physical. In the US, medical errors alone are responsible for anywhere from 44,000 to 98,000 preventable hospital deaths annually.[1] Adverse events and medical errors are common, and there is a high likelihood that every health care provider will be involved in one or more throughout the course of their clinical career.

Disclosing errors to patients and families and coping with the aftermath of errors personally and professionally are two of the more difficult aspects of being a health care provider. This chapter will explore a rationale for disclosure in health care and identify best practices each health care provider should take in the aftermath of an adverse event or medical error. Effective strategies to facilitate clear and accurate communication with patients and their families will be emphasized. In addition, the toll that adverse events and medical errors take on the health care provider as a "second victim" will be discussed. Recommendations for how to cope in these stressful professional circumstances, including a discussion of potentially helpful informal and formal support services and strategies, are outlined. Planning a structured approach when disclosing errors and a strategy to seek support ahead of time can help a health care provider better handle the stress associated with such events, enabling him or her to focus on fully supporting a patient recovering after a devastating adverse event or medical error.

THE RATIONALE FOR DISCLOSURE

> *It is a fundamental ethical requirement that a physician should at all times deal honestly and openly with patients. Patients have a right to know their past and present medical status and to be free of any mistaken beliefs concerning their conditions. Situations occasionally occur in which a patient suffers significant medical complications that may have resulted from the physician's mistake or judgment. In these situations, the physician is ethically required to inform the patient of all the facts necessary to ensure understanding of what has occurred. Only through full disclosure is a patient able to make informed decisions regarding future medical care.*
> Code of Medical Ethics, *American Medical Association*[2]

While the concept of disclosing adverse events and medical errors to patients is not a new one, it has gained increasing attention and acceptance in health care since 2000 with the publication of the Institute of Medicine's landmark report,[1] "To Err is Human: Building a Safer Health System," and the adoption of new patient safety and disclosure standards by the Joint Commission on Accreditation of Healthcare Organizations (JCAHO) a year later. At the most basic level, disclosure is rooted in ethical responsibilities to patients shared by all health care providers. Respect for patient autonomy and the preservation of informed consent are fundamental reasons why disclosure of unanticipated outcomes is necessary. Professional and moral obligations for health care providers to deal openly and honestly with patients also favor truthful communication. Despite this, many health care providers are reluctant to disclose adverse events and medical errors.

A common barrier to disclosure is the fear of litigation. Yet, the experiences of several prominent institutions with programs promoting open disclosure in concert with early resolution of malpractice claims paint a different picture. Disclosure, honesty, and transparency have been associated with reductions in liability payments, legal expenses, and in some cases even the number of claims and lawsuits filed.[3-5] Such proactive strategies are more likely to promote fair and just compensation of patients after an adverse event or medical error, defend reasonable medical care, and limit costly punitive claims. In fact, poor physician–patient communication lies at the heart of many malpractice claims.[6] A family's inability to obtain information, perceptions that some physicians had been misleading or dishonest, and the sense that other physicians would neither listen to nor answer their questions have all been described as key motivators in the decision to file suit.[7] Viewed in this light, disclosure is a unique opportunity to provide patients and their families with much needed information and formal acknowledgment of what they are going through and may also serve to diffuse tensions between patients, family members, and health care providers.

Litigation aside, fears of disciplinary action and the loss of reputation among patients and peers alike make disclosure feared by many health care providers. Morbidity and mortality conferences and peer review committees have long offered opportunities for physicians to review adverse outcomes, though they have historically been associated on some level with shame and blame. The paradigm of a "just culture" where errors can be discussed openly and nonjudgmentally without censure has been a mainstay in other high-reliability industries and is becoming increasingly accepted as a necessary foundation for modern health care. Done well, disclosure brings a new level of transparency and accountability to health care that patients appreciate and hospitals value as a part of ongoing quality improvement. In addition, while patients hope for ideal health care interactions, research has shown that most understand that medical errors sometimes occur.[8,9] When asked, patients actually maintain that disclosure enhances trust in their physicians' honesty and reassures them that they are seeing the whole picture of their care.

Significant variation exists among physicians in what information they choose to reveal to their patients after an error, underscoring a need for a standard approach to disclosure, not only to satisfy patient expectations but to uphold physician accountability.[10] Formal disclosure education with supervised practice is particularly beneficial to trainees, including resident physicians and medical students, increasing their comfort with and willingness to disclose errors in the future.[11,12]

Health care providers also worry that disclosure might cause additional and unnecessary distress to the patient. While powerful emotions of sadness, anxiety, and even anger are common after an error, the way in which a disclosure is made has a direct bearing on how patients react. Sometimes, the desire to portray an error in the best possible light by the physician not only hinders the free flow of information but creates the guise of evasiveness, increasing patient distrust of their providers.[8] Patients may be less likely to be upset if they perceive that an error has been disclosed honestly and compassionately and a sincere apology has been made.[8]

In summary, disclosure is a crucial part of the frank discourse between patients and their health care providers after an adverse event or medical error. It provides formal acknowledgement of the patient's suffering and validation of their emotional experience. It also offers a unique starting point from which health care providers can begin to learn from their errors, identify ways to prevent errors from occurring again, and find much needed professional support to move forward.

THE PROCESS OF DISCLOSURE

General Principles

Disclosure is appropriate when an adverse event or medical error has resulted in temporary or permanent harm, necessitated patient transfer to an ICU, or required additional surgery or other medical intervention. A simpler albeit more subjective gauge of appropriateness might be whether you would want to know about a specific adverse event or medical error if it happened to you or a member of your family. The fundamental principle guiding disclosure should be the patient's right to know about significant events that may impact their health and well-being. Disclosure of nonsignificant events that do not harm a patient should be guided by the provider's clinical judgment. Disclosure is best viewed as a proportional responsibility. The greater the harm or risk of harm caused by an event, the greater the duty to disclose the event to the patient.

Patients who have suffered an adverse event or medical error consistently seek the following things[8]:

- An explicit acknowledgment that an error has occurred
- An explanation of what went wrong and why
- An assessment of the clinical impact on their health
- An apology for what they are going through
- A description of how the error will be prevented in the future

Patients expect that their health care providers will be well prepared to discuss an adverse event or medical error, with empathy and caring. They seek shared dialogue, support, and follow-up as they recover from the event and as more information comes to light. They also want to know that providers have learned from the event and that processes have been improved. Yet, many disclosures fail to meet these fundamental needs and expectations.[13,14]

Preparing for Disclosure

Preparation before a disclosure ensures that an accurate and consistent message is communicated. When multiple providers are involved, every effort should be made to promote collaboration in shaping the disclosure conversation prior to any discussion with the patient or family. Residents and fellows should work in concert with their attending physician. Consensus should be reached beforehand on what basic information will be disclosed. Each provider should only disclose errors for which they bear personal responsibility. Physicians should not discuss errors made by other health care providers without involving those individuals in the conversation. It is helpful to anticipate questions the patient or family might ask and agree upon a set of uniform responses among providers. Simulating and practicing the disclosure conversation in a safe environment can build confidence and identify areas for improvement. Many institutions have developed disclosure coaching programs to aid with this process. Early consultation and inclusion of risk management and patient safety specialists can provide invaluable guidance and support in refining the disclosure conversation and understanding the true malpractice risk of the event or error.[15]

Whenever appropriate and possible, it may be helpful to bring the patient care team involved together (e.g., physicians, nurses, pharmacists, technicians, social workers, case managers) to verify the facts of the event and ensure an accurate and consistent message across the care team and multiple clinical services. Invaluable insight into the state of mind of the patient and family as well as their level of comprehension and medical literacy can be gained from the different perspectives of each member of the team. Cultural and language barriers can also be identified and addressed to best facilitate the conversation.

Determining which health care providers should participate in the actual disclosure conversation must take into account the provider's level of involvement in the event, their ability to provide a positive contribution to the discussion, and their emotional state. It is important to identify a provider who will lead the conversation, preferably someone with an established and trusting relationship with the patient. While this is usually an attending physician, nurses and other providers may also serve in this capacity depending on the nature of the event. When planning the disclosure conversation, one should recognize that a patient may benefit from the support of family and/or friends during the conversation and coordinate their presence accordingly. The involvement of a chaplain, social worker, patient advocate, or an interpreter, if a language barrier exists, may likewise be appropriate in many circumstances.

Communicating Error

Timely, honest, and sustained communication is essential after an adverse event or medical error. Ideally, this is a series of conversations. The first conversation should take place as soon as the patient is stable enough to understand the information presented and adequate preparation for the conversation has taken place. In some instances, an initial conversation may occur with an authorized member of the patient's family if the patient is unable to participate. Do not delay the first conversation pending a full analysis of the event.

In crafting the first conversation, it is crucial to remember that disclosure is not about claiming liability, making excuses, or criticizing the care of other health care providers. It is a formal encounter that focuses on the unambiguous exchange of clinical information, active listening and acknowledgment of patient and family questions and concerns, and identification of constructive solutions to address the patient's current situation and prevent future events, assuring them that you are always available to discuss this further and identifying who will be the primary contact for this is an important parting message. A structured approach to disclosure increases the likelihood that the patient's needs are adequately met. We have found the following guidelines to be helpful in improving the quality and success of a disclosure conversation (Table 14-1).

Throughout the disclosure conversation, providers should be seated at eye level with the patient. They should speak slowly and clearly. Ample opportunity for questions should be permitted. It is reasonable to ask if a patient's or family's needs are being met, both in terms of the information presented and the medical care provided. They should also be reassured and reminded that efforts to correct the event or error are underway and that they will be updated in a timely fashion through later conversations.

Documenting Error

The patient's medical record should contain accurate documentation of the event, including date, time, and place. The patient's medical condition immediately before and after the event followed by what medical interventions (e.g., diagnostic studies, medications, procedures, consultations, if appropriate) were initiated should be clearly described along with the patient's response to these interventions. Future treatment plans should be outlined.

Disclosure and other important medical care conversations with patients and their family should always be documented in the medical record, including time, date, and place of the discussion. The names and relationships of those present at the discussion, what was discussed, and patient/family responses should be described in detail. In this way, all subsequent members of the health care team will know what the patient and family were told, cementing transparency among the team with the patient.

TABLE 14-1 Guidelines for Conducting a Successful Disclosure

1. Begin the conversation with an explicit statement that an adverse event or medical error has occurred.
2. Describe the facts of the event clearly and compassionately in simple terms. Avoid medical jargon. Do not speculate or hypothesize if the exact cause of the event remains unknown.
3. Inform the patient that a review is necessary and underway to better understand the cause(s) of the event and that the patient will be updated as additional findings become available.
4. Advise the patient about potential clinical repercussions of the event on their health. Identify next steps in medical care and outline what treatment options are available and recommended.
5. Offer sincere expressions of regret or sympathy for the patient and family's suffering. If a medical error has occurred, apologize. An apology is an act of compassion and responsibility.
6. Ask the patient/family if they have further questions and answer them based on the facts available at the time of the conversation.
7. Reach out to the patient/family and emphasize a willingness to speak with them at any time. Designate one health care provider (e.g., attending physician) as a point of contact for future discussions and questions with the patient/family and make sure that they have a reliable means to contact that individual.
8. Identify who among the health care team will continue to be involved in the patient's care. If it is clear that an effective provider–patient relationship cannot be salvaged, transfer the patient's care to another provider.
9. Close the conversation with a summary of what has been discussed and repeat the key questions asked about the event.
10. Set up a definite time frame to meet again with the patient/family to communicate final results of the review along with a plan of what steps can be taken to prevent similar events from happening again in the future.

Providing Support for Patients After an Error

Preserving an open line of communication between patients, families, and health care providers is critical after a disclosure has taken place. It is common for patients to have other questions after the initial conversation, and these should be addressed in an honest and timely manner. Whereas some patients are content with knowing that an adverse event or medical error has occurred and that something is being done to address it, others may want additional, more detailed information as it becomes available. Additional emotional support and comfort can be found in chaplains, mental health clinicians, therapists, social workers, patient advocates, and other trained staff, and their involvement should be welcomed.

In many cases, it is reasonable and appropriate for a provider that has been directly involved in an adverse event or medical error to remain engaged in the clinical care of the victim. Doing so not only preserves the continuity of care but strengthens the therapeutic bond between providers and patients. Yet, there will also be times when a transition of care is necessary to restore trust and confidence in that bond. In conclusion, disclosing an error requires that physicians carefully plan how best to support the patient and families ahead of time, disclose the error openly and honestly, and listen and respond to the immediate and ongoing needs of the patient and family members.

CARING FOR THE SECOND VICTIM

Almost every physician and nurse has their story, their case, and their night. They remember the details as if it were yesterday, even if it was 10 or 20 years ago. They tell their stories with an intensity of emotion that brings tears to the eyes of both, the storyteller and the listener. Many have never shared their stories with anyone; some, with only a spouse or close friend. These stories usually end with expressions of shame, isolation, and lack of closure. The counsel received at the time of the incident, if any, included: "Stuff happens," "You can't dwell on it," "You'll just have to do it better the next time," and "Go back to work"... Given that the vast majority of errors are due to failures of bad systems and not bad people, providing support to clinicians and other staff at the sharp end of medical care is simply the respectful and compassionate thing to do.

James B. Conway, MD, *Institute for Healthcare Improvement*[16]

Traditionally, supporting the physical and emotional needs of patients and their families has been the single focus after an adverse event or medical error, without recognizing that health care providers can become "second victims," silent and forgotten.[17] For many providers, a serious medical error can rank among one of the worst experiences of their life, replete with profound emotions of sadness, anger, embarrassment, and fear.[18,19] Loss of self-confidence, reduced job satisfaction, difficulty sleeping, and heightened anxiety about committing future errors are common and can be debilitating.[20] Physicians are more likely to be distressed after serious errors if they have had a negative disclosure experience, are worried that they have a high risk of being sued, or feel unsupported after an error.

One of the greatest challenges faced by many physicians after an event is learning to forgive themselves for making the error.[8] No physician wants their decisions or actions to be inadvertently associated with causing patient harm. Guilt and self-blame can lead providers to isolate themselves, experience job burnout and emotional exhaustion, and even quit the practice of medicine altogether.[21] In the most severe circumstances, there have been reports of health care professionals taking their own lives in the aftermath of a medical error.[22]

The natural history of recovery after an adverse event or medical error by health care providers has been conceptualized based on qualitative interviews with physicians, nurses, and other health care providers.[23,24] In the immediate aftermath of an event, the provider struggles first to understand what has happened (chaos and accident response). They can be distracted in self-reflection, even while continuing to care for the patient in some cases. As the initial crisis stabilizes, the provider replays the event over and over in their mind, asking "what if" questions (intrusive reflections). This behavior cultivates a sense of inadequacy and self-isolation. The provider often searches for support from a trusted colleague, supervisor, friend, or family member (restoring personal integrity). They worry about the future of their career, what their colleagues will think of them, and whether they will ever be trusted to care for a patient again. As the full impact of the event sets in, the provider faces an uncertain future in which they might lose their job or medical license, or face litigation (enduring the inquisition). They search for reassurance and guidance from a trusted and "safe" figure (obtaining emotional first aid). Finally, the provider drops out, survives, or thrives (moving on). In the first of these, the provider finds a different job, works in a different location, or completely leaves the profession behind. In the second, the provider continues to work but is chronically haunted by the event. In the latter, the provider has turned the negative experience of the event into something positive, perhaps through practice changes at the personal, departmental, or even hospital level.

As evidenced by prior research, it is natural that most providers will feel high levels of stress and strong negative emotions after a serious adverse event or medical error.[25] Yet, choosing to seek support can be difficult, especially for physicians experienced in dealing with difficult and stressful situations common to the daily practice of medicine.[20,26] Generally, the social stigma that comes with engaging mental health care or institutional support systems (e.g., employee assistance programs) further encourages suffering in a veil of silence and anonymity. Providers often worry that the very act of seeking support will be documented in their employment record and adversely impact the future of their career. In addition, knowing what services are available, how to access them, and whether they are confidential in the case of a malpractice lawsuit are all formidable barriers. Finally, support, even when available, can be hard to accept. Whether it comes from being regularly accustomed to the role of caring for others or the fear of vulnerability, many physicians and other health care providers have mastered the denial of their own medical and emotional needs. Providers who isolate themselves or feel unsupported are likely to have the greatest difficulty recovering after an error.[20]

Regardless of these barriers, physicians and other "second victims" are seeking out and receiving support from a variety of informal and formal support services after medical errors (Table 14-2). As our knowledge and awareness of the second victim continues to mature, active strategies favoring early recognition and rapid intervention will help us ensure that these valuable members of our health care team are protected.

Informal Support

For physicians, speaking with a trusted physician colleague about the event is far more common practice than accessing traditional support mechanisms such as employee assistance programs and mental health services.[26] Shared culture, clinical experiences, and burdens of responsibility can create an honest and nonthreatening venue for discussing an event. This support is enhanced even more if the supporting physician has had a similar personal experience with an adverse event or medical error. Physicians may also seek support from a physician leader, such as a departmental chairperson. A similar reliance on trusted colleagues and managers for informal support is seen among nurses and other health care providers alike.

TABLE 14-2	Possible Support Systems for Second Victims
Formal Support Systems	Informal Support Systems
• Peer support system of trained clinical care providers, many of whom have previously experienced errors • Employee assistance program (EAP) • Patient safety and risk management programs • Community-based mental health programs • Psychiatrist or therapist • Chaplain	• Trusted colleague working in health care • Supervisor or attending physician • Spouse or partner • Family member • Close friend

Providers often share their experiences with their spouses or partners.[25] The unconditional acceptance underpinning this type of relationship, or that of a close friend, allows for open sharing and emotional vulnerability.

Formal Mental Health Support

Sometimes, informal discussion with trusted colleagues, spouses, partners, and close friends is not enough. Patient safety and risk management offices, where most of these events are initially reported, can be an invaluable source of support. Physicians and other health care providers who experience sleeplessness, depression, or anxiety after errors may benefit from meeting with trained mental health professionals or counselors. Employee assistance programs provide a wide range of services covering alcohol and substance abuse, addiction, conflicts in the workplace, stress management, and issues relating to marriage, parenthood, aging, and personal finances. Personnel staffing these comprehensive programs draw from backgrounds in clinical psychology, counseling, and social work. Though not geared specifically toward second victims of errors, these programs can provide much needed professional counseling and therapy, particularly after events associated with significant emotional distress and trauma. Consultation with a psychiatrist may be warranted in severe instances to consider medical and other specialized therapies. Comfort may also come from seeking the counsel of a spiritual or religious counselor, such as chaplain.

Peer Support Systems by Other Health Providers

A new formal support resource, a peer support system dedicated to caring for second victims, has come of age over the past decade in many hospitals across the US.[27,28] Drawing upon successful models originally designed to help first responders from law enforcement and emergency services cope with a traumatic event, peer support systems are different from traditional employee assistance and mental health programs in that they utilize clinical care providers to provide peer support, instead of mental health professionals. Peer supporters are respected providers within the institution, including physicians, who have been trained to identify second victims and those at risk of becoming one after an adverse event or medical error. Having other providers as peer supporters ensures that common emotional experiences felt after errors can truly be normalized and validated. Utilizing other physicians can also help to shift the emphasis from individual "shame and blame" to that of a "just culture," more effectively recognizing that entire systems and processes contribute to medical errors. Peer support also seeks to combat the isolation that second victims may feel through early, active, and ongoing engagement.

The approach of peer support is different from traditional therapy. Peer supporters are trained to listen and empathize, providing immediate emotional "first aid." Some peer supporters volunteer because they, too, were previously involved with an error and know how stressful the experience can be. Second victims may be referred for peer support through adverse event reporting, referral from patient safety or risk management, or self-referral.

Although medical errors are common within the entirety of the health care system, individual health care providers are unlikely to have an extensive experience with errors; a health care provider who has been involved with a medical error is often in a place of confusion and, potentially, chaos. Having an experienced guide describe what will happen in the aftermath of an error, how disclosure works, and how hospital practices related to errors operate can set accurate expectations for what to anticipate next.

To maintain confidentiality, peer supporters generally listen, but do not take notes. For a peer support system to be successful, it must:

• Create a safe environment.
• Be easily and reliably accessible immediately after the event.
• Maintain the confidentiality of the second victim.
• Convey empathy and reassurance in a nonjudgmental manner.
• Counteract the natural tendency toward isolation.
• Provide guidance and ongoing support, if desired, during the ensuing analysis of the event.
• Link second victims to additional professional resources when they are needed (e.g., employee assistance programs and mental health programs).

A key aim of peer support is to assure the provider that self-care is not selfish and is, instead, a crucial step to recovery and getting back to caring for others.

Peer supporters often educate providers about the processes by which adverse events and medical errors are analyzed, explaining what will occur in interviews with risk management, debriefings, root cause analyses, quality improvement meetings, and morbidity and mortality conferences. Sometimes, peer supporters or other colleagues offer to attend these meetings with second victims. Second victims should be periodically reassured that they are not alone and that they can depend on both their informal support networks and the peer support system to help them get through this challenging time.

Peer support is a cooperative effort. Every second victim is unique in their experiences and needs. The degree and nature of engagement will vary widely. Peer supporters should debrief regularly with other peer supporters and patient safety leaders to share ideas, discuss strategies, and develop best practices as to how to continue supporting our colleagues.

Finally, a tiered approach to second victim support balances the preferences of health care providers to "be among their own" with the responsibility to make the best use of limited mental health resources.[28] While the rendering of emotional "first aid" at the time of the adverse event or medical error by peer supporters is likely to meet the needs of most second victims, some may require more guidance and nurturing over weeks or months. When necessary, peer supporters also may escalate and expedite referral to employee assistance programs and other specialized services providing professional counseling, medical therapy, and longitudinal mental health care, if warranted.

CLINICAL VIGNETTE REVISITED

The patient underwent right-sided tube thoracostomy with radiographic improvement in the size of the pneumothorax. A brief meeting was convened between the physicians, nurses, and respiratory therapist involved in the patient's care. It was quickly determined that multiple attempts were made by the resident physician before the subclavian vein was successfully catheterized. Furthermore, a postinsertion chest film had not been ordered. The physicians met with the patient's family. After making introductions, the attending physician apologized and explained the nature of the adverse event and what was being done to correct it. He concluded by stating that they were looking further into the circumstances of the event and what could be done in the future to prevent it from happening again.

The resident physician was understandably distraught and spoke privately with both a colleague and his wife about how he was feeling after disclosing the error. He was also actively engaged by a member of the peer support team shortly after the incident, where they spoke at length about what would happen next. The peer supporter checked in regularly with the resident over the next 2 weeks. Eventually, they attended a patient safety debriefing and root cause analysis of the event together. Based on a review of central venous catheter insertion best practices, the resident physician developed a protocol empowering nurses observing catheter insertions to terminate the procedure if an operator exceeded more than three attempts without success. He also developed a web-based module to educate other trainees about safe and proper central venous catheterization in the months to follow.

Meanwhile, the patient was extubated a week after the adverse event. The thoracostomy tube was successfully removed and he was discharged home without any further complications. The team kept the patient and his family continuously apprised of the event analysis and the patient told them that he was pleased that efforts were being made to improve the safety of central venous catheter insertions in the ICU.

KEY POINTS

- Adverse events and medical errors are common.
- Disclosure promotes transparency, accountability, and validation of the patient's emotional experience after an adverse event or medical error.
- A structured approach to disclosure fosters clear and accurate communication between health care providers and patients.
- Health care providers can become second victims of an adverse event or medical error, sometimes with tragic consequences.
- Resources exist to identify, protect, and support second victims.

REFERENCES

1. Kohn L, Corrigan J, Donaldson M. *To Err is Human: Building a Safer Health System.* Washington, DC: National Academies Press; 2000.
2. American Medical Association. *Code of Medical Ethics of the American Medical Association: Current Opinions with Annotations, 2012–2013 edition.* Chicago, IL: American Medical Association; 2012.
3. Kraman SS, Hamm G. Risk management: extreme honesty may be the best policy. *Ann Intern Med.* 1999;131:963–7.
4. Boothman RC, Blackwell AC, Campbell DA, Jr., et al. A better approach to medical malpractice claims? The University of Michigan experience. *J Health Life Sci Law.* 2009;2:125–59.
5. Conway J, Federico F, Stewart K, et al. *Respectful Management of Serious Clinical Adverse Events. 2nd ed. IHI Innovation Series White Paper.* Cambridge, MA: Institute for Healthcare Improvement; 2011.
6. Levinson W, Roter DL, Mullooly JP, et al. Physician–patient communication. The relationship with malpractice claims among primary care physicians and surgeons. *JAMA.* 1997;277:553–9.
7. Hickson GB, Clayton EW, Githens PB, et al. Factors that prompted families to file medical malpractice claims following perinatal injuries. *JAMA.* 1992;267:1359–63.
8. Gallagher TH, Waterman AD, Ebers AG, et al. Patients' and physicians' attitudes regarding the disclosure of medical errors. *JAMA.* 2003;289:1001–7.

9. Burroughs TE, Waterman AD, Gallagher TH, et al. Patients' concerns about medical errors during hospitalization. *Jt Comm J Qual Patient Saf.* 2007;33:5–14.

10. Gallagher TH, Garbutt JM, Waterman AD, et al. Choosing your words carefully: how physicians would disclose harmful medical errors to patients. *Arch Intern Med.* 2006;166: 1585–93.

11. White AA, Gallagher TH, Krauss MJ, et al. The attitudes and experiences of trainees regarding disclosing medical errors to patients. *Acad Med.* 2008;83:250–6.

12. White AA, Bell SK, Krauss MJ, et al. How trainees would disclose medical errors: educational implications for training programmes. *Med Educ.* 2011;45:372–80.

13. Iedema R, Allen S, Britton K, et al. Patients' and family members' views on how clinicians enact and how they should enact incident disclosure: the "100 patient stories" qualitative study. *BMJ.* 2011;343:d4423.

14. Mazor KM, Greene SM, Roblin D, et al. More than words: patients' views on apology and disclosure when things go wrong in cancer care. *Patient Educ Couns.* 2013;90:341–6.

15. Loren DJ, Garbutt J, Dunagan WC, et al. Risk managers, physicians, and disclosure of harmful medical errors. *Jt Comm J Qual Patient Saf.* 2010;36:101–8.

16. Conway JB, Weingart SN. Leadership: assuring respect and compassion to clinicians involved in medical error. *Swiss Med Wkly.* 2009;139:3.

17. Wu AW. Medical error: the second victim. The doctor who makes the mistake needs help too. *BMJ.* 2000;320:726–7.

18. Lander LI, Connor JA, Shah RK, et al. Otolaryngologists' responses to errors and adverse events. *Laryngoscope.* 2006;116:1114–20.

19. O'Beirne M, Sterling P, Palacios-Derflingher L, et al. Emotional impact of patient safety incidents on family physicians and their office staff. *J Am Board Fam Med.* 2012;25:177–83.

20. Waterman AD, Garbutt J, Hazel E, et al. The emotional impact of medical errors on practicing physicians in the United States and Canada. *Jt Comm J Qual Patient Saf.* 2007;33: 467–76.

21. West CP, Huschka MM, Novotny PJ, et al. Association of perceived medical errors with resident distress and empathy: a prospective longitudinal study. *JAMA.* 2006;296:1071–8.

22. Cadwell SM, Hohenhaus SM. Medication errors and secondary victims. *J Emerg Nurs.* 2011;37:562–3.

23. Scott SD, Hirschinger LE, Cox KR, et al. The natural history of recovery for the healthcare provider "second victim" after adverse patient events. *Qual Saf Health Care.* 2009;18:325–30.

24. Luu S, Patel P, St-Martin L, et al. Waking up the next morning: surgeons' emotional reactions to adverse events. *Med Educ.* 2012;46:1179–88.

25. Newman MC. The emotional impact of mistakes on family physicians. *Arch Fam Med.* 1996;5:71–5.

26. Hu YY, Fix ML, Hevelone ND, et al. Physicians' needs in coping with emotional stressors: the case for peer support. *Arch Surg.* 2012;147:212–7.

27. van Pelt F. Peer support: healthcare professionals supporting each other after adverse medical events. *Qual Saf Health Care.* 2008;17:249–52.

28. Scott SD, Hirschinger LE, Cox KR, et al. Caring for our own: deploying a systemwide second victim rapid response team. *Jt Comm J Qual Patient Saf.* 2010;36:233–40.

15

Teamwork and Communication

Denise M. Murphy and James R. Duncan

CLINICAL VIGNETTE

During placement of a central line, a syringe labeled heparin 100 units/mL was filled with 1000 units/mL heparin. As a result, a child received approximately 2500 units of heparin when the catheter was flushed. The error was traced back to a breakdown in communication among team members. All members were experienced personnel but had only recently started working together. The person setting up the tray believed the heparin would be diluted before use. The physician who flushed the catheter believed the heparin had already been diluted.

INTRODUCTION

Teamwork is an essential part of modern health care. No single individual can create all the supplies needed for patient care, possess all the knowledge needed for their effective use, or provide continuous 24/7 coverage over an extended period. As a result, patient care depends on a vast network of people, processes, and technologies. Whitt et al. found that between 17 and 26 different frontline personnel cared for a patient during a typical hospitalization[1] and each of these frontline workers is supported by an even larger array of ancillary personnel and medical devices. The information needed to coordinate care grows exponentially as teams enlarge and the number of possible interventions increases. Viewed from this perspective, it is not surprising that breakdowns in communication and teamwork are the most common causes of untoward hospital events.[2]

Like safety and quality, communication and teamwork are properties of the system. Recruiting and retaining motivated, skilled individuals are no guarantee of good communication or effective teams. Rather, health care systems should be designed to promote and continually improve these traits. Although teamwork and communication are highly interdependent, this chapter will separately review the fundamental principles of each. The goal is to better understand the pathophysiology of dysfunctional teams and poor communication. The hope is that once diagnosed, these maladies can be remedied using tools and strategies for improvement.

MEMBERS OF THE PATIENT CARE TEAM

The nucleus of the patient care team is the patient and his/her support group. Certain illnesses and conditions exceed the capabilities of this core and prompt the patient to seek assistance from health care professionals. On arrival at the medical facility, the team rapidly expands and includes everyone the patient encounters along the journey. This often includes the hospital's parking lot attendants, receptionists, nurses, doctors, technologists, pharmacists, housekeepers, and a support group that includes lab technicians, administrators, and manufacturers of medical supplies. Patients expect all these team members to seamlessly coordinate their efforts. However, given the large number of people involved in even the simplest health care system, personnel are organized into multiple different small teams that work in different microsystems.[3] Hospitals are macroscopic systems where multiple different microsystems collaborate around patient care activities.

BENEFITS OF TEAMWORK

While performance at the individual level is determined by planning and execution,[4,5] teamwork requires coordinated execution of shared plans. In almost any clinical situation, high-performance teams greatly exceed the capabilities of individuals, no matter their skill, intelligence, or dedication.[6] Teams create robust plans by aggregating the knowledge spread across numerous individuals, especially in situations where there is no single best answer or course of action.[7,8] Such "wickedly complex problems" are best addressed by diverse teams who use their varying perspectives to analyze the situation and devise solutions.[9] For example, teams provide valuable insight into the vulnerabilities of the current system if asked to imagine there was a catastrophic event in their area and describe the circumstances that led up to that event.[10] Teams coordinate their actions and are capable of greater vigilance over extended periods by cross-checking one another or dividing attention to focus on different sources of information.[11]

Coordinated execution of shared plans requires team members to share their individual plans or mental models.[12] The resulting **shared mental models** describe the actions needed to transform inputs into outputs for each segment of the overall process. For each step, team members are able to observe each other's actions, and thus, actions are readily communicated. In contrast, the plans or mental models that drive those actions are held internally. Resolving the differences between each team member's mental model requires substantial investments in communication. As a result, the formation of high-performing teams is difficult.[13] Teams require time to coalesce, work through differences, and improve their performance (Fig. 15-1).

CHARACTERISTICS OF EFFECTIVE TEAMS

Teams start as a collection of individuals or informal workgroups. Performance typically declines during early stages of team development. This failure to immediately improve, while predictable, can lead individuals to ignore teammates and strike out on his/her own. While such behaviors might seem justified at the time, they lead to dysfunctional teams. Building teams starts with creating trust[13,15] and then proceeds through additional stages (Fig. 15-2).

Successful teams are built upon trust. Different definitions of trust include attributes such as confidence, integrity, and predictability. A modicum of trust accompanies every new interpersonal relationship and accounts for the honeymoon period that occurs with any new team. When trust is reinforced via demonstrations of integrity, intent, and capabilities, teamwork improves. However, trust can be lost more quickly than it is gained. This asymmetry helps explain the fragility of teams and the relative scarcity of high-performing teams. The time required to build trust also

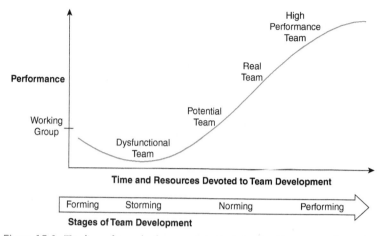

Figure 15-1. Timelines of team development. Individuals form working groups where actions are largely independent. Initial stages of team development typically lead to decreases in overall performance, and in some cases, it may be better to retain working groups rather than attempt to form teams. The accompanying stages of team development were first described by Tuckman.[14]

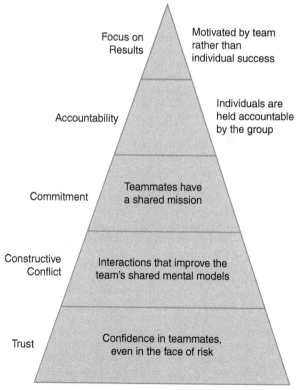

Figure 15-2. Factors influencing team development. Multiple authors emphasize the importance of trust as a prerequisite condition for creating effective teams.[13,15] Subsequent factors build on that foundation.

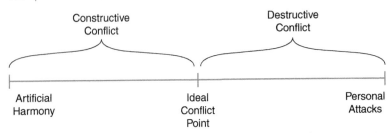

Figure 15-3. Conflict continuum. Lencioni identified conflict as a key factor in improving team performance but hypothesized that there is an ideal level of conflict.[13]

accounts for decreased organizational performance during periods of high employee turnover.[16,17]

Conflict is a key driver for improved performance. Constructive conflict prompts individuals to share and revise the mental models they use to solve the tasks at hand. High-performing teams possess shared mental models that include lessons learned from prior experiences and contingency plans for uncommon situations. While a moderate level of conflict is beneficial, too little or too much conflict is detrimental (Fig. 15-3). Too little conflict creates an artificial harmony and means that opportunities to improve mental models are missed. Too much conflict often degrades into personal attacks that degrade trust. Excessive conflict also diverts both time and energy from problem solving to conflict resolution.

Successful teams are committed to shared goals. This includes buy-in where individuals agree to a decision but do not naturally support it. Such buy-in does not signal group consensus or individual resignation. Rather, buy-in reflects an open-minded willingness to follow a path proposed by a teammate. The team's ability to disagree but commit must be matched by clarity of goals. Too often, discussion ends before teams develop a shared understanding of goals and their impact on each every member of the team. While clearly written goals reduce ambiguity, different viewpoints can persist. Lack of detail and linkage to real-world scenarios causes confusion. Even in cases of complete agreement, drift occurs over time and as goals are communicated throughout an organization.

In high-performance teams, team members hold each other accountable for the performance standards set by the group. Peer pressure and the fear of letting down a trusted teammate are strong motivators. They typically carry more weight within the organization than reprimands emanating from outside the team. Such accountability starts with the team's leader. The leader's actions must be congruent with the team's goals. Even small differences between the leader's actions and commitments undermine trust. The leader sets the tone and should invite feedback from team members. In this way, teams can begin overcoming the hesitancy that naturally accompanies the need to provide unflattering feedback.

Successful teams focus on results. They measure achievement by team success rather than individual honors. While any attempt to measure overall team performance can raise questions about which metric to use and how exactly it should be measured, there are no substitutes for measuring key indicators and sharing them with the team. Teams often establish their own means of measuring success. Over time, they refine their measurement methodologies and revise their goals.

Team Knowledge and Leadership

Studies of how teams learn, retain, and transfer knowledge suggest that teams learn through experience and store their knowledge in people, processes, and technology.[16] Performance suffers when useful knowledge is lost either through personnel turnover or forgetting past lessons. Written processes and technology are tools that promote knowledge retention. However, in contrast to other disciplines, health care teams rarely describe everyday tasks and the mental models used to perform those tasks in sufficient detail for a new team member to step in and immediately perform a complex task. Rather, health care retains a guild-like structure where key knowledge is held by individuals.[18] In contrast to the explicit knowledge found in written protocols and technology, implicit knowledge is passed from master to student via extended apprenticeships. While explicit descriptions promote knowledge transfer and teamwork via induction of shared mental models, attempts to transfer implicit knowledge is inefficient and often results to different team members possessing conflicting mental models.[12] A key advantage of embedding knowledge in technology is that device development creates an explicit description of the problem and solution. For example, surgeons once handcrafted enteric anastomoses, and now, they use stapling devices. The current devices benefit from an accumulating corpus of explicit knowledge and provide a more standardized, efficient, and effective solution. Teams lose a member's implicit knowledge when that individual leaves or retires. In contrast, the knowledge stored in written processes and technology is readily transferred across time and space to other team members and other teams. Such sharing often promotes acceleration of organizational learning.[16]

Members of high-functioning teams continually share and analyze information. These activities promote a shared understanding that has been termed "collective mindfulness."[19,20] Such awareness repeatedly compares predicted to observed performance. Predictable performance arises from standard work, especially when standard work is accompanied by explicit description of its steps and their rationale. In contrast, repeatedly using a nonstandard approach to standard work promotes a normalization of deviance.[21] Mindfulness identifies such variances and searches for an explanation. These approaches have been used to improve team performance in health care and other settings.[20,22]

Team members turn to named and unnamed leaders to organize work, resolve conflicts, provide examples, and monitor overall progress. Named leaders appear on organizational charts while unnamed leaders toil in the background. Since effective teams tend to be small (<10 members), all but the smallest organizations will have multiple opportunities for individuals to step into leadership roles. Like any complex behavior, the knowledge, skills, and abilities to lead are not innate qualities but rather learned through experience and training. A detailed discussion of leadership is beyond the scope of this chapter. Interested readers are referred to other texts on leadership[23,24] and leadership development.[25]

COMMUNICATION

Communication is an essential component of health care in general and teamwork in particular. Despite widespread acknowledgment of its importance, communication in health care is rarely defined. This occurs even though communication is a well-developed scientific discipline built upon rigorous theory.[26–28] A brief review of communication theory is provided to create a framework for understanding how breakdowns in communication occur and might be avoided.

Communication involves transmitting information across time and space. This includes conveying a physician's orders to the pharmacy or a procedure's risks, benefits, and alternatives to a patient. In each case, the sender attempts to communicate information to a recipient. Claude Shannon defined information by its ability to reduce uncertainty in the recipient.[26-28] In cases where the recipient is completely certain about a topic, there is no need to communicate. Predetermined instructions approach such certainty, and in those circumstances, communication focuses on when to begin executing those instructions. With standardized work, a long and complicated set of instructions can be reduced to "start now." Given that such certainty rarely exists in health care settings, a more common verbal exchange between experienced teammates is "start antibiotics on admission." The recipient then uses their pre-existing knowledge of patient variables, clinical settings, and prior examples to unpack the message and transform it into drug, dose, route, and schedule for a particular patient.

ENCODING, TRANSMITTING, DECODING

In each case, information was encoded by the sender, transmitted from sender to recipient, and then decoded by the recipient (Fig. 15-4). Since the sender wishes to remove uncertainty in the recipient, he/she must have some understanding of the recipient's mind-set. If the recipient only speaks Russian, a perfectly clear message in English will not reduce uncertainty in the recipient. Indeed, it is in the sender's best interest to translate the intended message into a format that will be properly decoded by the recipient. When communicating with patients, health care professionals need to avoid jargon and concepts that are not part of the patient's lexicon or established mental models.

Errors occur during each phase of the message's journey. Encoding and decoding errors arise when the sender and recipient possess different mental models. The vignette at the start of this chapter illustrates how small differences can have clear consequences. Errors also occur during transmission because noise is inevitably added to the message as it traverses the time and space separating the sender and recipient. Noisy procedure rooms and low-resolution fax machines are common examples.

Well-designed communication systems contain processes that detect errors and take corrective action. The most common error mitigation strategies involve redundancy. Redundancy occurs when the message is repeated in the setting of a noisy room. Redundancy also occurs within the message itself. This combats the noisy room

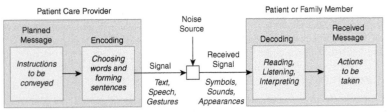

Figure 15-4. Communication schematic. When ill, patients or their family members face uncertainty about what might be done to treat their illness or alleviate its symptoms. Upon arriving upon a diagnosis, the provider attempts to convey this information. Those instructions are encoded into text, speech, or gestures and transmitted to the patient or family member. During transmission, noise is invariably added to the message. The patient or family member then decodes the message and uses the information to reduce their uncertainty.

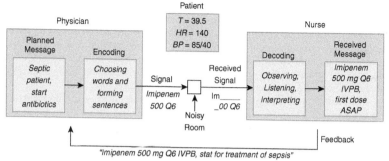

Figure 15-5. Communication and teamwork with shared mental models. Both the physician and nurse see a patient and review the vital signs. Each independently forms a mental model of a septic patient who needs immediate treatment. The physician gives a verbal order but a loud noise in the room means that the nurse only hears "im _____ hundred Q6." While in other circumstances, "im_____" might be interpreted as Imitrex, Imodium, or immobilization, given that she expected an order for antibiotics, she correctly decodes "im_____, _____hundred Q6" as "imipenem 500 Q6." The nurse then uses their mental model to add information regarding route and urgency. The nurse also provides feedback to acknowledge receipt of the message. The feedback message while longer than necessary serves two purposes. First, it convinces the physician that the original message was received and correctly interpreted. Second, it acknowledges a shared mental model that will be used as the basis for further communication about this patient's care. The steps for encoding and decoding the feedback message are omitted for the sake of clarity.

problem and also reduces encoding and decoding errors. An internally redundant message might state "heparin flush, 100 units/mL" where both the recipient and sender share a mental model that the standard concentration for heparin flush in this setting is 100 units/mL. The longer the message, the more likely it contains such internal redundancies. Shannon demonstrated this feature by reading a passage from a book, stopping mid sentence and asking a listener to guess the next word.[27,28]

While internal redundancy within the message is one means of improving communication, feedback is an even more effective strategy. By requiring that the recipient send a message back, the sender learns that the message was received and correctly decoded (Fig. 15-5). This is the philosophy behind strategies that require the recipient to read back the original message. This strategy still fails if the recipient simply parrots back the message phonetically. In this case, the message was not decoded by the recipient. It did not reduce uncertainty. A more effective strategy is to have the recipient generate a reply where the resulting message indicates a knowledgeable transformation of the original message's content. This is the philosophy of teach back strategies where the recipient issues a reply that makes sense to both parties.

BANDWIDTH

Communication requires bandwidth, defined as bits of information/second that can be transmitted through the communication channel. Bandwidth is commonly conserved by strategies that group information into chunks. Abbreviations are an example of this chunking strategy. However, chunking reduces message redundancy and thereby increases the probability of communication errors. This is especially true in situations where nonstandard abbreviations are used. The sender and receiver must have shared mental models of each chunk. Standard work is a chunking strategy where complex care plans can be created out of multiple predefined tasks. This strategy conserves communication bandwidth and is observed anytime teams must work under time pressure. In the prior example, the verbal order of "imipenem 500 Q6" is decoded to include urgency of obtaining the first dose, establishing intravenous (IV) access and standard procedure for administering the medication.

Bandwidth considerations also describe why error rates increase during efforts to rapidly transmit information through a constrained channel. In such situations, the channel can become completely filled with information flowing from the sender to the recipient. There is little to no bandwidth available for redundancy within the message and no bandwidth available for feedback. High-capacity channels allow sufficient bandwidth for feedback and message redundancy. Stated another way, time constraints lead to increased errors because the protective effects of feedback and redundancy are sacrificed. However, in emergent situations, the need for immediate action can supersede concerns about communication errors. The time and effort spent invested in creating standard work and fostering high-performing teams are clearly evident in such situations.

In summary, communication theory not only provides insight into the difficulty of conveying information but also suggests strategies for improving team performance. Aircraft carrier operations and other high-reliability organizations have long leveraged these strategies to improve outcomes.[19] The next section illustrates the challenges of applying this knowledge to patient care. The final section describes the results of different improvement strategies.

BARRIERS TO EFFECTIVE TEAMWORK AND COMMUNICATION

As stated earlier in the chapter, teamwork and communication are critical to error prevention. The study of accident causation and analyses conducted after serious safety events point to breakdown of teamwork, often associated with lack of effective leadership, human factors, and communication, as being commonly reported root causes of events resulting in patient harm (Table 15-1).

Barriers to team effectiveness referenced in this chapter include time constraints, poor communication, inflexible hierarchy, conflicting goals, personnel turnover, and differences in organizational culture. Human factors is discussed in Chapter 16.

TABLE 15-1	Top Three Identified Causes of Sentinel Events Reviewed by the Joint Commission by Year	
2010 N = 802	2011 N = 1243	2012 N = 901
Leadership = 710 (89%)	Human factors = 899 (70%)	Human factors = 614 (68%)
Human factors = 699 (87%)	Leadership = 815 (66%)	Leadership = 557 (62%)
Communication = 661 (82%)	Communication = 760 (61%)	Communication = 532 (59%)

People more easily relate to time barriers and interruptions but dysfunctional behaviors are harder to acknowledge and address. Organizational culture is understood through the attitudes, beliefs, and values that shape group behaviors and can strongly influence a group's ability to perform in a reliably safe manner. Detailed analysis of safety culture is found in Chapter 12 but here, it is discussed in the context of its impact on teamwork and communication. Cultures are also unique to local groups within the macrosystem and can differ from department to department.

For teams to thrive, they must be supported by not only local leadership but an organizational culture that promotes collaboration and honest, respectful communication. A commonly seen barrier is the traditional hierarchy of medicine, which can inhibit effective teamwork through promoting a division of labor (silos) where individuals are rewarded for solo performance instead of successful teamwork. This traditional culture also continues to foster a power distance and authority gradient, which erodes healthy teamwork. Power distance is defined as the acceptance by subordinates that power is distributed unequally, which is a barrier to the safety strategy "deference to expertise." This describes the idea that firsthand observation can often supersede the skill, knowledge, and abilities of off-site personnel who would otherwise be considered authorities on the subject. This realization motivates high-reliability organizations to move decisions to the front line whenever possible.[19]

The Agency for Healthcare Research and Quality (AHRQ) defines the authority gradient as the balance of decision-making power or the steepness of command hierarchy in a given situation. These concepts can translate as team members' reluctance to accept the alerts or insights of all teammates, deferring instead to an unspoken authority gradient. This phenomenon often allows those with more power to "rule" in a given situation even if there is known risk in that ruler's decision. Power distance and authority gradient may be the underlying issue seen in many cases where, during cause analysis interviews, concerned team members admit that they were afraid to voice their concerns, especially to anyone with more authority. In the 2005 study, Silence Kills, *VitalSmarts*, and the American Association of Critical-Care Nurses found that 84% of nurses and physicians reported observing colleagues taking dangerous shortcuts when working with patients, and yet, <10% were willing to speak up about their concerns.[29]

Residents and students encounter situations where speaking up about concerns is simply not the norm. In hierarchical cultures, where those less powerful perceive they will be ignored or even punished for "speaking up for safety," silence and divided loyalties can result in patient harm. This is especially true if medical staff and hospital employees have different agendas or divergent mental models.

A common example occurs when one team member suspects a foreign body may be unintentionally left in a wound. That member would request a radiograph to assess this possibility. The surgeon is anxious to complete the procedure because there is an urgent request to evaluate a patient in the emergency room. Each team member is attempting to optimize the situation to fit their mental model of what will best serve all patients in the system. Teamwork means communicating and balancing the competing agendas.

Competing priorities such as time constraints are often the cited reason for lack of compliance with safety policies. Policies and standard work are developed with the intent of ensuring that the patient's safety is never compromised for the convenience of their care providers. For this reason, high-performing teams often discuss or simulate these common situations before they occur and agree on a flexible, balanced approach to policy adherence that considers the needs of the patients first then all other team members.

Patients and families are a significant part of the equation and the most important members of the health care team. This requires our consideration, as providers, of their experience with power distance and authority gradient. In health care, physicians are generally placed at the top of the hierarchy with an inferred steep authority gradient relative to the patient and their family. Similar to but possibly even seen more in health care than other service industries, people tend to pause before questioning or complaining about the quality of their care to those delivering it. The cause for this lack of discussion may be patients' fear of some type of reprisal that could negatively impact their clinical care. People who are sick and frightened are in a vulnerable position, yet many clinicians are still reluctant to make changes that would balance the power in the patient–provider relationship. For example, inviting patients and family to be part of rounds where goals and plans of care are openly discussed might promote a subjective evaluation of our knowledge and practices by those we assume are less knowledgeable. The Joint Commission's National Patient Safety Goals and accreditation standards state that "an individual's involvement in care decisions is not only an identified right but also a source of accurate assessment and treatment information." These standards direct us to develop such partnerships with patients and break the traditional paradigm that has been more provider than patient focused.[30]

A *Health Affairs* policy brief provides a multidimensional framework for patient and family engagement in health and health care that outlines three levels of participation: consultation, involvement, and partnership/shared leadership. In consultation, the patient receives information about their diagnosis, involvement means the patient is asked about their preferences in developing a treatment plan, and true partnership is demonstrated by treatment decisions shaped by patient preferences, medical evidence, and clinical judgment. The framework includes factors influencing engagement such as patient beliefs about their role, health literacy, and education.[31]

Hierarchy presents yet another challenge to teamwork, which we will refer to as split hierarchy resulting in conflicting loyalties. Health care professionals, whether in academic medical centers or community hospitals, are often faced with dual organizational structures that result in different, possibly conflicting, goals and priorities. Infrastructure issues can affect resources, teamwork, and communication. Faculty members/attending physicians report to a departmental leader while nurses, technologists, and other staff take direction from the hospital's chain of command. Community hospitals' medical staff is often made up of physicians in private practice who find the hospital administration competing for time, resources, and even patients, which create financial challenges for both sides. Strategic goals and objectives may differ putting team members in a position of split loyalty and role confusion. For example, a school of medicine may set research and education as the top priority while the hospital is interested in driving volumes and services not aligned with the school's research agenda. Clinical researchers may find it hard to focus team partners on research tasks when those employees are mandated to meet productivity goals set by hospital supervisors.

Diverse communication styles are another potential barrier to safe teamwork. Gender, age, and cultural and language differences can often negatively impact team members' ability to deliver and/or receive accurate messages. Communication patterns are shaped by personal and professional education, training, and experience where role models, often unknowingly, teach us to be compatible or dysfunctional team players. Organizational culture type also plays an important role in how teams function. In hierarchical and, worse, pathologic cultures, problems or weaknesses are swept under the carpet for fear of a punitive response. Conversely, learning organizations adopt a collaborative culture that promotes open, honest communication and encourages those who speak up about risk.

From the perspective of any team member, effective communication is further hampered by lack of formal training in respectful assertion techniques. Assertion assumes that individuals will speak up and state their information or questions with appropriate persistence until there is clear resolution. Assertion is blocked by the same overall communication barriers of power distance, lack of shared mental model, lack of confidence, and past experiences (especially if intimidation has been part of one's experience). Employing standard methods of communication that provides the right amount/type of useful information and advocating for team members when intimidation is witnessed are helpful strategies that will be covered further in the table of error prevention tools at the end of this chapter.

CREATING MORE EFFECTIVE TEAMS

Teamwork training programs have been a force in improving reliability. Not only checklists and care bundles promote shared mental models but also they foster development of a safety culture. Over the last decade, beginning with the Institute for Healthcare Improvement's (IHI) 100,000 Lives Campaign (2005), teams have learned to bundle evidence-based prevention measures and use checklists to improve patient care. Implementation experience teaches us that bundles and checklists alone are not the answer to safer care because these tools were created for individuals that can decide to ignore or not fully implement them. Knowing what shapes individuals' willingness to comply with safety behaviors (human factors) and the influence of functional teams is a critical success factor in improving clinical quality and safety, an unending journey.

The Comprehensive Unit-Based Safety Program (CUSP) has been celebrated as a successful teamwork initiative that improved care for patients in intensive care units (ICUs) across the US. This effort integrated the focus on compliance with clinical bundles to reduce catheter-associated bloodstream infections (CLABSI) and the fundamental cultural issues that could promote adoption of safe practices. The combination of clinical and cultural interventions helped to bridge the divide or power distance among diverse patient care partners. Administrative leadership commitment, strong team leaders, and educated accountable team members worked together in hundreds of ICUs all over the country to realize an almost 40% reduction in CLABSI. The safety climate survey conducted in participating ICUs reported that the strongest predictor of clinical excellence (metric: zero CLABSI for 5 months or greater) was that caregivers felt comfortable speaking up if they perceived a problem with patient care.[32] ICU staff, physicians, and hospital administrators were trained on teamwork competencies, which included (1) mutual performance monitoring and adaptability [situational awareness], (2) supporting/backup behavior, (3) effective team leadership, (4) task-related assertiveness, (5) conflict resolution, and (6) closed-loop communication.[33] Other programs, such as TeamSTEPPS (Strategies and Tools to Enhance Performance and Patient Safety) and Team Performance Plus, have brought principles of high reliability to health care teams, emphasizing the positive effects of teamwork and communication.

Leader methods for reliability and safety behaviors demonstrated by use of error prevention tools are the foundation for improving the culture of safety, improved teamwork and communication, and reduction in harm. Error prevention tools are aimed at the causes for and types of human error (skill-based, knowledge-based, and rule-based). Examples and strategies for improving communication as well as assertiveness are summarized in Tables 15-2 to 15-5.

TABLE 15-2	Communication Guidelines for Nurses[34]

- Have I seen and assessed this patient myself before I call?
- Are there standing orders?
- Do I have at hand
  - The chart?
  - List of current meds, IV fluids, and labs?
  - Most recent vital signs?
  - If reporting lab work, date, and time, this test was done and results of previous tests for comparisons?
  - Code status?
- Have I read the most recent MD progress notes and notes from the nurse who worked the shift ahead of me?
- Have I discussed this call with my charge nurse?
- When ready to call,
  - Remember to identify self, unit, patient, and room number.
  - Know the admitting diagnosis and date of admission.
  - Briefly state the problem, what it is, when it happened or started, and how severe it is.
- What do I expect to happen as a result of this call?
- Document whom you spoke to, time of call, and summary of conversation.
- Engage and treat physician with respect.

WIKIS, WHITEBOARDS, AND OTHER ENABLING TECHNOLOGIES FOR SELF-ORGANIZING TEAMS

The traditional command and control model relied on centralized expertise and a hierarchical infrastructure to broadcast information to frontline teams. Collaborative models promote conversations as a means of sharing information with frontline staff. Dynamic situations such as managing a critically ill patient or working urgent/emergent patients into an existing schedule require ongoing reassessment and reformulation of plans. Whiteboards and similar technologies have long been used to manage dynamic systems. These vehicles allow multiple workers to continually update the posted information about the system's state. Recently, whiteboards and similar tools have been introduced into ICUs with encouraging results. While a series of one-to-one conversations were previously used to organize the care of critically ill patients,

TABLE 15-3	Key Elements for Improving Communication and Assertiveness

- Consider the goals for the conversation before starting to communicate.
- Get the person's attention by facing them and making eye contact.
- Introduce yourself if not known.
- Use the person's first name or formal title, whatever most appropriate.
- Ask knowable information.
- Explicitly ask for input.
- Provide information.
- Talk about next steps.
- Encourage ongoing monitoring and cross-checking.
- Always use a respectful tone and language

TABLE 15-4 Error Prevention Tools

Tool	Description	Example
STAR	**S**top, **T**hink, **A**ct, and **R**eview. This tool takes 2–3 s to perform, helps attention to detail, can reduce risk tenfold.	When prescribing high-risk medication, stop to review patient, desired drug, dose, and timing, type the order, review order, execute (hit "ok").
SBAR	**S**ituation, **B**ackground, **A**ssessment, **R**ecommendation, or **R**equest. Provides tool to organize thoughts and create standard, concise information handoff. Helps break down power distance or authority gradient when used at every organizational level	**Situation**: "Mrs. Nancy Drew in room 1130A has had a change in mental status in the last hour, appears disoriented." **Background**: "Mrs. Drew is 83 years old with history of PVD, postop day #1 from thrombo-embolectomy of left leg artery. She was lucid 45 min ago when I administered metoprolol and Zocor. She has no hx of dementia during this or any previous hospitalization." **Assessment**: "Vital signs look fine: Temp 37.1, P 72, BP 114/68, O_2 saturation 97% on room air. Accu-Chek reading 102. I'm concerned she may be having a stroke." **Recommendation**: "I'd like you to come see her right away. Is there something I should be doing in the meantime?"
Brief, Execute, Debrief	Process used by teams to prepare for, execute, and debrief after a procedure. Ensures situational awareness (everyone on the same page about what is about to happen and how it is to happen, to provide role clarity, and to gain agreement that procedure resulted in desired outcome). Script or boards can be used to standardize this process (e.g., ICU boards).	Traditional "time out" is the preprocedure briefing, which is expanded into discussion after procedure to share lessons learned and gain agreement that the desired outcome was achieved. Can be used in all procedure areas or at the bedside.

(Continued)

TABLE 15-4	Error Prevention Tools (*Continued*)

Tool	Description	Example
Peer Checking Peer Coaching	Everyone is responsible for practicing safe behaviors until they become habit. We're responsible for our own and our team members' behaviors. Organizational development courses such as "Crucial Conversations" provide scripting to assist staff in approaching team members for the purpose of reminding about safe behaviors (checking) and coaching when assistance is needed. Organizations with "Safety Coach" programs focus on the peer checking and peer coaching tools.	Poor compliance with hand hygiene and isolation precautions often provides opportunities for peer checking and peer coaching. Use of the tool ARCC helps escalate concerns in a calm, respectful manner. Remind people of the importance of safety behaviors and ask if there is any way you can assist to help them comply. Role modeling is the best method of peer checking and coaching. Tools that may also be useful include three-way repeat back and read back (answer, "that's correct."), phonetic ("that's Mr. Dridge...D-R-I-D-G-E") and numeric clarifications ("that's fifty: 5-0"), or asking clarifying questions ("I have a clarifying question"). Safety Coaches are team members trained to observe work behaviors and provide real-time feedback about practice and compliance with error prevention tools and reliability methods. These coaches are experts at the application of the peer checking and coaching tools.
Stop the Line	Stop all action when risk of harm is severe and imminent. Scripted so all team members understand the meaning of the phrase. Use low, respectful tone of voice. Used to ensure that all team members are on the same page about impending actions while providing alert that going forward without clarification could result in harm	During a rapid response team action, a team member realizes that there is an infusion bag hanging with penicillin added. The resident notes that the patient has an allergy arm band on with "penicillin" written in, as well as a note in the EMR allergy section. The resident immediately states, "Please stop the line, I need clarity." She then points to the infusion and the arm band to focus everyone's attention to what is likely the cause of the patient's deterioration.

TABLE 15-4	Error Prevention Tools (Continued)	
Tool	Description	Example
ARCC	**A**sk a question, make a **R**equest, voice a **C**oncern, then use **C**hain of command	Dr. Smith is about to enter the room of a patient on contact precautions for MRSA without donning protective garb. Resident Dr. Jones says, "Dr. Smith, can I help you with your gown and gloves?" (if still ignored...) "Dr. Smith, we've been asked to be meticulous with our isolation compliance...can I please help you with our garb?" (no action...) "Dr. Smith, I'm concerned about the many transplant patients on this unit and spreading MRSA." These steps usually result in compliance. If no action after these steps, discussion between the appropriate person and Dr. Smith's supervisor is warranted.
Red Rules	A red rule is a *safety imperative* that must be followed when the potential for harm is frequent and result of a mistake could be grave. Red rules are few but noncompliance generally results in serious corrective action. Red rules can be organizational or departmental or both.	Organizational red rule: use of two patient identifiers (e.g., name and date of birth) before any procedure or treatment where misidentification of a patient is likely to result in serious harm. ICU departmental red rule: no one is to walk past an alarming monitor without checking the monitor reading and observing the patient.
Great Catch Program	Great catches are celebrated when any member of the health care team go above and beyond their routine job duties to prevent harm or promote the safety culture.	Transporter stops the line when asked by RN to transport an oxygen-dependent patient to procedure area with low tank of O_2. Transporter is recognized not only for preventing harm to patient but also for speaking up for safety against an existing "power distance/authority gradient" on that unit.

TABLE 15-5	Team Methods to Improve Reliability and Communication	
Make safety a core value	Safety is made a visible priority by using our first words for patient safety and modeling that nothing is more important.	Start every meeting with a patient story. Link all decisions to safety. Encourage reporting of events and near misses and recognize those who speak up for safety.
Find and fix problems	Everyone highly alert for risk, problems identified before they result in harm. Sensitive to operations, present at the front line to help identify problems that make safe patient care difficult to deliver, solving causes of problems promptly.	Daily huddles provide a forum to find and fix problems as well as daily (or more frequent) rounds. Start the clock for safety issues means that high-risk or urgent problems are solved by a responsible person on a defined time line with appropriate follow-up to all those who need to know. Brief/Execute/Debrief is another tool to find and fix problems.
Daily safety huddle	Used daily to find and fix problems following standardized format and script. Huddles should be brief, approximately 15 min long. Expectation is set that key leaders attend in person or by phone.	Focus on what has occurred in the last 24 h that resulted in risk, how risk was mitigated, what might happen in next 24 h, and how will risk be mitigated. Includes responsible parties, timelines for action, and follow-up at next daily huddle (if not before).
Build and sustain accountability	Reliability is built through safe practice habits demonstrated by effective teams. Leaders and peers together must hold each other accountable for safety first.	Team leaders rounding to influence means they focus on a specific error prevention tool, asking others to demonstrate competency through discussion of application of tools in the practice setting. 5:1 feedback is a tool that promotes accountability through acknowledgment of best safety practices five times more than offering feedback about necessary performance improvement. This strategy builds trust through prompt and frequent recognition of positive behaviors and, subsequently, better acceptance by individuals receiving performance feedback when improvement is needed.

these whiteboards are a more efficient means of creating a shared mental model about the patient's condition and planned interventions. In addition, written information supports asynchronous communication where even though one's attention might be distracted for a period, the information remains accessible. In contrast, verbal communication requires attention and proper sequencing.

Electronic versions of these whiteboards promote even greater visibility of the system's state. Such transparency eliminates phone calls that were previously required to manage workflow and adjust staffing levels to accommodate schedule changes. Networked versions of electronic whiteboards constitute a type of wiki, where a wiki is a website that allows visitors to make changes, contributions, or corrections. Wikipedia.com is the best known example of a wiki. While subject matter experts will always have concerns about the accuracy and reliability of the information posted by large, diverse groups of authors, wikis are more responsive to rapidly changing events.[35-38] Wikis and whiteboards leverage the realization that frontline staff and other first person observers are the de facto experts when it comes to evaluating the local situation.

KEY POINTS

• Teamwork in patient care is essential. The team includes the patient, all care providers, and support personnel.
• Team performance depends on shared mental models and communication. Both benefit from experience working together as a team.
• Communication can be divided into three steps: message encoding, transmission, and decoding.
• Communication errors fall into common patterns. Redundancy, feedback, and constructing the message with the recipient in mind are proven prevention strategies.

REFERENCES

1. Whitt N, Harvey R, McLeod G, et al. How many health professionals does a patient see during an average hospital stay? *N Z Med J.* 2007;120(1253):U2517.
2. Commission J. *The Joint Commission Guide to Improving Staff Communication.* 2nd ed. Oakbrook Terrace, IL: Joint Commission Resources; 2008.
3. Nelson EC, Batalden PB, Huber TP, et al. Microsystems in health care: Part 1. Learning from high-performing front-line clinical units. *Jt Comm J Qual Improv.* 2002;28(9):472–93.
4. Reason JT. *Human Error.* New York, NY: Cambridge University Press; 1990.
5. Schmidt RA, Lee TD. *Motor Control and Learning: A Behavioral Emphasis.* 4th ed. Champaign, IL: Human Kinetics; 2005.
6. Wuchty S, Jones BF, Uzzi B. The increasing dominance of teams in production of knowledge. *Science.* 2007;316(5827):1036–9.
7. Tapscott D, Williams AD. *Wikinomics: How Mass Collaboration Changes Everything.* New York, NY: Portfolio; 2006.
8. Gleick J. *Chaos: Making a New Science.* New York, NY: Viking; 1987.
9. Surowiecki J. *The Wisdom of Crowds: Why the Many are Smarter than the Few and How Collective Wisdom Shapes Business, Economies, Societies, and Nations.* 1st ed. New York, NY: Doubleday; 2004.
10. Klein GA. *Streetlights and Shadows: Searching for the Keys to Adaptive Decision Making.* Boston, MA: The MIT Press; 2009.

11. The Better the Team, the Safer the World. Paper presented at: Conference on Group Interaction in High Risk Environments, Ruschlikon, Switzerland, 2004.
12. Senge PM. *The Fifth Discipline: The Art and Practice of the Learning Organization.* Revised and updated edition. New York, NY: Doubleday/Currency; 2006.
13. Lencioni P. *The Five Dysfunctions of a Team: A Leadership Fable.* 1st ed. San Francisco, CA: Jossey-Bass; 2002.
14. Tuckman BW. Developmental Sequence in Small Groups. *Psychol Bull.* 1965;63:384–99.
15. Covey SMR, Merrill RR. *The Speed of Trust: The One Thing that Changes Everything.* New York, NY: Free Press; 2006.
16. Argote L. *Organizational Learning: Creating, Retaining and Transferring Knowledge.* New York, NY: Springer; 2005.
17. Argote L, Epple D. Learning curves in manufacturing. *Science.* 1990;247(4945):920–4.
18. Emanuel L, Berwick DM, Conway J, et al. What exactly is patient safety? In: Henriksen K, Battles J, Keyes M, eds. *Advances in Patient Safety: New Directions and Alternative Approaches.* Rockville, MD: Agency for Healthcare Research and Quality; 2008.
19. Weick KE, Sutcliffe KM. *Managing the Unexpected: Assuring High Performance in an Age of Complexity.* 1st ed. San Francisco, CA: Jossey-Bass; 2001.
20. Liker JK. *The Toyota Way: 14 Management Principles from the World's Greatest Manufacturer.* New York, NY: McGraw-Hill; 2004.
21. Prielipp RC, Magro M, Morell RC, et al. The normalization of deviance: do we (un)knowingly accept doing the wrong thing? *Anesth Analg.* 2010;110(5):1499–502.
22. James BC, Savitz LA. How Intermountain trimmed health care costs through robust quality improvement efforts. *Health Aff (Millwood).* 2011;30(6):1185–91.
23. Deming WE. *Out of the Crisis.* 1st ed. Cambridge, MA: MIT Press; 2000.
24. Kotter JP. *Leading Change.* Boston, MA: Harvard Business Review Press; 2012.
25. Bennis WG. *On Becoming a Leader.* [Rev. ed.]. Cambridge, MA: Perseus Pub.; 2003.
26. Shannon CE, Weaver W. *The Mathematical Theory of Communication.* Urbana, IL: University of Illinois Press; 1949.
27. Gleick J. *The Information: A History, a Theory, a Flood.* 1st ed. New York, NY: Pantheon Books; 2011.
28. Pierce JR. *An Introduction to Information Theory: Symbols, Signals & Noise.* 2nd rev. ed New York, NY: Dover Publications; 1980.
29. Maxfield D, Grenny J, McMillan R, et al. *Silence Kills: The Seven Crucial Conversations for Healthcare.* 2005. http://www.aacn.org/WD/practice/docs/publicpolicy/silencekills.pdf. Accessed 9/24/13.
30. Methods DoSaS. *Standards Supporting the Provision of Culturally and Linguistically Appropriate Services.* 2009. http://www.jointcommission.org/assets/1/6/2009_CLASRelatedStandardsOME. pdf. Accessed 9/24/13.
31. Carman KL, Dardess P, Maurer M, et al. Patient and family engagement: a framework for understanding the elements and developing interventions and policies. *Health Aff (Millwood).* 2013;32(2):223–31.
32. Pronovost P, Needham D, Berenholtz S, et al. An intervention to decrease catheter-related bloodstream infections in the ICU. *N Engl J Med.* 2006;355(26):2725–32.
33. CUSP Toolkit. http://www.ahrq.gov/professionals/education/curriculum-tools/cusptoolkit/ index.html. Accessed 9/24/13.
34. *Practical Tactics that Improve Both Patient Safety and Patient Perceptions of Care.* Gulf Breeze, FL: Studer Group; 2007.
35. Tapscott D, Williams AD. *Wikinomics: How Mass Collaboration Changes Everything.* (Expanded ed.). New York, NY: Portfolio; 2008.
36. Tapscott D, Williams AD. *Macrowikinomics: Rebooting Business and the World.* New York, NY: Portfolio/Penguin; 2010.
37. Giles J. Internet encyclopaedias go head to head. *Nature.* 2005;438(7070):900–1.
38. Clauson KA, Polen HH, Boulos MN, et al. Scope, completeness, and accuracy of drug information in Wikipedia. *Ann Pharmacother.* 2008;42(12):1814–21.

16 Human Factors

Laurie Wolf and Sergio E. Trevino

CLINICAL VIGNETTE

Ms. W is a 50-year-old woman with lymphoma admitted for a stem cell transplant. She also has a history of atrial fibrillation with rapid ventricular rate for which she is on an esmolol drip and has a cardiac monitor. The monitor is located at the bedside, and the display of the cardiac rhythm can be viewed at the bedside but is also transmitted to the nurses' station. This evening, the patient had a peripherally inserted central catheter (PICC) line placed by the intravenous (IV) therapy service. While setting up her equipment to place the PICC line, the IV therapist accidentally bumped the bedside cardiac monitor, causing a cord on the back of the monitor to become unplugged. This caused the monitor to alarm. The IV therapist plugged the cord back into the back of the monitor, the alarm stopped, and the heart rhythm could again be seen at the bedside. The PICC line was then placed without incident. Later in the evening, one of the nurses noted that the patient's monitor was no longer transmitting to the nurses' station. She entered the patient's room, found her to be in asystole, and called a code. During the code, it was noted that the cord on the monitor had been plugged into the incorrect port. When the cord is plugged into this port, the heart rhythm can be viewed at the bedside but is not transmitted to the nurses' station. When it is plugged into the correct port, the rhythm can be viewed in both locations. The incorrect port was color-coded orange; the plug was green. However, the ports were not easily visible. Even if ports were visible and the color coding matched, the lighting was dim making visibility of color difficult.

- What human factors contributed to this event?
- How did the design of the equipment or room contribute to the event?
- How could the event be prevented in the future?

INTRODUCTION

Human Factors Engineering (HFE) (also called Ergonomics) is a discipline that conducts research regarding human psychological, social, physical, and biologic characteristics and works to apply that information with respect to the design, operation, or use of products or systems that optimize human performance, health, safety, and/or habitability.[1] The following is the definition most widely adopted by the HFE community, developed by the International Ergonomics Association[2]:

"Ergonomics (or human factors) is the scientific discipline concerned with the understanding of interactions among humans and other elements of a system, and the profession that applies theory, principles, data and methods to design in order to optimize human well-being and overall system performance."

The term human factors is sometimes used as a misnomer by attributing the cause of an error to a human action. However, the science of HFE rejects the premise that the human is primarily at fault and instead utilizes a systems approach to fully understand the circumstance that leads to an error.[3] In the clinical vignette, according to HFE, the cause of the error was the presence of two nonfunctioning ports, rather than the nurse's action (Fig. 16-1). The solution was focused on the system (the cardiac monitor) rather than the user (nurse). Systems are invented by humans and, hence, should be designed for humans to use them correctly. Any error that occurs by the user is thus attributable to the design of the system.[4]

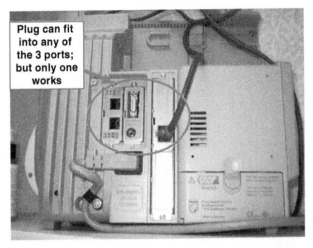

Plug can fit into any of the 3 ports; but only one works

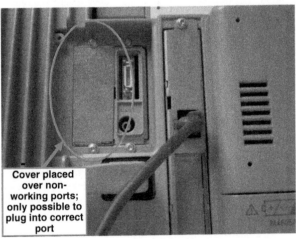

Cover placed over non-working ports; only possible to plug into correct port

Figure 16-1. HFE intervention on a cardiac monitor.

HFE began as a formal discipline after World War II, primarily in the military and aviation domains before moving into other industries in the 1970s.[4–6] Events in other industries such as the "Three Mile Island" nuclear accident in the US and the "Bhopal gas tragedy" in India resulted in several regulatory documents outlining how HFE must systematically be incorporated in system design. HFE has been utilized in health care to a small degree since the 1980s; however, HFE became more prominent in health care during the 1990s with the shift in culture away from "blaming the user" and the identification of active (user) and latent (systems) failures.[7]

There are three HFE core principles that have been applied to health care[8,9]:

1. Systems Orientation—Performance results from the interaction of a sociotechnical system instead of a single component (user).
2. Design Driven—Improvements directed toward the design of work environment, equipment, structures, and processes.
3. Person Centered—Systems should be designed to support the needs of the people using the system.

The foundation for HFE is based on the domains of physical, cognitive, and organizational (psychosocial) characteristics of people.[10] A few examples of these domains include:

- Cognitive Ergonomics—Includes mental workload, decision making, human–computer interaction, human reliability, stress, and training. These concepts can be used in health care to evaluate the usability of technology, design training systems, and user interfaces for information technology. Cognitive issues are critical when understanding incident or event reporting systems and analysis processes.
- Physical Ergonomics—Includes material handling, posture, repetition, workplace layout, and physical capabilities (all senses). These concepts can be used in health care to reduce worker and patient injuries and achieve optimal workplace (sound, lighting, glare, noise) and equipment layouts. Physical issues must be considered to achieve safe patient care.
- Organizational Ergonomics—Includes communication, job/work design, shift work, participatory design, teamwork, policies, procedures, and quality management. These concepts can be used in health care to design jobs that will reduce stress and burnout and improve patient and staff satisfaction. Organizational issues must be considered when designing patient care models to achieve appropriate work schedules and enhance worker performance and processes.

Factors that negatively affect human performance and can be addressed during an HFE assessment are shown in Table 16-1.

TABLE 16-1   Factors Affecting Human Performance

Fatigue	Noise	Shift work	Reliance on memory
Boredom	Heat	Illness and injuries	Reliance on vigilance
Frustration	Clutter	Interruptions	Poorly designed devices
Fear	Motion	Distractions	Poorly designed procedures
Stress	Lighting/glare	Unnatural workflow	

FRAMEWORKS AND MODELS

Applied Model

A systems approach for applying the domains of HFE into practice involves numerous disciplines, but for practical purposes, they can be grouped into three components: Organization, Human, and Environmental (Fig. 16-2). When an error or inefficiency occurs, it is usually the result of some combination of these components.

- Organization: Even when individual components of a system are designed with HFE in mind, it is still possible for an undesired outcome to occur if the design of the entire work system is not considered. Macroergonomics is a subdiscipline of HFE that studies the overall work system.[10] The study of macroergonomics concludes that for human factors to be effective, there is a need to integrate organization and management into the system design process.
- Human Capabilities and Limitations: A mismatch between physical abilities and job demands can lead to physical discomfort and injury. A mismatch with cognitive capabilities and perception abilities can lead to frustration and error.
  - Physical Capabilities: To understand the physical capabilities and limitations of humans requires knowledge of the size, strength, and physical activities of the person performing a specific task. Engineering anthropometry deals with the application of scientific physical measurement methods to develop engineering design standards. This field includes static and functional (dynamic) measurements of postural dimensions, forces, and energy expenditures. Numerous tables of data are available with various human populations that typically indicate the 5th, 50th, and 95th percentiles for dimensions such as standing height, seated height and width, leg length, etc.[6] Anthropometric data can be applied to the design of equipment and facilities to produce health care environments and processes that fit the physical capabilities of health care workers and their patients.

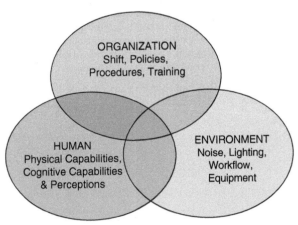

Figure 16-2. Practical application of a Human Factors Systems Approach.

○ Cognitive Capabilities: There are numerous considerations when understanding the mental processes that occur during a work task. Cognitive issues are a significant source of errors in health care.[11]

○ Perception: There are limitations with each of the five senses in recognition of various stimuli. Some common perceptual issues in health care are described in Table 16-2.

○ The design and implementation of technology into health care have raised numerous cognitive concerns such as usability of medical devices and cognitive workload. A health care worker is required to interact daily with multiple computer interfaces and information communication systems. Appropriate menu screen design and hierarchy access to information become critical as electronic medical records are becoming more complex and essential in communication. Another common problem is the overload of auditory and visual alarms that can lead to desensitization and ignoring alarms.

• Environment: The environment can be thought of in two categories. The first category includes the physical space where work is performed. This includes the immediate workstation, intermediate settings such as the building where work occurs, and more generally the community or city. The second category includes various aspects of the ambient environment such as illumination, noise, heat, cold, vibration, and pollution.

All of these environmental factors can interact to impact how one functions within the health care setting. For example, one intensive care unit (ICU) found that individuals frequently walked into the glass door to enter the unit. The hallway

TABLE 16-2	Common Perceptual Issues in Health care
Perceptual Limitation	Example
Auditory	The appropriate volume and frequency of alarms depend on ambient noise frequency and volumes. Auditory desensitization is common with frequent alarms.
Visual	Small font size and dim lighting make reading critical information difficult for aging eyes and creating the possibility of error.
Signal detection	Searching a monitor readout with information from several telemetry patients can be a monotonous, diligent task making it difficult to detect abnormal readings.
Pictures, icons, and menu selection	Electronic medical records can be difficult to navigate to find critical, timely information.
Information processing	Nurses can have over 10 tasks on their mind while simultaneously processing new information with more than three interruptions per hour in a constantly changing environment.[12]

entering the ICU was white. The glass door had a white label applied to the glass. The lack of contrast between the white lettering and the white background combined with the glare from the hallway lights made it very difficult to read the sign. Increasing the contrast of the label by utilizing a dark background and white letters increased the readability of the sign significantly.

SEIPS Model

An HFE model of person-centered sociotechnical systems that has been extensively used in health care is called Systems Engineering Initiative for Patient Safety (SEIPS). It was introduced by Carayon et al. in 2006[13] and developed at the University of Wisconsin. This model has been adopted by patient safety leaders and used to frame the design and analysis of research in the field. An updated version of the model has been proposed by Holden et al.[9] called SEIPS 2.0 (Fig. 16-3).

The structure of the SEIPS 2.0 model as depicted below proposes that a sociotechnical work system (LEFT) produces certain work processes (CENTER), which shape the outcomes (RIGHT). It includes feedback loops from the outcomes to the other two components, called adaptation (BOTTOM), in order to improve the outcomes.

- Work System—Composed of six interacting components: person(s), tasks, tools and technologies, organization, internal environment, and external environment. All components revolve around the Person, emphasizing that design should support the people involved including health care providers, patients, and family.
- Processes—This is the workflow and can be classified as physical, cognitive, or social/behavioral performance processes. There are different agents that lead in each process including professionals, patients, or a collaboration of both.
- Outcomes—The outcomes are the results from the work processes that reflect the goals of the different stakeholders including patients, health care professionals, and leaders of the organization. Outcomes of a process can be desirable or undesirable and immediate (proximal) or reflected in the future (distal).

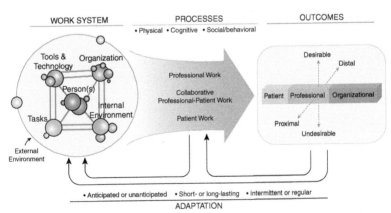

Figure 16-3. SEIPS 2.0 model by Holden et al. (From Holden RJ, et al. SEIPS 2.0: a human factors framework for studying and improving the work of healthcare professionals and patients. *Ergonomics.* 2013;56(11):1669–86.)

- Adaptation—Adaptation refers to changes due to feedback from the outcomes. Adaptations are inevitable in complex sociotechnical systems and can be intended or unintended, reactive or planned, and short or long lasting.

For a more detailed explanation of the SEIPS 2.0 model, please refer to the publication in *Ergonomics* by Holden et al.[9]

Published Examples of HFE Models at Work

There is significant published work about HFE models employed in different aspects of health care settings. A few of these are included to help obtain a better grasp of the effects of HFE in health care.

- Medical device purchases—HFE research was performed prior to the purchase of an infusion pump by a facility. Health care providers who use infusion pumps were videotaped using each of the candidate devices allowing for the selection of the safest and most person centered among four commercially available candidates.[14]
- ICU medication administration—This study used an HFE approach to evaluate potential medication administration failures and contributing factors. Focus groups of ICU nurses were utilized to identify the potential failure modes, contributing factors, and recovery processes used by nurses in the medication administration process. These findings can be utilized for process redesign.[15]
- Impact of bar-coded medication administration (BCMA)—An HFE assessment can describe and quantify the desirable and undesirable impact that the implementation of BCMA can have on a work process. This study found that a change to BCMA process had both desirable and undesirable effects.[16]

HUMAN FACTORS ASSESSMENT FORM

The assessment form in Table 16-3 is adapted from the Mayo Clinic Human Factors Analysis and Classification System (HFACS). This form can be used to assess a work area, or piece of equipment, or even to consider HFE issues that may have contributed to an adverse event. The assessment considers the impact of the following characteristics:

1. Environment/Layout
2. Environment/Conditions
3. Equipment (supplies, materials, availability)
4. Equipment Usability (hardware)
5. Equipment Usability (software)
6. Physical Capabilities and Limitations
7. Cognitive Capabilities and Limitations
8. Organization (policies and procedures)
9. Communication

For each of the above characteristics, the assessor can record the score of the block that best describes the condition of the situation being assessed. For example, if an audible alarm was missed at the nurse station during a shift change, the following scores could be considered:

- Environmental Layout = 2 (Environment allows task to be accomplished but achieved with difficulty and many not be accurate.)
- Environmental Conditions = 2 (Noise levels can cause misperceptions.)

TABLE 16-3 Human Factors Engineering Assessment Form

Date:

Describe what is being assessed, i.e., nurse station, IV pump, desk, med room:

Instructions: For each "Human Factors Characteristic," record the score of the block that best describes the condition of the situation being assessed. List opportunities for improvement.

Human Factors Characteristic	5 Points Outstanding No errors, no problems	4 Points Excellent No errors, task on time	3 Points Good Ask completed when needed	2 Points Marginal Adequate performance	1 Points Poor Task inadequate or late	0 Points Unacceptable Task not achieved, errors	Score
Environment/ Layout: Does the general environment encourage optimal performance?	Physical layout is optimal with no physical barriers. The environment enables tasks to be achieved with ease and comfort.	Physical environment promotes a task to be done correctly (orderly, clean good layout).	The environment allows the task to be adequately accomplished with minimal interference.	The environment allows the task to be accomplished, but it was achieved with difficulty and may not be accurate.	Extreme physical barriers exist, but the task can be minimally accomplished. (Performance or quality is compromised.)	Physical layout makes it impossible to accomplish the task.	
Environment/ Conditions: Are environmental conditions such as noise, lighting, temperature appropriate?	Optimal lighting, noise, and temperature levels exist to ensure the task is successful.	Conditions such as lighting, noise, and temperature levels allow task to be achieved.	Lighting, noise, and temperature levels are tolerable and do not interfere with the required task.	Lighting, noise, and temperature levels are uncomfortable or can cause visual or verbal misperception.	Lighting, noise, or temperature levels make it difficult to achieve the task and/or detect errors.	Extreme lighting, noise, or temperature conditions make it impossible to accomplish the task.	

Equipment, Supplies, Materials Availability: Right equipment, right time, right place?	Equipment, supplies and materials are always available, convenient, easy to obtain, and in good working order. Tasks can be achieved accurately and on schedule.	Equipment, supplies and materials are where they need to be, when they are needed to perform the desired task at all times.	Equipment, supplies and materials were obtained with moderate difficulty but did not interfere with completion or timeliness of the task.	Task was completed but was not finished on time or not completely successful due to lack of proper supplies or equipment.	Task was not adequately completed or was done incorrectly due to unavailability or distance of correct equipment or supplies.	Equipment necessary to perform a task is unavailable or not working properly, making it impossible to achieve the task.
Equipment Usability (Hardware) Is equipment easy to use?	Controls and displays are easy to use, understandable, and have obvious interactions. Incorrect usage is impossible.	Controls, displays and labels are easy to understand with minimal training.	If controls and/or displays are misinterpreted or used incorrectly, it allows the worker to detect a mistake and change it before an error occurs.	Operator can get used to controls and/or displays with extensive training and continued practice. Equipment has been modified (i.e., labels to clarify operation).	Equipment required extensive training and constant practice to remember how to use it. Displays do not indicate normal or abnormal status. Mistakes are not detected.	Traditional expectations (such as red is "bad," or up is "on") are violated in the layout of controls. Displays do not alert user causing errors to go undetected.

(Continued)

TABLE 16-3	Human Factors Engineering Assessment Form (Continued)					
Equipment Usability (Software) Is equipment easy to understand?	Equipment interaction is not only easy to understand, but is impossible to use incorrectly (i.e., guardrails on IV pump). Software will predict the users needs and suggest appropriate actions.	Equipment is easy to use and has warnings or alerts to identify errors.	If an incorrect entry is made it is detected and displayed and can be corrected easily before an error is made.	The worker has modified the equipment (figured out a "workaround" to better fit their needs).	Equipment required extensive training and constant practice to remember how to use it.	Critical warnings do not alert user, causing errors to go undetected.
Physical Capability and Limitations: Is task within the physical abilities of the user (lift, push, pull, see, hear, touch)?	All tasks can be performed without causing physical stress or fatigue. If capabilities must be exceeded, then an adaptive device is always available (i.e., Lift device, magnifying glass, protective gear)	Pushing, pulling, lifting, walking can be achieved with minimal stress. Rest breaks are possible when needed.	A healthy worker can achieve the tasks and still have energy at the end of the work shift.	A worker is tired and hungry at the end of the work shift. Feeling like there is never enough time in the day to get the work done.	Completing the task causes exhaustion or physical discomfort. No rest breaks or breaks for food or water are possible. Taking a pain reliever at the start or end of the day is helpful.	The task is physically impossible to achieve and does not get done, or is done incorrectly.

(Continued)

Mental Capability and Limitations: Is task within the mental abilities of the worker?	Tasks receive proper attention with minimal distraction without the worker feeling rushed, frustrated or stressed.	Memory aids are built into the process so the worker can remember several tasks without interruptions causing mistakes.	When workload is high there are easy to use memory aids available to make sure nothing is forgotten.	Tasks are completed but in a confused fashion with frequent interruptions and opportunity for error. Worker may have to call in a forgotten task to the next shift.	Too many things to remember and frequent interruptions make completing tasks very difficult. By the end of the shift, worker has feeling that things were forgotten.	Distractions and excessive workload cause frustration and result in long shifts and incomplete, inaccurate work.
Organization, Policy, Procedures: Do the organization, policies, coworkers, and management allow tasks to be successful?	Management and Health Service Organization (HSO) policies allow the required tasks to be completed as needed with patient/employee safety as the highest priority.	HSO beliefs and policies reinforce safe practice and rewards, patient/employee safety, and quality behavior.	Policies are reviewed periodically with staff. Daily work tasks are in alignment with policies. Management support is recognized by the staff.	Policies are not reviewed or used in the actual work day. New education initiatives are tolerated as "flavor of the month."	The chain of command is confusing and the HSO mission is unclear. It is well known that written policies do not reflect the actual activities in the work area.	Bending the rules is encouraged by supervisors and coworkers. Incentives exist to cut corners. Help is unavailable when training is needed.

TABLE 16-3 Human Factors Engineering Assessment Form (*Continued*)

Communication: Is information available and unambiguous as needed?	Communication at all levels is excellent. Handoffs between shifts and locations are seamless with no ambiguity.	Communication is good with standard briefings between handoffs. If an assignment is unclear, help is easily available.	Handoffs occur with standard terminology. Questions are tolerated and resolution can be obtained with minimal difficulty.	Communication is minimal. Questions are tolerated but resolution is difficult and time consuming to obtain.	Assignments come from several sources and are often conflicting and confusing. Minimal support is available for clarification. Speaking up about an error is uncomfortable and cumbersome.	Communication is confusing without any standard briefings. Supervisors or contacts are unavailable for clarification. Speaking up about an error is not tolerated.

Opportunities for Improvement:

Overall Human Factors Rating: **Average**

(Adapted from: Mayo Clinic Human Factors Analysis and Classification System (HFACS); Perrow C. *Normal Accidents*, 1984; Ciavarelli A. Human factors checklist. *An Aircraft Accident Investigation Tool*, 2002.)

- Equipment/Supplies = 4 (Equipment needed was available, just couldn't be heard.)
- Equipment Usability = 4 (Audible display was easy to understand, just couldn't be heard.)

In this example, it shows the environmental conditions were more responsible for the missed alarm than the usability or human characteristics (like physical or mental capabilities).

This assessment form can be used proactively to predict what may contribute to an error or reactively after an error has occurred. During error debriefings, the form can ensure many aspects of human factors are considered during the discovery/diagnostic phase to achieve an understanding of causation.

CONCLUSION

HFE provides the opportunity for health care workers to identify challenges with performing a task without assuming it is their fault. Often, the designers of a technology do not realize the frequency of interruptions, multitasking, and complexity of the environment where the task is performed. Introducing the rigor of HFE into health care will allow greater systemic solutions to some of the challenges in the health care environment.[4]

KEY POINTS

- Human factors should be incorporated into system design.
- Minimize "work-arounds" in the process.
- Avoid mental, physical, or sensory overload.
- If you can't "design-out" potential mistakes, make the status visible.
- Human error is inevitable; design systems that make it easy to do the right action and hard to do the wrong action.

REFERENCES

1. Stramler JH. *The Dictionary for Human Factors/ergonomics.* Boca Raton, FL: CRC Press; 1993;xiii:413.
2. IEA. *What is Ergonomics?* 2000 [cited December 3, 2013]. http://www.iea.cc/whats/index.html
3. Russ AL, et al. The science of human factors: separating fact from fiction. *BMJ Qual Saf.* 2013;22(10):802–8.
4. Cafazzo JA, St-Cyr O. From discovery to design: the evolution of human factors in healthcare. *Healthc Q.* 2012;15:24–9.
5. Wilson JR, Corlett EN. *Evaluation of Human Work.* 3rd ed. Boca Raton, FL: Taylor & Francis; 2005;xix:1026.
6. McCormick EJ, Sanders MS. *Human Factors in Engineering and Design.* 5th ed. New York, NY: McGraw-Hill; 1982;viii:615.
7. Reason J. Understanding adverse events: human factors. *Qual Health Care.* 1995;4(2):80–9.
8. Dul J, et al. A strategy for human factors/ergonomics: developing the discipline and profession. *Ergonomics.* 2012;55(4):377–95.
9. Holden RJ, et al. SEIPS 2.0: a human factors framework for studying and improving the work of healthcare professionals and patients. *Ergonomics.* 2013;56(11):1669–86.

10. Carayon P. *Handbook of Human Factors and Ergonomics in Health Care and Patient Safety.* Human Factors and Ergonomics. Mahwah, NJ: Lawrence Erlbaum Associates; 2007;xiv:995.

11. Bisantz AM, Burns CM, Fairbanks RJ. *Cognitive Systems Engineering in Health Care.* Boca Raton, FL: CRC Press; 2014:224. https://www.crcpress.com/Cognitive-Systems-Engineering-in-Health-Care/Bisantz-Burns-Fairbanks/9781466587960#googlePreview Container.

12. Wolf LD, et al. Describing nurses' work: combining quantitative and qualitative analysis. *Hum Factors.* 2006;48(1):5–14.

13. Carayon P, et al. Work system design for patient safety: the SEIPS model. *Qual Saf Health Care.* 2006;15(Suppl 1):i50–8.

14. Nemeth C, et al. Between choice and chance: the role of human factors in acute care equipment decisions. *J Patient Saf.* 2009;5(2):114–21.

15. Faye H, et al. Involving intensive care unit nurses in a proactive risk assessment of the medication management process. *Jt Comm J Qual Patient Saf.* 2010;36(8):376–84.

16. Holden RJ, et al. That's nice, but what does IT do? Evaluating the impact of bar coded medication administration by measuring changes in the process of care. *Int J Ind Ergon.* 2011;41(4):370–9.

17 Cognition and Decision Making

Bryan Kane and Christopher Carpenter

CLINICAL VIGNETTE

Dr. P is a previously healthy 80-year-old retired medical school professor, who lives at home with his wife of 55 years and plays tennis twice weekly. He takes a daily aspirin and medication for his hypertension but denies any prior hospitalizations or surgeries. He presents to the emergency department (ED) after a syncopal episode while walking from his car to the tennis court. Witnesses noted no seizure-like activity, postsyncope confusion, or other sequelae from the fainting episode. He is awake and alert with no fall-related injuries. He notes no pain or any other complaint on physical exam. His workup is unremarkable, including a normal chest x-ray, electrocardiogram, hemoglobin, chemistries, and cardiac enzymes. While assessing a level I patient and whisking another patient with an ST-segment elevation myocardial infarction to the cardiac catheterization lab, the ED physician contemplates the most likely and immediately life-threatening diagnostic possibilities. The last three syncope patients that she managed were ultimately diagnosed with pulmonary embolism (PE), one at the time of autopsy 2 days after discharge. However, the Choosing Wisely Campaign has heightened clinician's attention to the phenomenon of overdiagnosis and pseudodiagnosis. Therefore, after determining that the patient is at moderate risk for PE with a validated risk stratification rule, the ED physician orders a ventilation–perfusion (V/Q) scan rather than a PE protocol computed tomography (CT) noting significantly reduced radiation dose to the patient via the former study. Before obtaining the V/Q scan, the patient inquires about whether the V/Q scan identifies aortic dissection since his younger brother died of one last year. You discuss the limitations of V/Q for non-PE diagnoses and the risks of CT with the professor who opts for the CT scan, which subsequently demonstrates a type I aortic dissection for which you promptly call thoracic surgery.

- How do health care providers assimilate information to guide decision making?
- What cognitive errors and factors lead to suboptimal clinical decisions?
- How can structured clinical decision making reduce diagnostic and therapeutic error in chaotic environments?

INTRODUCTION

Cognitive errors in medicine are neither infrequent nor restricted to the hectic ED where errors leading to delayed diagnosis are the most frequent subtype.[1–4] The lay press is recognizing the imperfections in physician decision making with increasing frequency.[5-8] Unfortunately, traditional medical school, resident, and continuing medical education neglect the "black box" of cognitive reasoning.[9] Incorporating decision making into medical education at any level is challenging because the "black box" of cognitive concepts lacks objective tests of presence and nobody has demonstrated the ability to efficiently reduce error or alter physician's behavior by understanding these constructs.[10-12] Further, traditional medical education through such delivery systems as "Morbidity and Mortality" conferences focuses on a lack of professional acumen on the physician's part.[13] Conference participants often receive feedback that a missed diagnosis is the worst error a doctor can make.[14] On the other hand, health care providers receive little objective, evidence-based internal or external feedback on their practice behavior, leading to an environment where overtesting may receive positive re-enforcement. For example, excessive testing is associated with increased revenue and decreased malpractice risk reinforcing the mind-set that higher resource utilization equates to higher-quality medical care.[15,16] Diagnostic failure represents one major oversight of the Institute of Medicine (IOM) report *To Err Is Human*.[17,18] For example, the term "medication error" appears 70 times in the IOM report in contrast to the term "diagnostic error," which appears only twice.[19]

The first step to understanding the intellectual process that occurs between the initial patient contact (a constellation of symptoms, risk factors, and available tests) and identification of the etiology is to review decision-making models. The study of cognitive reasoning continues to evolve with an expanding awareness that effective patient safety strategies and curricula require an understanding of the cognitive models that traditionally fall within the realm of psychologists.[20-22]

CLINICAL DECISION-MAKING MODELS

Philosophers, cognitive psychologists, and decision-making experts catalog and define multiple constructs for misleading pathways to achieving "truth" (http://www.fallacyfiles.org/taxonomy.html). We summarize these logical fallacies in Table 17-1. Most early research about decision making occurred in nonmedical fields, but over the last decade, these theories have moved into the fields of medicine and medical education.[9,10] Acquisition of professional expertise in music, athletics, writing, or other skill-based tasks like medical decision making requires appropriate mentoring and deliberate practice.[23,24] Health care providers' understanding of their internal decision-making process, what they are thinking while they are thinking, is called **metacognition**.[25] One component of metacognition is understanding the conscious and subconscious framework upon which clinical reasoning occurs.

A variety of cognitive process theoretical constructs exist, though proving their existence and measuring their prevalence and impact are challenging.[20,26] In decision-dense, time-deprived environments like the ED, recognition-primed decision making is believed to be most prevalent (Fig. 17-1).[27] The "cognitive checkpoint" in Figure 17-1 is the determination of whether the patient fits into a previously defined pattern. This model and other decision-making constructs also fit into the dual-process model of reasoning[26] (Fig. 17-2). The dual-process model consists of two subtypes that have different confounders and paths to aptitude: System 1 and System 2. **System 1** is driven by underlying intuition, which is often subconscious and nonanalytical. When disease is recognized using System 1, the diagnosis is made without recognized awareness using the unconscious thought theory.[26,28] System 1 is referred to as "Augenblink" or "blink of an eye" by some cognitive psychology authors.[29]

TABLE 17-1 Subtypes of Logical Fallacies

Logical Fallacy Type Subtypes	Descriptor	Example(s)
Propositional Affirming the consequent Denying the antecedent Affirming a disjunct Denying a conjunct Improper transposition	Logical relations between propositions as a whole with truth-functional connectives	Today is Sunday and it is raining.
Probabilistic Base rate neglect Gambler's fallacy Multiple comparisons fallacy	Outcome rate based upon conceived likelihood premise	
Syllogistic Illicit process Exclusive premises Four-term fallacy	Rationale with two premises (syllogism) and one conclusion	All chest pain is lethal. No chest pain is benign.
Modal	Relationship in logic and modalities of possibility to necessity, past and future truth, or knowledge and belief	If the patient is old, then she must be dying. If the ST segments are elevated, then it has to be a myocardial infarction (MI).
Bad reasons	The conclusion is false because the argument provided is bad, unproven, or incomplete.	Chest x-rays are inaccurate for aortic dissection so the patient cannot have a dissection.
One-sidedness Quoting out of context	Presents only evidence favoring preferred or posited conclusion, ignoring evidence against this conclusion	A 20-year-old previously healthy motor vehicle accident victim with chest pain, an increasingly elevated troponin, and a nondiagnostic ECG cannot have coronary disease when eventual imaging demonstrates coronary dissection.
Ambiguity Amphiboly Accent Equivocation	Feature of language when a word or phrase has >1 meaning causing form of reasoning to appear validating	

(Continued)

TABLE 17-1	Subtypes of Logical Fallacies (*Continued*)	

Logical Fallacy Type Subtypes	Descriptor	Example(s)
Accident	Application of generalization without considering exceptions	Most severely intoxicated patients with altered mental status are not injured; patient X is very drunk and disoriented; therefore, patient X is not injured.
Appeal to ignorance	Absence of evidence is evidence of absence.	No randomized controlled trials demonstrate any lifesaving benefit for parachutes; therefore, jumping out of an airplane with a parachute is not beneficial.
Red herring Straw man Genetic fallacy Bandwagon fallacy Emotional appeal Guilt by association Appeal to consequences Two wrongs make a right	Rationale that distracts the decision maker from the key issue via introduction of irrelevance	Female patient with right lower quadrant pain and 7 wbc in urine microscopy must have UTI.
Composition	Attributing properties of a portion to the whole, assuming that the attribute of the part applies all levels of the whole	Human body is made of cells that are invisible; therefore, the body is invisible.
Non causa pro causa Regression fallacy Texas sharpshooter fallacy Cum hoc, ergo propter hoc Post hoc, ergo propter hoc	Noncause for cause in which causality is erroneously inferred without good reason	Attributing domestic violence–related diffuse bodily bruises to inadvertent trip over garden hose weeks ago
Black or white	Logic based upon erroneous constructive dilemma or disjunctive premise	Chest pain is either acute myocardial infarction (AMI) or pneumothorax; the chest x-ray is normal, so this chest pain is an AMI.
Vagueness Fake precision Slippery slope	Existence of borderline examples that do not clearly belong or not belong to a category	

TABLE 17-1 Subtypes of Logical Fallacies (*Continued*)

Logical Fallacy Type / Subtypes	Descriptor	Example(s)
Begging the question Loaded words Question-begging analogy	Circular form of logic in which the conclusion appears as one of the premises to support the conclusion	CT is the gold standard to diagnose PE begging the question that the PIOPED-II estimate of CT sensitivity (93%) is an underestimate of the true 100% sensitivity of CT for PE.
Special pleading	Argument for a special exception to a rule of thumb based upon an irrelevant characteristic that does not define an exception	Emergency physicians deliver babies; therefore, emergency physicians should practice office-based obstetrics.
Weak analogy Unrepresentative sample Anecdotal fallacy	Erroneous or unlikely conclusions based on comparisons or context not strong enough for the argument	Clogged arteries require surgery to prevent disease; therefore, clogged highways should be cleared to prevent motor vehicle trauma.

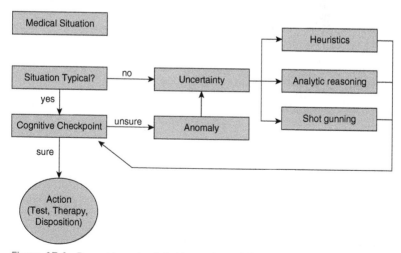

Figure 17-1. Recognition-primed decision making. (Adapted from Klein G, Orasanu J, Calderwood R. *Decision Making in Action: Models and Methods.* Norwood, NJ: Ablex Publishing; 1993.)

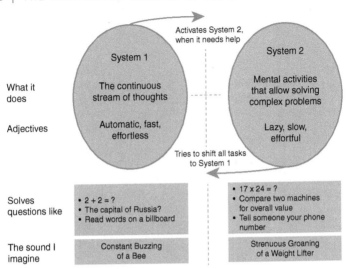

Figure 17-2. Dual-process decision model. (From Campbell SG, Croskerry P, Bond WF. Profiles in patient safety: a "perfect storm" in the emergency department. *Acad Emerg Med.* 2007;14(8):743–9.)

Experienced providers will often successfully use clinical gestalt to achieve a diagnosis, which less experienced providers can only achieve through the use of Evidence-Based Medicine (EBM) checklists.[30,31]

System 1 thinking can lead to overconfidence and has multiple potential "blind spots." It is possible that these deficiencies can be mitigated by experience, but completion of residency training may be insufficient.[32,33] Traditionally, the majority of cognitive errors were attributed to System 1 problems, although recent research questions this theory.[34,35] The automaticity of System 1 can be confounded by emotion, intrinsic cognitive biases, and personality.[36] Examples of personality issues skewing System I decision making to err include overconfidence,[37] risk tolerance,[38] motivation, and cultural milieu. On the other hand, **System 2** is the rational and methodologic approach to appraising a medical situation within the context of textbooks and research while re-evaluating accuracy based upon evolving test results and therapeutic response. These influences sometimes yield irrational behavior that is called dysrationalia.[26,39] The two systems are not mutually exclusive. In fact, effective System 1 decision making requires System 2 oversight—recognizing when the initial pattern does not fit with the evolving medical situation and altering the diagnostic/therapeutic plan accordingly. System 2 is more time and resource intense than System 1 and is not immune to error. Decision-maker characteristics like cognitive indolence and fatigue as well as ambient environmental conditions like task distractions impede reliable System 2 processes. Disruptions to System 2 decision making increase the risk of System 1 error by reducing the effectiveness of System 2.[26]

Experts define a variety of subtypes of clinical decision-making error from Table 17-1, which we include in Table 17-2.[36] Anchoring bias, confirmation bias,

TABLE 17-2	Classification Nomenclature for Cognitive Errors in Medicine

Error of overattachment to a particular diagnosis

Anchoring	The tendency to fixate on specific features of a presentation too early in the diagnostic process and subsequent failure to adjust
Confirmation bias	The tendency to look for confirming evidence to support the hypothesis, rather than to look for disconfirming evidence to refute it
Premature closure	Accepting a diagnosis before it has been fully verified

Error due to failure to consider alternative diagnoses

Multiple alternatives bias	Irrational inertia against optimizing choice among competing alternatives
Representativeness restraint	Restraint from considering a particular diagnosis for a patient because the presentation is not sufficiently representative of the class
Search satisficing	The tendency to call off a search once something is found and not considering additional findings or diagnoses
Sutton's slip	Fixation on the most obvious answer or interpretation
Unpacking principle	Being influenced by the way in which the facts are presented
Vertical line failure	Rigidity and inflexibility in the approach to clinical problems (not thinking laterally)

Error due to inheriting someone else's thinking

Triage cueing	A predisposition toward a particular decision as a result of a judgment made by care givers early in the patient care process
Diagnosis momentum	The tendency for a particular diagnosis to become established in spite of other evidence
Framing effect	A decision being influenced by the way in which the scenario is presented or "framed"
Ascertainment effect	When thinking is preshaped by expectations

Errors in prevalence perception or estimation

Availability bias	The tendency for things to be judged more frequently if they come readily to mind
Base rate neglect	Failing to adequately take into account the prevalence of a particular disease
Gambler's fallacy	The belief that a sequence of similar diagnoses will reverse (belief that the same thing won't happen again)

(Continued)

TABLE 17-2	Classification Nomenclature for Cognitive Errors in Medicine (Continued)
Hindsight bias	Once the outcome is known, an underestimation (illusion of failure) or overestimation (illusion of control) of the calibration of the original decision
Playing the odds	Deciding that a patient does not have a particular disease on the basis of a likelihood judgment (frequency gambling)
Posterior probability error	Having a judgment unduly influenced by what is known to have been the case before
Order effects	Focusing on information given at the beginning or end of a history, to the neglect of the "stuff in the middle"

Error involving patient characteristics or presentation context

Fundamental attribution error	Attributing the blame for a circumstance or event to the patient's personal qualities rather than the situation
Gender bias	When the decision made is influenced unduly by the patient's gender or the gender of the decision maker
Psych out error	A variety of biases associated with the health care provider's perception of the psychiatric patient
Yin-yang out	Presumption that extensive prior investigation has ruled out any serious diagnosis

Error associated with physician affect or personality

Commission bias	Tendency toward action rather than inaction
Omission bias	Tendency toward inaction rather than action
Outcome bias	Choosing a course of action according to a desired outcome; avoiding possibilities that would suggest an undesired outcome
Visceral bias	Making decisions influenced by personal (positive or negative) feeling toward patient (affective bias)
Over confidence/ underconfidence	Being overconfident in (more likely) or underconfident in the efficacy of decision that we make
Belief bias	The tendency to accept only things that fit in with our belief systems
Ego bias	In this context, a systematic overestimation of the prognosis for one's own patients
Sunk costs	Unwillingness to give up a diagnosis in which we have invested considerable effort
Zebra retreat	Reticence to pursue a rare diagnosis for a variety of reasons

From Campbell SG, Croskerry P, Bond WF. Profiles in patient safety: a "perfect storm" in the emergency department. *Acad Emerg Med.* 2007;14(8):743–9.

availability bias, base rate neglect, and triage cueing are particularly prevalent. Strategies to understand individual clinician's cognitive biases profile include simulation and efforts to capture cognitive processes during clinical shifts.[22,40,41]

IMPACT OF FLAWED CLINICAL DECISION MAKING ON PATIENT SAFETY

Eliminating diagnostic errors is unrealistic given the complexities of disease processes, test availability and inherent inaccuracy, as well as heterogeneous patients and medical providers at the interface of a constantly evolving health care system.[42] However, reducing cognitive errors mandates understanding the prevalence, precipitants, and consequences. Early patient safety researchers used retrospective chart reviews that made it difficult to detect cognitive process failures, particularly in diagnostics.[18] In contrast, medication and procedural errors are usually clearly visible. Diagnostic errors remain an underappreciated cause of medical errors. For example, the contemporary Institute for Healthcare Improvement (IHI) Global Trigger Tool does not identify diagnostic errors.[18,43] Nonetheless, there is a growing body of evidence pointing toward cognitive errors as a tangible target for patient safety–focused quality improvement efforts.

One prospective ED-based study of almost 2000 visits found that one-fifth of reported errors were diagnostic errors.[1] Another retrospective ED study found that half (50%) of unexpected deaths within 7 days were related to the ED visit and up to 60% may be related to cognitive error. Barriers ED physicians experience found in this cohort include interpretation, coexisting substance abuse/intoxication, and patient characteristics such as severity of disease, psychiatric or neurologic illness, and poor medical literacy.[44] The use of EBM or heuristic checklists is a possible solution,[31] but here, the potential to select the wrong checklist, known as confirmation bias, is a significant potential error.[45] A study of closed malpractice claims found that the overwhelming cause of the claims was cognitive error (96%). Systems issues such as handoff communications, workload, and supervision were found to combine with incomplete examinations and inappropriate test ordering or interpretation to create the situations where harm to patients and subsequent lawsuits occurred. Of note, most cases in this series found that multiple errors occurred.[2]

As noted by Elstein,[46] diagnostic errors also occur outside the ED. A survey of 310 clinicians from 22 institutions suggested that clinicians of all specialties occasionally recognize problems with cognitive processes. In this study, 583 diagnostic errors were reported, including 28% rated as "major" with the most common missed or delayed diagnoses including PE, drug reactions, cancer, stroke, and acute coronary syndromes.[3]

COGNITIVE DISPOSITIONS TO RESPOND

Cognitive dispositions to respond (CDR) can be thought of as how we as humans intrinsically process information in order to arrive at a decision. CDR are intended to be nonpejorative.[47] Since it is sometimes challenging to separate cognition from our emotional state, CDR are often linked with affective dispositions to respond (ADR). The Morsani Medical College of Medicine (University of South Florida) trains its medical students with the pneumonic HALT: Hungry, Angry, Late, Tired. These and other environmental and intrinsic factors, including physical, emotional, and psychiatric, can impact a physician's overall disposition to respond or ability to make a decision.[48] In the end, an understanding of both CDR and ADR, as well as their interplay, is a vital part of understanding how medical decision-making errors occur.

Since physicians cannot "know everything" about a patients disease (or health), the ability to be completely rational is limited. One proposed solution is to limit information and have "bounded rationality"[49] and understand economic motivators[50] as a way to make decisions with incomplete or imperfect information. The issue then lies in where to place the boundary between sufficient and insufficient information, as its placement can lead directly to error.

Individual CDRs are the means by which they acquire, analyze, and interpret these information thresholds. Table 17-2 summarizes many CDRs and groups similar types of flawed thinking together.[36] By understanding the variety of cognitive errors in medical reasoning, physicians can incorporate shared decision making. For example, a chest pain patient in the ED could be shown a card depicting their personal risk of acute coronary syndrome to reduce prevalence perception errors.[51]

Traditional medical training vehicles such as the Morbidity and Mortality conference create a cognitive environment in which the missed diagnosis is considered much worse than overtesting or overutilization of resources.[52] Based upon a theory whereby complex medical decisions evolved in an award-based environment, the error management theory (EMT) implies that efforts to improve clinical decision making face a challenge much greater than altering medical education.[53] Fundamentally, EMT seeks to explain, often in a Darwinian sense, how bias in decision making can in the long run lead to improved outcomes. Under EMT, improving the overall quality and reliability of clinical decision making will require each physician to unlearn potentially dangerous behaviors that were previously rewarded. The challenge for patient safety advocates is to find interventions that overwhelm the reward-based learned behavior. While recent attempts to improve clinical decision making have been unsuccessful,[12] efforts should continue.

SPECIAL SITUATIONS

Fatigue and Patient Handoffs

Fatigue is a well-recognized cause of errors and subsequent patient safety issues.[54,55] Starting with the Bell Commission in 1989 and ultimately culminating with widespread Accreditation Council for Graduate Medical Education (ACGME) regulations in 2003, physicians in training have had temporal restrictions placed upon them as a means to address this issue. Recent articles have noted that the decrease in clinical responsibilities has led to an increase in reported errors.[56] This substantiates prior study with earlier versions of the duty hour rules where medication safety was not improved, but rather trended in a less safe direction.[57] Early speculation that the lack of increased patient safety stemmed from an increased number of handoffs was recently confirmed in a study that was terminated early.[58] Handoffs in health care allow for multiple cognitive errors.[59] The most obvious transition of care related to cognitive misstep from Table 17-2 is "inheriting someone else's thinking" errors. Recognizing the importance of handoff communication, the Joint Commission in 2007 focused on handoff communication as a National Patient Safety Goal. The SBAR (Situation, Background, Assessment, Recommendation) model was recommended.[60] The ACGME has also recognized the importance of handoff communication as a potential threat to patient safety. The "Clinical Learning Environment

Review" visits which the ACGME now conduct focus on the following six areas: Patient Safety, Quality Improvement, Supervision, Duty Hours Oversight/Fatigue Management and Mitigation, Transitions in Care, and Professionalism (https://www. acgme.org/acgmeweb/Portals/0/PDFs/CLER/CLER_Brochure.pdf). An institutional approach to improving this aspect of patient care has recently been described.[61]

Procedures and Patient Safety

Procedural safety as it relates to patient safety has received recent increased attention. Traditionally, physicians have focused on the technical aspects of performing the procedure. For example, one study of lumbar puncture noted 26 major steps, none of which had to do with patient selection,[62] disease probability,[63] test–treatment thresholds,[64] or other decisions made prior to performing the procedure.[65] Recently, external organizations such as the Joint Commission seek to mitigate cognitive errors such as diagnosis momentum (i.e., "the chest tube tray is on the right side so that must be the side the patient requires the thoracostomy") using a "time out" as part of a "Universal Protocol" (http://www.jointcommission.org/standards_information/up.aspx). As another example, the IHI Central Lines bundle focuses on the cognitive decisions made before and after, rather than during, the procedure. Despite educational theory, which defines competency as a continuum that moves from unconscious incompetence to unconscious competence, the ACGME has traditionally defined procedural competence by a number of procedures performed (http://www.gordontraining.com/free-workplace-articles/learning-a-new-skill-is-easier-said-than-done/).[66] The ACGME has recently moved for all residency training from the Core Competencies to the Next Accreditation System (NAS), often referred to as the Milestones Project (https://www.acgme.org/acgmeweb/tabid/430/ProgramandInstitutionalAccreditation/NextAccreditationSystem/Milestones.aspx). A stated goal of the Milestones Project is to codify specific skills that need to be demonstrated. While this includes the number of expected procedures, there is now also an emphasis on the decisions to perform the procedure (https://www.acgme.org/acgmeweb/Portals/0/PDFs/Milestones/EmergencyMedicineMilestones.pdf). Some specialties have chosen to describe the highest level of competence in this framework as an "Entrustable Professional Activity (EPA)," denoting that a learner can perform the procedure without expert oversight (https://www.acgme.org/acgmeweb/Portals/0/PDFs/Milestones/MilestonesFAQ.pdf).

Critical Thinking in an Emergency

Rapid, urgent, or emergent decision making occurs in many parts of health care, including but not limited to the operating room, labor and delivery room, and intensive care units. In the ED, challenges unique to these types of environments have been described (Table 17-3).[67] Shift work intensifies the handoff issues just discussed and, with the advent of an increasing use of the "hospitalist" model of care, is relevant not just to the ED but also to internal medicine, pediatrics, general/trauma surgery, and obstetrics/gynecology (OB/GYN), among others. Throughout the inpatient segment of the health care system, the round-the-clock nature culture may create not just fatigue but "shift work syndrome." As health care, especially inpatient health care, becomes more fragmented, the traditional long-term physician relationship and the more rational, from a cognitive perspective, benefits that come with it may become rarer.

TABLE 17-3	Unique Operating Characteristics of the Emergency Department Predisposing to Medical Error

High levels of diagnostic uncertainty

High-decision density

High-cognitive load

High levels of activity

Inexperience of some physicians and nurses

Interruptions and distractions

Uneven and abbreviated care

Narrow time windows

Shift work

Shift changes

Compromised teamwork

Poor feedback

From Croskerry P, Sinclair D. Emergency medicine: a practice prone to error? *CJEM*. 2001;3(4):271–6.

KEY POINTS

1. Diagnostic error is underemphasized. Traditional medical education focuses on only part of the problem and missed diagnosis and tends to minimize type 1 or false-positive errors.
2. Humans use System 1 ("blink of an eye"), and System 2 processes to yield clinical decisions. System 1 may be more prone to error, but the two systems are interdependent.
3. Human CDR are numerous. Evolving toward a safer health care environment using these theoretical constructs remains a challenge and will involve behavioral modifications to unlearn reward-based, ingrained situational responses.
4. In order to improve decision making and patient safety, special attention should be given to the periprocedural time period, to provider fatigue and subsequent patient handoffs, and the ED as a decision-dense environment.

ONLINE RESOURCES

1. Types of logical fallacy: http://www.fallacyfiles.org/taxonomy.html
2. Society for Medical Decision Making: http://www.smdm.org/
3. The Brunswick Society: http://www.brunswik.org/
4. Decision Analysis Society: https://www.informs.org/Community/DAS
5. Society for Judgment and Decision Making: http://www.sjdm.org/
6. Center for Adaptive Behavior and Cognition: http://www.mpib-berlin.mpg.de/en/research/adaptive-behavior-and-cognition

REFERENCES

1. Fordyce J, Blank FSJ, Pekow P, et al. Errors in a busy emergency department. *Ann Emerg Med.* 2003;42(3):324–33.
2. Kachalia A, Gandhi TK, Puopolo AL, et al. Missed and delayed diagnoses in the emergency department: a study of closed malpractice claims from 4 liability insurers. *Ann Emerg Med.* 2007;49(2):196–205.
3. Schiff GD, Hasan O, Kim S, et al. Diagnostic error in medicine: analysis of 583 physician-reported errors. *Arch Intern Med.* 2009;169(20):1881–7.
4. Tehrani AS, Lee H, Mathews SC, et al. 25-Year summary of US malpractice claims for diagnostic errors 1986–2010: an analysis from the National Practitioner Data Bank. *BMJ Qual Saf.* 2013;22(8):672–80.
5. Gigerenzer G. *Calculated Risks: How to Know When Numbers Deceive You.* New York City, NY: Simon & Schuster; 2002.
6. Groopman J. *How Doctors Think.* New York City, NY: Houghton Mifflin; 2007.
7. Newman DH. *Hippocrates' Shadow: Secrets from the House of Medicine.* New York City, NY: Scribner; 2008.
8. Wen L, Kosowsky J. *When Doctors Don't Listen: How to Avoid Misdiagnosis and Unnecessary Tests.* New York City, NY: St. Martin's Press; 2012.
9. Sandhu H, Carpenter C. Clinical Decision making: Opening the black box of cognitive reasoning. *Ann Emerg Med.* 2006;48(6):713–22.
10. Bowen JL. Educational strategies to promote clinical diagnostic reasoning. *N Engl J Med.* 2006;355(21):2217–25.
11. Graber ML. Educational strategies to reduce diagnostic error: can you teach this stuff? *Adv Health Sci Educ Theory Pract.* 2009;14(Suppl 1):63–9.
12. Sherbino J, Kulasegaram K, Howey E, et al. Ineffectiveness of cognitive forcing strategies to reduce biases in diagnostic reasoning: a controlled trial. *CJEM.* 2014;16(1):34–40.
13. Orlander JD, Barber TW, Fincke BG. The morbidity and mortality conference: the delicate nature of learning from error. *Acad Med.* 2002;77(10):1001–6.
14. Deis JN, Smith KM, Warren MD, et al. Transforming the morbidity and mortality conference into an instrument for system wide improvement. In: Henrikson K, Battles JB, Keyes MA, Grady ML, eds. *Advances in Patient Safety: New Directions and Alternative Approaches. Vol 2: Culture and Redesign.* Rockville, MD: Agency for Healthcare Research & Quality; 2008.
15. Brownlee S. *Overtreated: Why too Much Medicine is Making us Sicker and Poorer.* New York, NY: Bloomsbury; 2007.
16. Welch HG, Schwartz L, Woloshin S. *Overdiagnosed: Making People Sick in the Pursuit of Health.* Boston, MA: Beacon Press; 2011.
17. Kohn LT, Corrigan JM, Donaldson MS. *To Err Is Human: Building a Safer Health Care System.* Washington, DC: National Academy Press; 1999.
18. Croskerry P. Perspectives on diagnostic failure and patient safety. *Healthc Q.* 2012;15 Spec No:50–6.
19. Wachter RM. Why diagnostic errors don't get any respect--and what can be done about them. *Health Aff.* 2010;29(9):1605–10.
20. Norman G. Research in clinical reasoning: past history and current trends. *Med Educ.* 2005;39(4):418–27.
21. Croskerry P. From mindless to mindful practice—cognitive bias and clinical decision making. *N Engl J Med.* 2013;368(26):2445–8.
22. Ericsson KA. An expert-performance perspective of research on medical expertise: the study of clinical performance. *Med Educ.* 2007;41(12):1124–30.
23. Ericsson KA. Deliberate practice and the acquisition and maintenance of expert performance in medicine and related domains. *Acad Med.* 2004;79(10 Suppl):S70–81.
24. Ericsson KA. Deliberate practice and acquisition of expert performance: a general overview. *Acad Emerg Med.* 2008;15(11):988–94.
25. Marcum JA. An integrated model of clinical reasoning: dual-process theory of cognition and metacognition. *J Eval Clin Pract.* 2012;18(5):954–61.

26. Croskerry P. Critical thinking and reasoning in emergency medicine. In: Croskerry P, Cosby KS, Schenkel SM, Wears RL, eds. *Patient Safety in Emergency Medicine*. Philadelphia, PA: Lippincott Williams & Wilkins; 2009:213–8.

27. Weingart SD. Critical decision making in chaotic environments. In: Croskerry P, Cosby KS, Schenkel SM, Wears RL, eds. *Patient Safety in Emergency Medicine*. Philadelphia, PA: Lippincott Williams & Wilkins; 2009:209–12.

28. Dijksterhuis A, Meurs T. Where creativity resides: the generative power of unconscious thought. *Conscious Cogn*. 2006;15(1):135–46.

29. Gladwell M. *Blink: The Power of Thinking Without Thinking*. New York, NY: Little Brown & Company; 2005.

30. Penaloza A, Verschuren F, Meyer G, et al. Comparison of the unstructured clinician gestalt, the wells score, and the revised geneva score to estimate pretest probability for suspected pulmonary embolism. *Ann Emerg Med*. 2013;62(2):117–24.

31. Ely JW, Graber ML, Croskerry P. Checklists to reduce diagnostic errors. *Acad Med*. 2011;86(3):307–13.

32. Christakis NA, Lamont EB. Extent and determinants of error in doctors' prognoses in terminally ill patients: prospective cohort study. *BMJ*. 2000;320(7233):469–72.

33. Berk WA, Welch RD, Levy PD, et al. The effect of clinical experience on the error rate of emergency physicians. *Ann Emerg Med*. 2008;52(5):497–501.

34. Croskerry P. Cognitive and affective dispositions to respond. In: Croskerry P, Cosby KS, Schenkel SM, Wears RL eds. *Patient Safety in Emergency Medicine*. Philadelphia, PA: Lippincott Williams & Wilkins; 2009:219–27.

35. Sherbino J, Dore KL, Wood TJ, et al. The relationship between response time and diagnostic accuracy. *Acad Med*. 2012;87(6):785–91.

36. Campbell SG, Croskerry P, Bond WF. Profiles in patient safety: a "perfect storm" in the emergency department. *Acad Emerg Med*. 2007;14(8):743–49.

37. Croskerry P, Norman G. Overconfidence in clinical decision making. *Am J Med*. 2008;121(5 Suppl):S24–9.

38. Tubbs EP, Broeckel-Elrod JA, et al. Risk taking and tolerance of uncertainty: implications for surgeons. *J Surg Res*. 2006;131(1):1–6.

39. Stanovich KE. Dysrationalia: a new specific learning disability. *J Learn Disabil*. 1993;26(8):501–15.

40. Bond WF, Kuhn G, Binstadt E, et al. The use of simulation in the development of individual cognitive expertise in emergency medicine. *Acad Emerg Med*. 2008;15(11):1037–45.

41. McLellan L, Tully MP, Dornan T. How could undergraduate education prepare new graduates to be safer prescribers? *Br J Clin Pharmacol*. 2012;74(4):605–13.

42. Graber ML, Gordon R, Franklin N. Reducing diagnostic errors in medicine: what's the goal? *Acad Med*. 2002;77(10):981–92.

43. Classen DC, Resar R, Griffen F, et al. 'Global trigger tool' shows that adverse events in hospitals may be ten times greater than previously measured. *Health Aff*. 2011;30(4):581–9.

44. Sklar DP, Crandall CS, Loeliger E, et al. Unanticipated death after discharge home from the emergency department. *Ann Emerg Med*. 2007;49(6):735–45.

45. Pines JM. Profiles in patient safety: confirmation bias in emergency medicine. *Acad Emerg Med*. 2006;13(1):90–4.

46. Elstein AS. Thinking about diagnostic thinking: a 30-year perspective. *Adv Health Sci Educ Theory Pract*. 2009;14(Suppl 1):7–18.

47. Croskerry P. Achieving quality in clinical decision making: cognitive strategies and detection of bias. *Acad Emerg Med*. 2002;9(11):1184–204.

48. Croskerry P, Abbass AA, Wu AW. How doctors feel: affective issues in patients' safety. *Lancet*. 2008;372(9645):1205–6.

49. Marewski JN, Gigerenzer G. Heuristic decision making in medicine. *Dialogues Clin Neurosci*. 2012;14(1):77–89.

50. Brennan TJ, Lo AW. An evolutionary model of bounded rationality and intelligence. *PLoS One*. 2012;7(11):e50310.

51. Hess EP, Knoedler MA, Shah ND, et al. The chest pain choice decision aid: a randomized trial. *Circ Cardiovasc Qual Outcomes.* 2012;5(3):251–9.

52. Kaldjian LC, Forman-Hoffman VL, Jones EW, et al. Do faculty and resident physicians discuss their medical errors? *J Med Ethics.* 2008;34(10):717–22.

53. Johnson DD, Blumstein DT, Fowler JH, et al. The evolution of error: error management, cognitive constraints, and adaptive decision-making biases. *Trends Ecol Evol.* 2013;28(8):474–81.

54. Croskerry P, Singhal G, Mamede S. Cognitive debiasing 1: origins of bias and theory of debiasing. *BMJ Qual Saf.* 2013;22(Suppl 2):ii58–64.

55. Keers RN, Williams SD, Cooke J, et al. Causes of medication administration errors in hospitals: a systematic review of quantitative and qualitative evidence. *Drug Saf.* 2013;36(11):1045–67.

56. Sen S, Kranzler HR, Didwania AK, et al. Effects of the 2011 duty hour reforms on interns and their patients: a prospective longitudinal cohort study. *JAMA Intern Med.* 2013;173(8):657–62.

57. Landrigan CP, Fahrenkopf AM, Lewin D, et al. Effects of the accreditation council for graduate medical education duty hour limits on sleep, work hours, and safety. *Pediatrics.* 2008;122(2):250–8.

58. Desai SV, Feldman L, Brown L, et al. Effect of the 2011 vs. 2003 duty hour regulation-compliant models on sleep duration, trainee education, and continuity of patient care among internal medicine house staff: a randomized trial. *JAMA Intern Med.* 2013;173(8):649–55.

59. Perry S. Transitions in care: safety in dynamic environments. In: Croskerry P, Cosby KS, Schenkel SM, Wears RL, eds. *Patient Safety in Emergency Medicine.* Philadelphia, PA: Lippincott Williams & Wilkins; 2009:201–4.

60. Haig KM, Sutton S, Whittington JC. SBAR: a shared mental model for improving communication between clinicians. *Jt Comm J Qual Patient Saf.* 2006;32(3):167–75.

61. DeRienzo CM, Frush K, Barfield ME, et al. Handoffs in the era of duty hours reform: a focused review and strategy to address changes in the Accreditation Council for Graduate Medical Education Common Program Requirements. *Acad Med.* 2012;87(4):403–10.

62. Mark DG, Hung YY, Offerman SR, et al. Nontraumatic subarachnoid hemorrhage in the setting of negative cranial computed tomography results: external validation of a clinical and imaging prediction rule. *Ann Emerg Med.* 2013;62(1):1–10.

63. Perry JJ, Stiell IG, Sivilotti ML, et al. Sensitivity of computed tomography performed within six hours of onset of headache for diagnosis of subarachnoid haemorrhage: prospective cohort study. *BMJ.* 2011;343:d4277.

64. Pines JM, Carpenter CR, Raja AS, et al. Diagnostic testing in emergency care. In: Pines JM, Carpenter C, Raja AS, Schuur JD, eds. *Evidence-Based Emergency Care: Diagnostic Testing and Clinical Decision Rules.* 2nd ed. Oxford, UK: Wiley-Blackwell; 2013:3–10.

65. Lammers RL, Temple KJ, Wagner MJ, et al. Competence of new emergency medicine residents in the performance of lumbar punctures. *Acad Emerg Med.* 2005;12(7):622–8.

66. Flower J. In the mush. *Physician Exec.* 1999;25(1):64–6.

67. Croskerry P, Sinclair D. Emergency medicine: a practice prone to error? *CJEM.* 2001;3(4):271–6.

18 Tools to Improve Patient Safety

James J. Fehr and Jason C. Wagner

CLINICAL VIGNETTE

A healthy 4-year-old child is scheduled for surgical repair of a left inguinal hernia. The surgeon obtains informed consent and marks the surgical site in the preoperative holding area. The child is taken to the operating room (OR) and anesthetized, and the surgical field is prepared. Both inguinal areas are prepped and draped, and a time out is performed prior to the incision. As the time out occurs, music is playing, conversations are ongoing, and a ringing phone is answered. The team does not notice that the preoperative marking was inadvertently cleaned off during the sterile prep. The surgical incision is made in the right inguinal area. Following dissection, no hernia sac is identified. The surgeon reviews the clinical documentation and the error is discovered.

Questions:
• Why did wrong-sided surgery occur?
• What could prevent this from ever happening again?

INTRODUCTION

Early accounts of adverse patient care events stemmed from analyses of the events that led to medical malpractice claims.[1] Further descriptions of adverse events in hospitalized patients revealed the widespread extent of these problems.[2,3] The increased focus on the causative factors of adverse events in hospitalized patients and the methods for addressing them has spurred the entire medical industry toward greater engagement in improving the health care environment. Over the past several decades, there has been a drive to improve the safety of patients and a requirement for better tools to teach optimal safety practices to physicians, to improve clinical care, and to measure performance and outcomes. Numerous organizations have spearheaded this effort including the Joint Commission, the Agency for Healthcare Research and Quality (AHRQ), and the Institute for Healthcare Improvement (IHI). The focus of the Joint Commission in the 2013 National Patient Safety Goals for hospitals is to make sure that patients are identified correctly, improve staff communication, use medicines safely, prevent infection, identify patient safety risks, and prevent surgical mistakes.[4] This has resulted in the development of numerous tools to educate health care providers and consumers about the complex issues surrounding patient safety and to assist clinicians in their management of increasingly complicated patients. Some of these tools are straightforward, some of the techniques are elaborate, but they all serve a common goal: to reduce medical errors to zero, thereby saving hundreds of thousands of lives over the next decade and alleviating a substantial amount of misery through the prevention of injury and adverse events.

The United States of America has the most expensive health care in the world, but the results fare poorly when compared with other developed nations. This results gap is sustained even when controlling for socioeconomic status.[5] In the quest to reduce the cost of health care, address health care disparities, and improve patient safety, a broad range of approaches have been pursued. This chapter will review some of the lessons being applied to the medical field that have been drawn from other disciplines, which must operate with a razor-thin margin of error, such as the nuclear power and aviation industries. Tools to improve patient safety that have been inspired from these industries and adapted for clinicians include checklists, medical simulation, and crisis resource management (CRM). Preflight checklists are standard procedure for airline pilots and are integrated into the daily management of nuclear power plants. They are increasingly being applied to the health care sector, from the OR to the intensive care unit, to reduce the adverse events associated with high-risk procedures. Flight simulators are also utilized in aviation to train new pilots, assess experienced pilots, and train on new equipment. The principles of crew resource management were first developed from an evaluation of airline crashes that occurred in the 1970s. This technique involves raising the situational awareness of all of the individuals who compose a team and fostering a sense of ownership of the tasks at hand and developing clear and effective communication.

This chapter will explore some of these tools and the way they are currently impacting patient safety. It will examine how checklists have been created to prevent the physician from making simple avoidable errors with potential severe ramifications such as wrong side surgery. Simulation will be explored as a platform for teaching patient safety, training teams, and assessing performance. The principles of CRM will be described as an approach to optimize team performance. In the final analysis, however, the availability of useful and effective tools is of no benefit if they are not utilized or are applied incorrectly. And while valuable lessons can be garnered from other industries, in the field of medicine, the physicians and other care providers do not go down with the ship; it is the patient and their family who bears the risk associated with adverse events. Therefore, for physicians and other health care providers, it is a moral imperative to always incorporate tools that can improve patient safety at every level of practice.

CHECKLISTS

The preflight checklist has long been the standard before any pilot takes off in any aircraft from a single-engine craft as simple as a Piper Cub all the way up to the B-2 Stealth Bomber. Despite the rapid adoption of checklists in other industries, medicine has been resistant to the routine use of checklists to avoid common errors. A major impetus was the publication of Gawande's *The Checklist Manifesto* in 2009, which made the New York Times Best Seller list and led to a public outcry for the medical field to adopt checklists.[6] A convergence of public and institutional awareness of the problems of patient safety and the availability of tools such as checklists that can improve safety has led to a steady increase in the integration of checklists for processes ranging from simple procedures to the complex management of medical crises. A 2013 expert consensus of patient safety strategies strongly encouraged checklists as patient safety strategies ready for immediate adoption by clinicians.[7] In particular, these were perioperative and anesthesia checklists to reduce perioperative events and checklists to reduce central line–associated bloodstream infections.

Checklists have been utilized for central line placement to assure that all line placements followed standard recommendations from the Center for Disease Control. In a study at Johns Hopkins, the bedside nurse completed a five-question checklist (Fig. 18-1), which recorded if the person placing the line followed evidence-based practice for sterile placement of central lines.[8] Prior to the introduction of the checklists, their data demonstrated a 62% compliance with infection control guidelines. Following the intervention, there was a reduction in the central line infection rate from 11.3/1000 catheter days to zero during the study period. Checklists have also been shown to improve patient outcome in situations more complex than simple procedures. A study involving eight hospitals in eight countries conducted by the

| Catheter-related Blood Stream Infection |
| Care Team Checklist |

Purpose:	To work as a team to decrease patient harm from catheter-related blood stream infections
When:	During all central venous or central arterial line insertions or re-wires
By whom:	Bedside nurse

1. Today's date ____ / ____ / _____
   month day year

2. Procedure: ☐ New line   ☐ Rewire

3. Is the procedure: ☐ Elective   ☐ Emergent

4.   Yes   No   Don't know

Before the procedure, did the housestaff:
Wash hands (chlorhexidine or soap) immediately prior   ☐   ☐   ☐
Sterilize procedure site   ☐   ☐   ☐
Drape entire patient in a sterile fashion   ☐   ☐   ☐

During the procedure, did the housestaff:
Use sterile gloves   ☐   ☐   ☐
Use hat, mask and sterile gown   ☐   ☐   ☐
Maintain a sterile field   ☐   ☐   ☐

Did all personnel assisting with procedure follow
the above precautions   ☐   ☐   ☐

After the procedure:
Was a sterile dressing applied to the site   ☐   ☐   ☐

Please return completed form to the designated location in your ICU.

Figure 18-1. Central line checklist. (From: Berenholtz SM, Pronovost PJ, Lipsett PA, et al. Eliminating catheter-related bloodstream infections in the intensive care unit. *Crit Care Med.* 2004;32:2014–20.)

TABLE 18-1 Elements of the Surgical Safety Checklist[a]

Sign in

Before induction of anesthesia, members of the team (at least the nurse and an anesthesia professional) orally confirm that

The patient has verified his or her identity, the surgical site and procedure, and consent

The surgical site is marked or site marking is not applicable

The pulse oximeter is on the patient and functioning

All members of the team are aware of whether the patient has a known allergy

The patient's airway and risk of aspiration have been evaluated and appropriate equipment and assistance are available

If there is a risk of blood loss of at least 500 mL (or 7 mL/kg of body weight, in children), appropriate access and fluids are available

Time out

Before skin incision, the entire team (nurses, surgeons, anesthesia professionals, and any others participating in the care of the patient) orally

Confirms that all team members have been introduced by name and role

Confirms the patient's identity, surgical site, and procedure

Reviews the anticipated critical events

Surgeon reviews critical and unexpected steps, operative duration, and anticipated blood loss

Anesthesia staff review concerns specific to the patient

Nursing staff review confirmation of sterility, equipment availability, and other concerns

Confirms that prophylactic antibiotics have been administered ≤60 min before incision is made or that antibiotics are not indicated

Confirms that all essential imaging results for the correct patient are displayed in the operating room

Sign out

Before the patient leaves the operating room

Nurse reviews items aloud with the team

Name of the procedure as recorded

That the needle, sponge, and instrument counts are complete (or not applicable)

That the specimen (if any) is correctly labeled, including with the patient's name

Whether there are any issues with equipment to be addressed

The surgeon, nurse, and anesthesia professional review aloud the key concerns for the recovery and care of the patient

---

[a]From: Haynes AB, Weiser TG, Berry WR, et al. A surgical safety checklist to reduce morbidity and mortality in a global population. *N Engl J Med.* 2009;360:491–9.

Safe Surgery Saves Lives Study Group demonstrates the impact of a Surgical Safety Checklist (Table 18-1) on patient safety in surgery. Between October 2007 and September 2008, there was a reduction in perioperative death rate from 1.5% to 0.8% as well as a reduction in inpatient complications from 11% to 7%.[9]

Beyond preplanning for surgical cases, checklists improve patient outcomes when implemented to handle crises in the OR. In a 2011 pilot study, Ziewacz et al. showed a sixfold reduction in failure to adhere to critical steps in the management of a variety of simulated rare surgical situations. Failure to adhere to the critical steps was 24% without and 4% with the checklist. An example of the cases used and checklist are shown in Figure 18-2.[10] Expansion of this pilot study by Arriaga et al. in 2013 demonstrated a similar reduction in failures to comply with critical steps from 23% without the use of checklists to 6% when checklists were used.[11]

Since clear reductions in morbidity and mortality have been demonstrated, it is imperative to implement checklists into daily practice. The use of checklists has minimal costs to hospitals such as for the initial training and a small amount of time

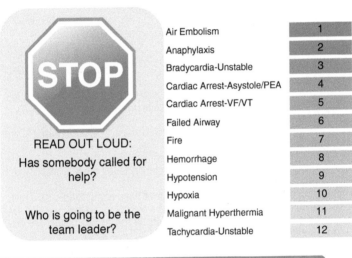

Figure 18-2. OR critical event checklist. Panel A shows the cover of the OR critical event checklist that directs users to the correct checklist. Panel B demonstrates the Air Embolism management checklist. (From: Ziewacz JE, Arriaga AF, Bader AM, et al. Crisis checklists for the operating room: development and pilot testing. *J Am Coll Surg*. 2011;213:212–9.)

before, during, and after each situation in which the checklist is used. These costs in dollars and time are easily made up for by the decrease in medical errors, which result in longer and increasingly unreimbursed hospital stays and increased demands on health care worker's time. Such demands are not insignificant, as "checklist fatigue" can result in nonapplication of this simple and effective method. In the perioperative arena, nurses, surgeons, and anesthesiologists can all agree that checklists reduce human error and improve human safety but admit that it is not used for every procedure in every OR.[12]

SIMULATION

Simulation is an educational approach that provides an opportunity to learn and practice complex medical care without putting any patients at risk. There are numerous tools and techniques utilized in the realm of simulation including task trainers, standardized patients, computer-controlled mannequins, and computer programs. This approach can be varied depending on the state of the learner, the provider's experience, and the clinical situations encountered. Simulation can focus on team training, CRM, and the education and assessment of individuals and teams.

A simulation can expose new learners to basic knowledge such as using good hand washing techniques and calling for help in emergencies. Patient safety concepts can be integrated throughout all levels of the simulation education. For example, early learners can be trained to introduce themselves upon meeting patients. These concepts can be reinforced during the training of more experienced providers as new layers are integrated into the training. Basic components of medical care can be approached through simulation including bag mask ventilation, basic life support, and patient interview practice. As students progress through their studies, simulation can focus on more advanced techniques such as effective cardiopulmonary resuscitation, advanced airway management, and effective communication techniques.

In a recent expert consensus, simulation exercise and team training have been encouraged as patient safety strategies ready for immediate adoption.[7] Simulation has been used to enhance team training in emergency department settings[13] and has been used to evaluate anesthesiologists' nontechnical skills (ANTS) of task management, teamwork, situational awareness, and decision making.[14] It has been used to evaluate latent safety threats to patients from new teams working in new health care facilities and in neonatal intensive care units.[15,16] Such work allows the identification and correction of these latent threats before patient exposure. Simulation has also been used to demonstrate the efficacy of checklists and performance improvement during simulated crisis.[11]

CRISIS RESOURCE MANAGEMENT

The roots of simulation, like checklists, did not start in medicine but rather grew from the aviation industry with the discovery that the majority of aircraft mishaps were not due to equipment failure or lack of experience but rather to the inability of the crew to harness their resources when needed at a critical moment. From this awareness, the aviation simulation model of Crew Resource Management grew in the 1980s as a joint venture between the private airline industry, NASA, and the US military.[17] This has since been adopted by medicine as CRM. Like aviation, medicine offers a dynamic environment where multiple problems can occur spontaneously or compound each other. Medicine shares another commonality with aviation in that groups of individuals (crews) often work together toward common goals. The decision-making process and behaviors are often the same whether the team consists of health care providers focusing on a decompensating patient or pilots struggling to avert a crashing plane.

In CRM, each discipline in health care is considered a crew. Teams are comprised of crews working together. Therefore, an OR case may consist of individual crews of surgeons, an anesthesiologist, OR nurses, and a surgical technician. The entire collection of crews is the assembled team taking on the presented case. While a large percentage of simulation education involves training individuals or groups from the same "crew," the crux of CRM involves integrating the crews into teams. Integration of the team allows the individuals of a crew and the crews themselves to not only practice their specific skills and contributions to the case but more importantly allows the crews to develop the critical components of teamwork and communication necessary to achieve a good patient outcome. Another side benefit is that individuals from one crew often learn to appreciate the skills and knowledge that another crew's members bring to the health care team.

The key principles of CRM as established by Gaba[18] and Salas and modified by Carne[19] are:

- Know your environment.
- Anticipate leadership and role clarity.
- Communicate effectively.
- Call for help early.
- Allocate attention wisely—avoid fixation.
- Distribute the workload—monitor and support team members.

Typically, CRM consists of three main components: didactics, simulation scenarios, and debriefing. The didactic portion is frequently the first component of CRM education but can also be inserted between simulation sessions as a component of the debriefing. When done ahead of time, the didactic component should be reasonably concise with small digestible amounts of information. This information is then immediately put to work in the simulation sessions where the team begins to integrate the new information into their simulated practice. The final and often most overlooked portion of CRM simulation is the debriefing. Typically done in between simulation scenarios and often involving video and audio recordings, the debriefing allows team members to see what was done well and what could use improvement in any given scenario. Digital recordings are an invaluable tool in these scenarios as they leave little room for disagreement when things go poorly while allowing the entire team to witness actions done well. To get the most out of simulation, allow for 2–3 minutes of debriefing time for every minute of simulation time. During CRM debriefing, keep in mind that the emphasis is not on the individual cognitive tasks or skills but instead on the management behaviors critical to CRM. It is the teamwork and crew interactions that must be most closely monitored and critiqued.

Finally, it must be asked, "Does CRM simulation training make a difference in patient outcomes?" This is difficult to answer as the situations where CRM is most meaningful are often low-occurrence high-acuity situations. These events by their very nature make it difficult to accumulate enough real-world cases to appropriately power a study demonstrating a clinical benefit. Dozens of studies have shown that based on survey data from simulated settings, learners feel much more comfortable after CRM training. There are also multiple studies demonstrating improved teamwork characteristics after CRM sessions. While these measures take place in the simulated world, data suggest that we practice like we play so should expect similar results in the real world.

The AHRQ has developed the TeamSTEPPS (Strategies and Tools to Enhance Performance and Patient Safety) course as a teamwork training system for advancing patient safety in organizations. The goal of TeamSTEPPS is to produce highly effective teams that effectively utilize available resources, information, and team members to produce optimal patient outcomes. It is evidence based and created in collaboration between AHRQ and the Department of Defense.

CONCLUSION

Medicine has advanced more in the past 150 years than it had in the previous 2 millennia. Great advancements, however, have created greater challenges in identifying and managing events that result in patient injury and death. Estimates of a million injuries and 100,000 annual deaths from adverse events make medical errors the sixth leading cause of death in the US. Recent data suggest that these numbers have not decreased substantially in the last decade.[20] Numerous tools and techniques have been developed in response to increasing focus from a growing number of stakeholders. These include checklists, time outs, team training, and simulation-based education and assessment. Checklists have demonstrated a reduction of morbidity and mortality when utilized for central line placement as well as for preoperative surgical preparation.[21] Despite the supportive evidence for using checklists to optimize patient safety, there is evidence that checklists are not uniformly used and "never events" continue to occur.[22] Examples of sentinel events that should never occur include wrong-sided surgery, retained objects following procedures, and discharging an infant to the wrong family. Unfortunately, these events continue to occur. Of the 6994 sentinel events reported from 2004 to 2012, there were 928 wrong-patient, wrong-site, or wrong procedures performed, 773 events with an unintended retention of a foreign body, and 3 infants discharged home to the wrong family.[23] These events do not represent an historical phenomenon that is gradually disappearing. Of the 928 wrong-site procedures, 93 happened in 2010, 152 in 2011, and 109 in 2012. A similar pattern occurs for all reported sentinel events and suggests that patient safety is a major public health problem that is only beginning to be addressed. An analysis of 9744 surgical never events from 1990 to 2010 demonstrated a 6.6% mortality permanent injury in 33% and temporary injury in 59% of the patients. The costs of medical malpractice claims for surgical never events during this period were estimated to be over $1.3 billion dollars.[24] These events are preventable and would be prevented if practitioners followed existing recommendations for care during procedures including utilizing checklists, providing leadership to protect patients, and assuring effective communication. Medicine has had a weak tradition of focusing on patient safety. Future physicians and health care providers will need to balance increasingly limited resources with the imperative to optimize patient safety. Effective evidence-based tools must be utilized to achieve these goals and to live up to the intent of nonmaleficence enshrined by the Hippocratic Oath: *Primum non nocere*, First Do No Harm.

KEY POINTS

- Numerous tools are available to address the ubiquitous problem of patient safety including checklists, simulation, and team training. These tools are uniformly useless if not utilized.
- Checklists have been shown to reduce morbidity and mortality.
- Properly performed time outs prior to procedures reduce medical errors.
- Simulation is an educational method of reflection, repetition, and movement toward mastery.
- Simulation provides an arena for practice without exposing patients to the risk of injury.
- CRM training strives to create teams, which use all available resources with situational awareness, adaptability, leadership, and effective communication.
- TeamSTEPPS is a team training system intended to develop highly functioning teams producing optimal patient outcomes.

ONLINE RESOURCES

The following is a nonexhaustive list of online resources for further information about tools for patient safety:

1. AHRQ: http://www.ahrq.gov/professionals/quality-patient-safety/index.html
2. AHRQ TeamSTEPPS: http://teamstepps.ahrq.gov/
3. IHI: http://www.ihi.org/explore/patientsafety/Pages/default.aspx
4. Institute for Safe Medication Practices: www.ismp.org
5. The Joint Commission: http://www.jointcommission.org/topics/patient_safety.aspx
6. The Leapfrog Group: http://www.leapfroggroup.org/
7. Society for Pediatric Anesthesia: http://www.pedsanesthesia.org/
8. Quality Net [Center for Medicare & Medicaid Services]: https://www.qualitynet.org/
9. The World Health Organization Safe Surgery Program: http://www.safesurg.org/

REFERENCES

1. Couch NP, Tilney NL, Rayner AA, et al. The high cost of low frequency events: the anatomy and economics of surgical mishaps. *N Engl J Med.* 1981;304:634–7.
2. Brennan TA, Leape LL, Laird NM, et al. Incidence of adverse events and negligence in hospitalized patients. Results of the Harvard Medical Practice Study I. *N Engl J Med.* 1991;324:370–6.
3. Leape LL, Brennan TA, Laird N, et al. Incidence of adverse events and negligence in hospitalized patients. Results of the Harvard Medical Practice Study II. *N Engl J Med.* 1991;324:377–84.
4. Parker J. *Meeting the Joint Commission's 2013 National Patient Safety Goals.* Oakbrook Terrace, IL: The Joint Commission; 2012.
5. Murray CJL, Frenk J. Ranking 37th—measuring the performance of the US health care system. *N Engl J Med.* 2010;362:98–9.
6. Gawande A. *The Checklist Manifesto: How to Get Things Right.* New York, NY: Henry Holt; 2011.
7. Shekelle PG, Pronovost PJ, Wachter RM, et al. The top patient safety strategies that can be encouraged for adoption now. *Ann Int Med.* 2013;158(5 Part 2):365–8.

8. Berenholtz SM, Pronovost PJ, Lipsett PA, et al. Eliminating catheter-related bloodstream infections in the intensive care unit. *Crit Care Med.* 2004;32:2014–20.

9. Haynes AB, Weiser TG, Berry WR, et al. A surgical safety checklist to reduce morbidity and mortality in a global population. *N Engl J Med.* 2009;360:491–9.

10. Ziewacz JE, Arriaga AF, Bader AM, et al. Crisis checklists for the operating room: development and pilot testing. *J Am Coll Surg.* 2011;213:212–9.

11. Arriaga AF, Bader AM, Wong JM, et al. Simulation-based trial of surgical-crisis checklists. *N Engl J Med.* 2013;368:246–53.

12. O'Connor P, Reddin C, O'Sullivan M, et al. Surgical checklists: the human factor. *Patient Saf Surg.* 2013;7:14.

13. Shapiro MJ, Morey JC, Small SD, et al. Simulation based teamwork training for emergency department staff: does it improve clinical team performance when added to an existing didactic teamwork curriculum? *Qual Saf Health Care.* 2004;13:417–21.

14. Flin R, Patey R, Glavin R, et al. Anaesthetists' non-technical skills. *Br J Anesth.* 2010;105(1):38–44.

15. Geis GL, Pio B, Pendergrass TL, et al. Simulation to assess the safety of new healthcare teams and new facilities. *Sim Healthc.* 2011;6:125–33.

16. Wetzel EA, Lang TR, Pendergrass TL, et al. Identification of latent safety threats using high-fidelity simulation-based training with multidisciplinary neonatology teams. *Jt Comm J Qual Patient Saf.* 2013;39(6):268–73.

17. Gaba DM, Howard SK, Fish KJ, et al. Simulation-based training in anesthesia crisis resource management (ACRM): a decade of experience. *Simul Gaming.* 2001;32:175–93.

18. Gaba DM, Fish KJ, Howard SK. *Crisis Management in Anesthesiology.* New York, NY: Churchill Livingston; 1994.

19. Carne B, Kennedy M, Gray T. Review article: crisis resource management in emergency medicine. *Emer Med Australas.* 2012;24:7–13.

20. Landrigan CP, Parry GJ, Bones CB, et al. Temporal trends in rates of patient harm resulting from medical care. *N Engl J Med.* 2010;363:2124–34.

21. Pronovost P, Needham D, Berenholtz S, et al. An intervention to decrease catheter-related bloodstream infections in the ICU. *N Engl J Med.* 2006;355:2725–32.

22. Ring DC, Herndon JH, Meyer GS. Case 34–2010: a 65-year-old woman with an incorrect operation on the left hand. *N Engl J Med.* 2010;363:1950–7.

23. The Joint Commission. Sentinel event statistics as of December 31, 2012. http://www.joint-commission.org/assets/1/18/2004_4Q_2012_SE_Stats_Summary.pdf. Accessed 12/13/15.

24. Mehtsun WT, Ibrahim AM, Diener-West M, et al. Surgical never events in the United States. *Surgery.* 2013;153:465–72.

19

Surgery and Procedural Areas

Paul Santiago, Kathleen S. Bandt, Peter Vila, and Brian Nussenbaum

CLINICAL VIGNETTE

Ms. G is a 34-year-old woman with a 4-year history of progressive thoracic back pain with associated right leg numbness and weakness. Her past medical history is significant for a history of bipolar disorder. She has a reputation for poor compliance with her medical care. She is currently being treated for type II diabetes, hypertension, and hyperlipidemia. Workup of her spinal complaints reveals a large thoracic disc herniation with spinal cord compression. Ms. G has a 10th grade education and relies on her family to help make decisions. She is anxious about having surgery but is also quite concerned about the weakness in her right leg and her difficulty walking. She frequently asks whether surgery is "necessary."

- What difficulties might there be in obtaining informed consent in this case?
- What are the essential steps in obtaining informed consent?
- What other types of adverse events may occur during the perioperative period?

INTRODUCTION

Over $400 billion are spent annually on surgical procedures in the US.[1] These are performed in a variety of health care settings, ranging from outpatient offices to tertiary care centers. More so than any other form of medical intervention, surgical intervention represents a form of controlled "harm" to the patient. This "harm" is meant to ultimately result in a desired outcome for the patient. However, surgical interventions/procedures can result in unintended complications that may not benefit the patient either in the short or long term. It is fundamental to the physician–patient relationship that patients are made aware of these risks, in order for the patient to determine if they are willing to accept these risks in light of the potential benefits. This chapter will cover some of the issues regarding the process of educating patients or their representatives regarding the risks and benefits associated with medical interventions in general, as well as reviewing some of the more common perioperative complications, including thromboembolic events, wrong-site surgery (WSS), and retained foreign objects. Also, a brief discussion of processes that are being developed to decrease the occurrence of these events will be included. Currently reported rates of perioperative/periprocedural complications are in the range 3–17% and are felt to be underreported.[1] Clearly, there is a significant "cost" in both harm to patients and resources to the health care system associated with care provided in surgical and procedural areas. Both patients and health care providers need to be aware of these costs and work to contain them.

Informed Consent

It is rare for a patient not to have questions regarding the goals of a particular treatment and potential consequences of this treatment. The discussion of "risks and benefits" is a common interaction between health care providers and patients. Most patients, however, have little information upon which to base their decisions. Furthermore, the source of most of their information is a member of the health care team providing the treatment, resulting in inherent bias. The goal of pretreatment counseling is not only to educate the patient about their treatment but also to obtain a patient's permission for the treatment in question to be rendered. The extent to which all potential complications or potential adverse events are discussed with a patient may vary from case to case. The following is a brief introduction to the history of informed consent and general guidelines to obtaining informed consent under a variety of circumstances.

The concept of formal informed consent is a relatively recent one, although there are abundant historical references to discussions between physicians and patients regarding treatment. One such case involved the battlefield care provided to General Thomas "Stonewall" Jackson. In 1863, General Jackson sustained a severe injury to his left arm. There is documentation of a face-to-face discussion between the general and his surgeon, the intended procedure was discussed (amputation), and verbal consent was obtained.[2] No mention is made of potential complications associated with the procedure. While, in fact, General Jackson survived the procedure, he died of pneumonia 8 days later. The term "informed consent" first entered the medical lexicon in the early 1960s during the malpractice case Natanson v. Kline (1960).[3] Ms. Natanson was referred to Dr. Kline for radiation treatment for breast cancer. Radiation therapy was at that time in its infancy, and the standards for effective treatment with minimal injury to surrounding tissue were yet to be established. As a consequence of Dr. Kline's treatment, Ms. Natanson went on to develop necrosis of her chest wall adjacent to the site of treatment. Ms. Natanson alleged that Dr. Kline did not inform her of this potential risk and had she known that significant injury to her chest was a potential risk associated with the treatment, she would not have consented to the procedure. After several appeals, the Kansas State Supreme court issued the following ruling: "The duty of the physician to disclose however is limited to those disclosures which a reasonable medical professional would make under the same circumstances. How the physician [executes his responsibility] to the patient…is a question of medical judgment." The definitions of a reasonable medical professional and good judgment were left vague and have been the basis of litigation since. The ruling, however, represents a major shift in the consent process. Prior to this, legal matters regarding consent were focused mainly on a patient's right to refuse treatment rather than their right to be informed about their treatment (Schloendorff v. Society of New York Hospital, 1914).[4]

Components of Informed Consent

While there is no absolute standard for what constitutes informed consent, some general principles are widely accepted. Among the most basic of these standards, with the exception of emergency consent, is that a discussion of the treatment goals and the potential for complications/adverse events must occur. It must not be assumed that the patient understands a priori that there are risks associated with treatment. Secondly, record must be made of this discussion and entered into the medical record. To this end, most practitioners have adopted the use of standardized forms to document this discussion. Use of such standardized forms does not replace the requirement for discussion with the patient prior to treatment. At a minimum, this discussion should cover the following:

• The patient's diagnosis and the anticipated course of the disease/condition.
• The nature of the proposed treatment or procedure.
• The most commonly associated risks and benefits of the proposed treatment or procedure.
• Alternatives to the proposed procedure and their associated risk and benefits, including the option of no further treatment.
• The discussion should occur in lay language and the individual seeking consent must verify that the patient understands the language being used.
• The person providing consent must be given the opportunity to ask questions. The person obtaining consent must make the effort to ascertain what is important for the person obtaining consent to understand, as this will vary from person to person.

Who May Provide Informed Consent

Any adult of legal age and of sound mind may provide consent for treatment. Patients who are obtunded, unconscious, encephalopathic, psychotic, or otherwise impaired may not provide consent for treatment. Unless the absence of treatment represents significant risk to the patient, treatment cannot proceed until either a patient is able to provide consent or an acceptable alternate can be found. The exact hierarchy of who may provide consent for a patient unable to do so for himself varies from state to state, but the following list is typical of the list used in many jurisdictions:

1. Legal power of attorney
2. Patient's spouse
3. Patient's adult child*
4. Patient's parent*
5. Patient's sibling*
6. Patient's adult grandchild or other adult relative*
7. Close friend of the patient*
8. Legal guardian of the patient's estate

Special Considerations
Cognitively Impaired Patients

There is a spectrum of cognitive impairment. While some individuals with mild cognitive impairment are unable to live independently, many patients with mild cognitive impairment are capable of and should make decisions with respect to their health care. It is important to establish whether a patient makes these types of decisions independently or with the aid of a guardian/legal power of attorney. When in doubt, it is best to solicit the aid of available family members. Every effort should be made to include the patient in discussions regarding their care to the extent that the patient is able to participate.

Pediatric Patients

Patients old enough to express understanding and voice an opinion pertaining to medical treatment must be included in the process for obtaining informed consent. While, legally, informed consent is obtained from a child's or youth's guardian, ethically, assent should be obtained from the minor during the informed consent process.

---

*Agreement must be reached between members of equal priority

Lack of assent should prompt delay of treatment for nonemergent procedures. Under certain circumstances, minors can be treated as adults with respect to consent for medical treatment. "Emancipated" minors represent a special class of patient. The criteria defining an emancipated minor vary from state to state. In general, minors living independently or with children of their own are considered "emancipated." In some states, minors, who would otherwise rely on parents or guardians to provide consent in most matters, may provide consent independent of their parents/guardians under certain circumstances, particularly with respect to treatment for pregnancy and sexually transmitted diseases.

Patients Whose Primary Language Is Not English

A licensed, approved medical interpreter should be involved whenever attempting to obtain informed consent from a non-English–speaking patient. Family members should not be used for this purpose under nonemergent circumstances, unless the patient is unable to participate in the consent process. In most hospitals, interpreter services are readily available or can be contacted by telephone.

The Unconscious Patient

The groundwork for treating a patient unable to provide consent and for whom no one is available to provide consent was established at the turn of the 20th century. Mary Schloendorff consented to an exam under anesthesia to determine if a fibroid tumor was malignant.[4] She did not provide consent for removal of the tumor. While under anesthesia, her surgeon determined that the tumor was indeed malignant and removed the tumor. Ms. Schloendorff proceeded to sue the hospital and not her surgeon. While the case had a significant impact on the immunity of charitable organizations to be sued for the actions of its employees, the case also had an impact on the ability of physicians to use their judgment in the care of an unconsentable patient. In Schloendorff v. Society of New York Hospital (1914), the court ruled: "Every human being of adult years and sound mind has a right to determine what shall be done with his own body…This is true except in cases of emergency where the patient is unconscious and where it is necessary to operate before consent can be obtained." Emergent consent is obtained by two physicians agreeing that a procedure is required to treat an emergent condition for an unresponsive patient, when all reasonable measures to contact next of kin have been exhausted. At that point, both physicians sign the consent form, document necessity for the procedure and what efforts were made to reach next of kin, and then proceed with surgical intervention.

COMPLICATIONS FROM INVASIVE PROCEDURES

The intention of the informed consent process is to inform patients and their families of the reasonably expected risks and benefits associated with a particular treatment. In most cases, it is impossible to predict which patients will experience what complication. Certain complications, however, occur frequently enough and are felt to have a significant enough impact on patient outcome that they deserve special consideration and have come to be referred to as "never events." The intended consequence of this designation is to provide patients with "safer" care and better outcomes. The impact of these measures on patient outcomes remains to be established.

The term "never events" has been used by the Center for Medicare and Medicaid Services (CMS) to describe conditions for which reimbursement of medical costs incurred as a consequence of these "never events" will be withheld.[5] The goal is to

TABLE 19-1	Center for Medicare and Medicaid Services 2013 List of Non-reimbursable Serious Hospital-Acquired Conditions (HAC)[5]

- Fall leading to injury
- Catheter-associated urinary tract infection (UTI)
- Vascular catheter–associated infection
- Surgical site infection (SSI) after coronary artery bypass grafting (CABG), bariatric or orthopedic surgery or after placement of a cardiac implantable electronic device
- Deep vein thrombosis/pulmonary embolism (DVT/PE) after total hip or knee replacement
- Death or disability associated with diabetic ketoacidosis, nonketotic hyperosmolar coma, hypoglycemic coma, secondary diabetes with ketoacidosis or hyperosmolarity
- Foreign object retained after surgery
- Air embolism
- Blood incompatibility
- Stage III or IV pressure ulcer
- Iatrogenic pneumothorax during venous catheterization

promote the delivery of "safer" care to patients by incentivizing to hospitals to establish quality and safety programs (Table 19-1). A review of some of the most commonly encountered adverse events follows.

Central Line–Associated Bloodstream Infections

Placement of a central venous catheter (CVC) is one of the most commonly performed invasive procedures. In the surgical patient, these catheters can be used to monitor central venous pressure, administer antibiotics/medications, provide a route for fluid resuscitation/transfusion, provide nutritional support, and allow for blood draws. Because these catheters are often in place for extended periods of time and frequently accessed, they are at significant risk for infection. Infections associated with CVCs have been estimated to result in excess of 2 billion dollars per year in additional health care costs.[6] The incidence for this type of infection is often tracked as the incidence of infection over a certain number of line days. Using this method of tracking, the incidence of catheter-related bloodstream infections has been reported to range from 0.1 to 2.7/1000 line days and is highly dependent on the type of catheter.[7] Short-term central venous catheters, such as those commonly used perioperatively, have the highest rate of infection. The most common organisms involved are staphylococci. Infection is felt to occur both due to extra- and intraluminal migration of bacteria and yeast along the catheter. Tunneling of long-term catheters decreases the risk of extraluminal spread. Treatment generally consists of removal of the line and a course of intravenous (IV) antibiotics but is dependent on the causative organism and the type of line affected. Prevention remains the mainstay of treatment. Numerous studies have demonstrated that strict adherence to standardized treatment protocols can result in a significant decrease in the rate of CVC infections rates. These protocols and care bundles provide both behavioral and treatment guidelines.[6] Please refer to Table 19-2 for a summary of these guidelines.[8] See Chapter 9 for more information about central line–associated blood stream infections.

TABLE 19-2	Recommended Practices for Prevention of Central Venous Catheter–Related Bloodstream Infection[8]

- Limit insertion to trained personnel.
- Avoid use of the femoral vein.
- Use subclavian vein in lieu of the internal jugular or femoral vein depending upon risk of injury during insertion.
- Use a central venous catheter with the minimum number of lumens required for patient care.
- Complete hand hygiene prior to insertion, assessment, or dressing change of catheter exit site.
- Do not administer systemic antimicrobial prophylaxis.
- Use chlorhexidine/silver sulfadiazine or a minocycline-/rifampin-impregnated central venous catheters when the local rate of central line–associated bloodstream infection is not declining despite education of optimal insertion and maintenance practices.
- Use of >0.5% chlorhexidine plus alcohol for preparation of skin before insertion.
- Use maximum sterile barrier precautions, including cap, mask, sterile gown, sterile gloves, and a sterile full-body drape for insertion and during guidewire exchange.
- Place semipermeable transparent or gauze dressing over insertion site.
- Gauze favored when exit site is bloody or moist.
- Restrict application of antimicrobial ointment to exit sites of hemodialysis catheters and only then when approved for use by catheter manufacturer.
- Assess exit site daily.
- Exchange exit site dressing whenever damp, loosened, or soiled.
- Replace gauze dressings every 2 days.
- Replace semipermeable transparent dressings every 7 days.
- When adherence to aseptic technique was compromised during insertion, replace the catheter as soon as possible.
- Do not routinely replace central venous catheters to prevent infection.
- Remove any intravascular catheter as soon as it is no longer required for patient care.

Venous Thromboembolism

The incidence of deep vein thrombosis (DVT) in critically ill patients is quite high. Surgical intervention itself is felt to be an independent risk factor for the development of DVT. Chemo- and mechanical prophylaxis can substantially reduce DVT rates but does not eliminate the problem. Approximately 1/3 of the nearly 200,000 deaths associated annually with venous thromboembolism (VTE) occur in postoperative patients, and while approximately 50% of trauma patient may be found to have DVT, it appears that only 5% of trauma patients may develop symptomatic VTE.[9–11] In both cases, the use of mechanical and chemoprophylaxis has become the standard of care. Some surgical and trauma patients despite being at high risk for the development of DVT/ VTE are also at high risk for the development of hemorrhagic complications from pharmacologic prophylaxis. The increased risk of hemorrhage for these patients while on anticoagulation therapy varies in the literature and depends on the exact nature of the injury and the method of treatment. Inferior Vena Cava (IVC) filters are not currently recommended for primary VTE prevention in general, abdominal-pelvic or trauma surgery patients.[9] IVC filters may be used for inpatients with VTE in whom anticoagulation therapy cannot be started, must be stopped, or is insufficient to protect patients from a clinical significant PE, but only provide protection from large thromboembolic events and do not treat the underlying disease.[12] Additionally, not all filters are ultimately retrievable. An indwelling IVC filter commits patients to lifelong anticoagulation therapy, if there are no contraindications to anticoagulation, and the potential for filter thrombosis.[12] Judicious use should be made of IVC filters, particularly in young patients, nonterminally ill patients, and patients at high risk for fall, as they may require lifelong anticoagulation/antiplatelet therapy. Despite all of the above, early mobilization and mechanical/pharmacologic prophylaxis are the standard of care for surgical and trauma patients, and there is abundant support in the literature that this standard has an impact upon the rate of DVT.[9,13-15] For more information about VTE prevention, see Chapter 8, Preventable Harm.

Falls

Up to 1 in 5 patients fall at least once during their hospital stay.[16,17] These falls lead to injuries, increased length of stay, and increased medical expenditure. It has been argued extensively in the public arena as to whether or not falls are preventable in the inpatient setting. The reactionary response to the financial implications of an inpatient fall being considered a nonreimbursable event frequently led providers to either chemically or physically restrain a patient considered a "fall risk" but who would otherwise not meet restraint criteria. This excessive use of both chemical and physical restraints may themselves lead to untoward and unintended consequences including higher thromboembolic complications due to immobility and/or delayed recovery due to prolonged sedation as well as functional loss, delirium, and pressure ulcers.[16] A recent systematic review identified that, at best, up to 20% of inpatient falls could be prevented.[17] Unfortunately, no intervention has been shown to reduce the risk of serious injury following an inpatient fall. For more information about fall prevention, see Chapter 8, Preventable Harm.

Surgical Site Infections

Surgical site infections (SSIs) are the third most common nosocomial infections, representing approximately 15% of all hospital-acquired infections overall. In surgical patients, SSIs represent the most common hospital-acquired infection at 38% of the total. Of these, 2/3 are defined as superficial SSIs and 1/3 represent deep SSIs. SSIs are associated with significant morbidity and mortality for patients who develop them. SSIs extend hospital stays by up to a week after routine surgical procedures and contribute to a significant increase in health care costs for patients.[18] A heightened awareness of postoperative wound infections and measures to prevent them can have useful results including meticulous attention to proper surgical technique and postoperative wound care, but overuse of antibiotics may contribute to bacterial resistance and/or secondary infections including *Clostridium difficile* colitis. Additionally, patient comorbidities often contribute to complications with wound healing, including diabetes and prior exposure to radiation therapy. To say that all SSIs are preventable is unlikely, but strict adherence to best practices should be the norm regardless of reimbursement. For more information about Surgical site infections, see Chapter 9, Health Care-Associated Infections.

Retained Sponges and Instruments

Various terms exist for the scenario when an object is left in the patient after a surgical procedure, including retained foreign bodies, retained foreign objects, retained surgical instruments, or, as used here, retained sponges and instruments (RSI). No matter which term is used, however, all can agree that whenever this situation occurs, there is resulting harm to patients, with physical, emotional, social, and financial implications. In addition, surgeons can be held legally responsible for its occurrence, even in the face of the nursing staff admitting liability.[19] Beginning in 2002, the National Quality Forum (NQF), a nonprofit organization tasked with the improvement of health care quality measurement and reporting, released a list of serious reportable events (SREs). The "unintended retention of a foreign object in a patient after surgery or other invasive procedure," or RSI, is one of these events.[20] In addition, the Centers for Medicare and Medicaid Services have decided since 2007 to not reimburse for any part of the surgical procedure in the case of RSI. Despite multiple studies and interventions put into place to reduce the incidence of RSI, such as counting of sponges and instruments, for example, these "never events" continue to occur.

The incidence of RSI has been estimated to range from 1 in 5500 to 1 in 18,760 inpatient operations per year.[21–23] In a landmark study by Gawande et al. of 54 patients with RSI, 37 (69%) required reoperation, and 1 died (2%). The most common risk factors for the occurrence of RSI included emergent surgery, unexpected change in the surgical procedure, and high body mass index (BMI). The time course for the detection of RSI was highly variable, with a range from postoperative day 0 to over 6 years after the procedure, and the median time of detection was postoperative day 21.[22] Lincourt et al. replicated this study, examining cases of RSI from 1996 through 2005 at a large academic medical center.[24] Over this time period, 37 cases of RSI occurred, with 25 patients (83%) requiring reoperation. This study found additional risk factors for RSI, including the reporting of an incorrect count and the total number of major procedures. A similar study by Cima et al. of 34 cases of RSI from 2003 to 2006 at a large academic medical center largely replicated these findings; however, in this study, none of the cases of RSI resulted from emergent cases, multiple surgical teams, or late procedures.[23] Tables 19-3 and 19-4 summarize the characteristics and risk factors for RSI after a surgical procedure.

A large review of over 9000 malpractice claims filed in Massachusetts during the years 1988–1994 revealed that the most common procedures resulting in RSI were procedures with an open body cavity, with 40 cases of RSI total. Together, obstetrics/gynecology procedures (23 out of 40 cases) and general surgery (12 out of 40 cases) accounted for over 80% of the claims, with two laminectomies, a Caldwell-Luc (sinus surgery), and two coronary artery bypass grafts comprising the remaining claims.[19] Other studies have reported consistent findings, with the most common locations for RSI including the abdomen or pelvis (47–54%), thorax (7.4–23%), or vagina (22%).[22,24]

The surgical count is a widely used method of screening for RSI. The protocol standardized by the Association of Perioperative Registered Nurses (AORN) involves an initial count (before the procedure), interim counts (throughout the procedure), the closing count (at the end of the procedure before the skin is closed), and the reconciliation count (after all instruments have been removed from the field and the surgical site is closed). These are performed by the circulating nurse and surgical technologist, and any discrepancies in the count are communicated to the surgeon.[25]

In a study of counts during elective general surgery cases, the authors found that on average about 17 counts occurred per case, and discrepancies in the count occurred once per eight cases, or once per 14 hours of operative time. When a discrepancy occurred, the most common reason was due to a misplaced object (59%), meaning the item was unintentionally lost, ending up anywhere from in the trash to inside the patient (however, no RSI was detected during this study). A documentation

TABLE 19-3 Characteristics of Cases of RSI after a Surgical Procedure

	Number of cases	
Characteristic	n	%
Type of retained object (n = 118)[22–24]		
Sponge	60	51
Clamp	18	15
Other	24	20
Outcomes (n = 84)[22,24]		
Reoperation	62	74
Readmission/prolonged hospital stay	40	48
Death	1	1
Correct count reported at conclusion of procedure (n = 118)[22–24]	NR	80

NR, not reported.

TABLE 19-4 Risk Factors for RSI after a Surgical Procedure

Characteristic	Risk Ratio (95% CI)	P Value
Incorrect count reported[24]	16.3 (1.3–19.8)	0.02
Emergent operation[22]	8.8 (2.4–31.9)	<0.001
Unexpected change in operation[22]	4.1 (1.4–12.4)	0.01
Multiple surgical teams[22]	3.4 (0.8–14.1)	0.10
Change in nursing staff during procedure[22]	1.9 (0.7–5.4)	0.24
Total number of surgical procedures[24]	1.6 (1.1–2.3)	0.008
BMI (per 1-unit increment)[22]	1.1 (1.0–1.2)	0.01
Estimated volume of blood loss (per 100 mL increment)[22]	1.0 (1.0–1.0)	0.19
Count performed[22]	0.6 (0.03–13.9)	0.76
Female sex[22]	0.4 (0.1–1.3)	0.13
Unexpected change in operative procedure[24]	NR	>0.05
Length of case[24]	NR	>0.05
Procedure performed after 5:00 PM[24]	NR	>0.05

NR, not reported.

error was the next most common reason (38%), and a pure miscount was rare (3%). A change in either the circulating nurse or the surgical technologist during the procedure resulted in a threefold higher risk of a discrepancy.[26]

Because the surgical count is subject to human error and thus is an imperfect process, some have questioned its efficacy. One should note that in patients with RSI, the count was documented as correct 88% of the time, which was not statistically significantly different from study controls with no RSI (92%).[22] In a study of coronary bypass surgeries in New York State, Egorova et al. showed that the specificity of a normal count in the detection of RSI was 99.3%, with a negative predictive value of approximately 100%. In contrast, the sensitivity of a discrepancy in the count was 77%, with a positive predictive value of 1.6%.[21]

Additional measures such as sponge counters, bar-coding sponges, radiofrequency (RF) identification technology, and x-ray or CT screening have been proposed to minimize the incidence of RSI. While low-cost measures such as sponge counters (bags to hold sponges) have been widely adopted but not rigorously studied, other methods have been shown to be useful in the published literature. A randomized, controlled trial comparing a traditional counting protocol to bar-coded sponge counting found that while the use of bar-coded sponges led to increased counting time (9 minutes vs. 12 minutes per case), their use also led to an increase in the detection of a discrepant count.[27]

RF technology has shown excellent diagnostic accuracy in cadaver[28,29] and preliminary human studies,[30] with a detection rate of 100%. However, before wide adoption of RF sponges, cost-effectiveness analyses in addition to randomized, controlled trials are needed to justify the increased cost. Even with preliminary data showing excellent results, it is still possible to miss retained sponges by scanning incorrectly or scanning too early before all sponges have been used.[29] In addition, the Food and Drug Administration (FDA) has pointed out the potential risk for RF technology interfering with other electronic medical devices, such as pacemakers and implantable cardioverter–defibrillators (ICDs).[31]

The use of routine postoperative x-rays, although expensive, was shown to have found 59% of RSI detected, all in patients with a correctly reported count. Unfortunately, x-ray imaging alone is not sufficient to capture all cases of RSI, as the foreign body was not detected in 6 out of 18 patients in this same study. Reasons that x-ray imaging may not be successful, as suggested by the authors, included poor image quality, multiple foreign objects in the field, and failure to communicate the reason for obtaining the image to the radiologist.[23] In addition, there is evidence that performing routine intraoperative x-rays would not be cost-effective. One cost-effective study showed that even if we assume that x-rays have 100% sensitivity for the detection of sponges, the cost of preventing one retained surgical sponge would be >$1.3 million per sponge.[32]

Although the occurrence of RSI is uncommon, it can have a devastating impact on the patient and health care provider alike. New methods are currently under development to serve as an adjunct to the surgical count, but no method has yet proven to be without its disadvantages. Making RSI truly a "never event" while operating under a realistic budget may prove to be a formidable challenge. In spite of its faults, it is important to take the surgical count seriously and not allow one's ego to stand in the way of providing safe surgery.

Wrong-Site Surgery, Time Outs, and Checklists

Wrong-site surgery (WSS) deeply resonates with patients, the public, the media, and other health care providers as an adverse event for which there is simply no excuse.

These events have been written about in the lay press in addition to top medical journals. Surgery performed on the wrong body part, surgery performed on the wrong patient, and wrong surgical procedure performed on a patient are all surgical never events as defined by the NQF. These types of events are typically categorized together as wrong-site surgeries since they share common root causes and prevention interventions.

Although the true incidence of WSS is difficult to measure, these adverse events accounted for 13% (928/6994) of reported sentinel events to the Joint Commission from 2004 to 2012.[33] In 2011, Kaiser Health News reported that the Joint Commission officials estimated that WSS occurs 40 times each week in US hospitals and clinics.[34] Studies using data from malpractice insurers and surveys show wide variations in the estimated incidence, particularly between spine surgeries and other sites.[35–39] Even though there have been several interventions and initiatives to prevent WSS, the incidence seems to be increasing. It is unclear if this is related to a true increase or improved event reporting.[33]

There are several factors that contribute to WSS events. These factors can be categorized into human factors, patient factors, procedure factors, and system factors.[40] Once the decision is made to perform an operation, the complexities of the process to get that patient into the operating room and start surgery provide several layers at risk for errors to be made that could lead to a WSS.[41] The Joint Commission Center for Transforming Healthcare identified 29 main causes of WSS throughout the preoperative surgical continuum, which included scheduling ($n = 4$), pre-op holding ($n = 12$), operating room ($n = 8$), and organization culture ($n = 5$).[42] The Joint Commission additionally reported in 2012 that of 879 cases of WSS, the 3 most common root causes were related to leadership, communication, and human factors.[43]

In 2003, the Joint Commission introduced Universal Protocol (UP) for prevention of WSS. UP included a briefing (occurs immediately upon patient arrival into the operating room) and time out (occurs after the patient is prepped and draped and prior to incision), which emphasized preoperative verifications, site marking, and other standardized confirmations.[44] Shortly after being introduced, UP was mandated by the Joint Commission for hospital accreditation. The next major effort to prevent WSS was the Safe Surgery Saves Lives Initiative from the World Health Organization (WHO), which aimed to reduce the number of surgical-related deaths and complications worldwide. It is important to understand that this effort did not intend to just decrease the incidence of WSS, but all surgical-related deaths and complications. A Surgical Safety Checklist was created by multidisciplinary and interdisciplinary groups with the hypothesis that improved team communication and consistency of care would reduce complications and deaths related to surgery.[45] After being studied in a wide range of hospital practice environments worldwide, use of the WHO Surgical Safety Checklist significantly decreased deaths, SSIs, unplanned reoperations, and complications.[46] These data also translated favorably to urgent operations.[47] This effort has now been expanded to surgical crisis checklists and customized checklists that are procedure specific.[48,49] Other surgical checklists have also been well tested, including the Surgical Patient Safety System (SURPASS), a multidisciplinary checklist that follows the surgical pathway from admission to discharge.[50]

The data regarding whether UP and checklist interventions have decreased the incidence of WSS are equivocal.[36,51–54] Simply introducing a surgical checklist will not necessarily make an impact unless there is training, teamwork, and engagement of the involved health care providers.[55] As stated by Dr. Martin Makary "The moral hazard of the Universal Protocol is that we rely on it in place of ourselves. Although I agree that Universal Protocol compliance is important, it is not the magic wand of Merlin."[56]

KEY POINTS

- With the exception of emergency consent, informed consent must include a discussion of treatment goals along with the potential for adverse events to occur. There are special considerations for obtaining informed consent for cognitively impaired patients, pediatric patients, patients whose primary language is not English, and unconscious patients.
- Surgical "never events" are defined by the NQF and include errors in surgical care, which are identifiable, are preventable, and have serious consequences to patients.
- Adherence to best practices can minimize the occurrence of several serious complications from invasive procedures.
- The occurrence of RSI is uncommon, but it can have a devastating impact on the patient and health care provider. Several risk factors have been identified for RSI. New methods are currently under development to serve as an adjunct to the surgical count.
- There have been significant efforts to decrease the incidence of WSS. Causes for WSS are multifactorial and related to the continuum of the perioperative process rather than just what happens in the operating room. Regular use of surgical safety checklists will hopefully decrease the incidence of WSS and other surgical complications.

ONLINE RESOURCES

1. The Joint Commission Center for Transforming Healthcare: www.centerfortransforminghealthcare.org
2. Checklists: www.projectcheck.org

REFERENCES

1. Eappen S, Lane BH, Rosenberg B, et al. Relationship between occurrence of surgical complications and hospital finances. *JAMA*. 2013;309:1599–606.
2. Cleary B. The Death of Jackson. Web blog post. *Opinionator*. The New York Times Company; 2013.
3. Irma Natanson v. John R. Kline and St. Francis Hospital and School of Nursing, Inc. 187 Kan. 186; 354 P2s 670; 1960 Kan. Lexis 398. 1960.
4. Mary Schloendorff v. Society of New York Hospital. 211 N.Y. 125, 105 NE 92. 1914.
5. Centers for Medicare and Medicaid Services. Hospital acquired condition factsheet. http://www.cms.gov/Medicare/Medicare-Fee-for-Service-Payment/HospitalAcqCond/downloads/HACFactsheet.pdf. Accessed 9/12/12.
6. Shah H, Bosch W, Thompson KM, et al. Intravascular catheter-related bloodstream infection. *Neurohospitalist*. 2013;3:144–51.
7. Maki DG, Kluger DM, Crnich CJ. The risk of bloodstream infection in adults with different intravascular devices: a systematic review of 200 published prospective studies. *Mayo Clin Proc*. 2006;81(9):1159–71.
8. O'Grady NP, et al. Guidelines for the prevention of intravascular catheter-related infections. *Am J Infect Control*. 2011;39(4 Suppl 1):S1–34.
9. Gould MK, et al. Prevention of VTE in nonorthopedic surgical patients: antithrombotic therapy and prevention of thrombosis, 9th ed: American College of Chest Physicians Evidence-Based Clinical Practice Guidelines. *Chest*. 2012;141(2 Suppl):e227S–77.
10. Horlander KT, Mannino DM, Leeper KV. Pulmonary embolism mortality in the United States, 1979-1998: an analysis using multiple-cause mortality data. *Arch Intern Med*. 2003;163(14):1711–17.

11. Geerts WH, Code KI, Jay RM, et al. A prospective study of venous thromboembolism after major trauma. *N Engl J Med.* 1994;331(24):1601–6.
12. Kaufman JA, Kinney TB, Streiff MB, et al. Guidelines for the use of retrievable and convertible vena cava filters: report from the Society of Interventional Radiology multidisciplinary consensus conference. *J Vasc Interv Radiol.* 2006;17(3):449–59.
13. Mont MA, et al. Preventing venous thromboembolic disease in patients undergoing elective hip and knee arthroplasty. *J Am Acad Orthop Surg.* 2011;19:768–76.
14. Baglin T. Defining the population in need of thromboprophylaxis—making hospitals safer. *Br J Haematol.* 2010;149:805–12.
15. Kaboli PJ, Brenner A, Dunn AS. Prevention of venous thromboembolism in medical and surgical patients. *Cleve Clin J Med.* 2005;72(Suppl 1):S7–13.
16. Frank C, Hodgetts G, Puxty J. Safety and efficacy of physical restraints for the elderly. Review of the evidence. *Can Fam Physician.* 1996;42:2402–9.
17. Oliver D, et al. Strategies to prevent falls and fractures in hospitals and care homes and effect of cognitive impairment: systematic review and meta-analyses. *BMJ.* 2007;334:82.
18. Cruse PJ, Foord R. The epidemiology of wound infection. A 10-year prospective study of 62,939 wounds. *Surg Clin North Am* 1980;60:27–40.
19. Kaiser CW, Friedman S, Spurling KP, et al. The retained surgical sponge. *Ann Surg.* 1996;224:79–84.
20. National Quality Forum. *Serious Reportable Events In Healthcare—2011 Update: A Consensus Report.* Washington, DC: Author; 2011.
21. Egorova NN, Moskowitz A, Gelijns A, et al. Managing the prevention of retained surgical instruments—what is the value of counting? *Ann Surg.* 2008;247:13–8.
22. Gawande AA, Studdert DM, Orav EJ, et al. Risk factors for retained instruments and sponges after surgery. *New Engl J Med.* 2003;348:229–35.
23. Cima RR, Kollengode A, Garnatz J, et al. Incidence and characteristics of potential and actual retained foreign object events in surgical patients. *J Am Coll Surg.* 2008;207:80–7.
24. Lincourt AE, Harrell A, Cristiano J, et al. Retained foreign bodies after surgery. *J Surg Res.* 2007;138:170–4.
25. AORN Recommended Practices Committee. Recommended practices for sponge, sharps, and instrument counts. *AORN J.* 2006;83:418, 421–6, 429–33.
26. Greenberg CC, Regenbogen SE, Lipsitz SR, et al. The frequency and significance of discrepancies in the surgical count. *Ann Surg.* 2008;248:337–41.
27. Greenberg CC, Diaz-Flores R, Lipsitz SR, et al. Bar-coding surgical sponges to improve safety—a randomized controlled trial. *Ann Surg.* 2008;247:612–6.
28. Fabian CE. Electronic tagging of surgical sponges to prevent their accidental retention. *Surgery.* 2005;137:298–301.
29. Macario A, Morris D, Morris S. Initial clinical evaluation of a handheld device for detecting retained surgical gauze sponges using radiofrequency identification technology. *Arch Surg.* 2006;141:659–62.
30. Steelman VM. Sensitivity of detection of radiofrequency surgical sponges: a prospective, cross-over study. *Am J Surg.* 2011;201:233–7.
31. Radiation-Emitting Products. U.S. Food and Drug Administration. 2013. http://www.fda.gov/Radiation-EmittingProducts/RadiationSafety/ElectromagneticCompatibilityEMC/ucm116647.htm. Accessed 6/9/14.
32. Regenbogen SE, Greenberg CC, Resch SC, et al. Prevention of retained surgical sponges: a decision-analytic model predicting relative cost-effectiveness. *Surgery.* 2009;145:527–535.
33. www.jointcommission.org/sentinel_event.aspx
34. www.kaiserhealthnews.org/stories/2011/june/21/wrong-site-surgery-errors.aspx?p=1
35. Devine J, et al. Avoiding wrong site surgery: a systematic review. *Spine.* 2010;35(9 Suppl):S28–36.
36. Kwaan MR, et al. Incidence, patterns, and prevention of wrong site surgery. *Arch Surg.* 2006;141:353–7.
37. Meinberg EG, Stern PJ. Incidence of wrong site surgery among hand surgeons. *J Bone Joint Surg Am.* 2003;85:193–7.

38. Mody MG, et al. The prevalence of wrong site surgery among spine surgeons. *Spine.* 2008;33:194–8.

39. Jhawar BS, Mitsis D, Duggal N. Wrong sided and wrong level neurosurgery: a national survey. *J Neurosurg Spine.* 2007;7:467–72.

40. Seiden SC, Barach P. Wrong side/wrong site, wrong procedure, and wrong patient adverse events: are they preventable? *Arch Surg.* 2006;141:931–9.

41. Clarke JR, et al. Wrong site surgery: can we prevent it? *Adv Surg.* 2008;42:13–31.

42. www.centerfortransforminghealthcare.org/…/CTH_wrong_site_surgery

43. www.jointcommission.org/sentinel_event_statistics/

44. www.jointcommission.org/facts_about_the_universal_protocol/

45. Weiser TG, et al. Perspectives in quality: designing the WHO surgical safety checklist. *Int J Qual Health Care.* 2010;22:365–70.

46. Haynes AB, et al. A surgical safety checklist to reduce morbidity and mortality in a global population. *N Engl J Med.* 2009;360:491–9.

47. Weiser TG, et al. Effect of a 19-item surgical safety checklist during urgent operations in a global patient population. *Ann Surg.* 2010;251:976–80.

48. Arriaga AF, et al. Simulation-based trial of surgical crisis checklists. *N Engl J Med.* 2013;368:246–53.

49. www.projectcheck.org/checklists.html

50. deVries EN, et al. Effect of a comprehensive surgical safety system on patient outcomes. *N Engl J Med.* 2010;363:1928–37.

51. Stahel PF, et al. Wrong site and wrong patient procedures in the universal protocol era: analysis of a prospective database of physician reported outcomes. *Arch Surg.* 2010;145:978–84.

52. Urbach DR, et al. Introduction of surgical safety checklists in Ontario, Canada. *N Engl J Med.* 2014;370:1029–38.

53. Mahar P, et al. Interventions for reducing wrong site surgery and invasive procedures. *Cochrane Database Syst Rev.* 2012;12:1–51.

54. Vachhani JA, Klopfenstein JD. Incidence of neurosurgical wrong site surgery before and after implementation of the universal protocol. *Neurosurgery.* 2013;72:590–5.

55. Leape LL. The checklist conundrum. *N Engl J Med.* 2014;370:1063–4.

56. Makary MA. The hazard of more reporting in quality measurement: comment on "Wrong site and wrong patient procedures in the universal protocol era." *Arch Surg.* 2010;145:984.

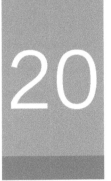

20 Establishing a Patient Safety/Quality Improvement Program in Obstetrics

Kate Mitchell and George A. Macones

CLINICAL VIGNETTE

Ms. C was a 22-year-old woman who was pregnant for the first time. At 38 weeks, 2 days gestation (determined by first trimester ultrasound), she was admitted for induction of labor for severe pre-eclampsia. At admission, Leopold measurements revealed an estimated fetal weight of 3900 g. Ms. C's pregnancy was only complicated by anemia (iron deficiency and sickle cell trait). She was induced with misoprostol and augmented with oxytocin. She progressed to complete cervical dilation. At time of delivery, the neonate was noted to show the "turtle sign," in which the neonate's head appeared retracted. The neonate subsequently had shoulder dystocia that lasted for 1.5 minutes and was relieved by the McRoberts maneuver, suprapubic pressure, and, ultimately, the Woods maneuver. Ms. C had a second-degree laceration that was repaired in layers, with the use of local anesthesia. She had an estimated blood loss of 400 mL.

The newborn's actual weight was 3245 g, and his Apgar scores at 1 and 5 minutes were 7 and 8, respectively. The newborn's cord gases were as follows: pH 7.2, pCO_2 63 mm Hg, HCO_3 22 mEq/L, and base deficit 5.5 mEq/L. The shoulder dystocia was diagnosed as left shoulder anterior. The pediatric team also noted that the newborn had an asymmetric Moro reflex (right < left) at the time of delivery. This finding suggests that a brachial plexus injury occurred. The events were disclosed to Ms. C, and a disclosure note was written and placed in the chart.

Ms. C's systolic blood pressure (BP) was 130–140 off magnesium prophylaxis, and she was discharged home on postpartum day (PPD) #2 with no additional BP medication and a follow-up appointment in 4–6 weeks.

Ms. C presented to the Pregnancy Assessment Center (PAC) on PPD#5 after her BP at home was 180/90. She had severe range BPs initially in PAC, but no neurologic symptoms and normal labs, and her BPs became normal to mild, so magnesium was not initiated. Ms. C was given nifedipine XL 30 mg to achieve BP control. She stayed overnight to ensure good BP control and was discharged on PPD#6.

- Could anything have been done prenatally to prevent the elevation in Ms. C's BP that led to her induction of labor?
- Could anything have been done immediately postpartum to prevent the readmission?

INTRODUCTION

Patient safety/quality improvement (PS/QI) in obstetrics is unique in that it not only involves the care of the pregnant mother but also must consider the safety and well-being of the fetus. The management of one patient directly affects the outcome of the other. Numerous programs have been established over the years to improve the teamwork and collaboration of all members of the care team in labor and delivery, including the obstetricians, neonatologists, anesthesiologists, and nurses.[1]

The American College of Obstetrics and Gynecology (ACOG) has been committed to PS and quality throughout the care continuum. Although inpatient issues initially took first priority in PS efforts nationwide, ambulatory PS has been given its own set of standards. In 2003, ACOG developed a set of principles and objectives that they ask all obstetrician–gynecologists to adopt in their clinical practice or hospital.

The objectives are to:

• encourage a culture of PS
• implement recommended safe medication practices
• reduce the likelihood of surgical errors
• improve communication with health care providers
• improve communication with patients
• establish a partnership with patients to improve safety
• make safety a priority in every aspect of practice[2]

Adverse Outcomes in Obstetrics and Gynecology

According to ACOG, the rate of pre-eclampsia in the US has increased 25% in the last two decades, and this hypertensive disorder is the leading cause of maternal mortality in the US and worldwide. The 2011 Child Health USA reported that the rate of maternal death related to eclampsia and pre-eclampsia was 1.5/100,000 live births, and the Centers for Disease Control and Prevention (CDC) reported that 9.9% of all pregnancy-related deaths in the US from 2006 to 2009 were due to eclampsia and pre-eclampsia. There is no clear-cut way to identify those women with pre-eclampsia who are at increased risk for adverse outcomes. Safe delivery and management of the mother and baby with pre-eclampsia depend on the appropriate management of the systolic and diastolic BPs during the prenatal, intrapartum, and postpartum periods. This involves close surveillance at each prenatal visit and aggressive treatment of the hypertension as soon as it arises. The only "cure" that exists for pre-eclampsia is delivery of the baby once all the risks to the mom and the baby have been considered.[3]

Review of the Current State/Inventory

A current state inventory is the only way to evaluate how an obstetric service is doing in terms of preventable harm, safety, and quality. This will allow the service to identify steps the PS/QI program can take to improve. The following information on outcomes of interest should be collected and evaluated: information on patient complaints, claims, serious/sentinel events, peer-review referrals from hospitals or other departments, infection control data, morbidity and mortality (M&M) cases, and quality assurance/QI criteria.

The obstetric service should next assess which of the following recommended activities are already in place:

• Peer-review committee to select M&M cases
• Analysis of events according to PS/QI criteria or trigger tools

- Event reporting system
- Medication error reporting
- Infection surveillance
- Ongoing efforts to promote a culture of PS and transparency
- Collection of staff perceptions of, and suggestions for improving, PS
- Determination of staff willingness to report errors

The department can begin its analysis of events with their PS officer and should always cooperate with and participate in any hospital event analysis processes such as debriefings and root cause analysis. By looking into how adverse events are reported and investigated, as well as into the details of the discussion, it will often be possible to find suggestions for improvements that can be extended to providers. These suggestions can only add to the understanding of the existing environment and inform the department about interventions and processes most likely to be successful (Fig. 20-1).

PS/QI Infrastructure

After determining the priorities and identifying strategies are already being implemented in the department, the challenges are to provide an infrastructure to support the collection and analysis of events and outcomes and to assure that learning points or remediation will follow from that analysis. As in any successful organization, leadership is key to setting the tone, culture, and overall PS environment for success.

Patient Safety Team

ACOG suggests that the team should include representation from each service that is affected. This guideline ensures that all important stakeholders are involved in the process of identification, discussion, and possible action for process improvement. For example, such a team would include an obstetrician, obstetrician anesthesiologist, neonatologist/pediatrician, and obstetric and pediatric nurses. Each of these representatives should have some component of leadership and technical expertise and should be involved in the day-to-day process of the clinical unit.[4]

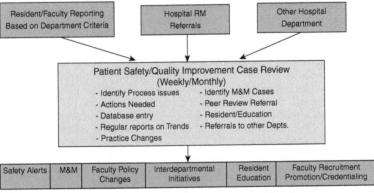

Patient Safety/Quality Improvement Process

Figure 20-1. WUSM Department of OB/GYN improvement process diagram.

Patient Safety Officer

Department leadership must identify one or two key individuals as the PS/QI team leader(s). These key staff should have special training in PS to guide the discussion of events from a mere anecdotal/reactive approach to a more global view of processes and systems. This person must be capable of doing and saying the challenging things when necessary but also of encouraging an informal way for staff to communicate concerns, problems, or errors. These individuals will hold respect within the department on a clinical and academic level as well as among peers outside of the department. The staff/individuals must be credible and nonjudgmental, and they should be comfortable asking questions in a nonaccusatory manner.[4] The PS officer will be the starting point for the PS/QI team that will form within the department and thus must be able to manage all the resources of the team involved, encourage team behavior, and sometimes help resolve team conflicts. He or she speaks for the group that is analyzing each case as well as for the department. This person will lay the groundwork for ongoing discussions on any given topic or case and set the tone for the initial discussion, analysis, and ongoing conversations that will result from identification of cases. The department leadership must support this role and be committed to fostering a safe environment in which all feel free to openly discuss adverse events, errors, and outcomes. Clear leadership has been shown to improve PS that benefits providers, staff, the medical institution, and, most importantly, the patient.[4]

Patient Safety Coordinator

Accountability is a vital piece of the PS/QI infrastructure. This includes accountability to the providers of the care, the staff that participated in the care, and the patient herself. Many safety or quality teams may include a PS coordinator to help ensure accountability. This person is a caregiver with either a clinical background or PS background who participates in the case discussion and keeps each member of the committee/team on task to ensure that identified process improvements are made. This person's primary role is to aid in the identification and implementation of interventions to decrease medical errors and enhance PS through systematic care process and outcome evaluation in the Department of OB/GYN. The PS coordinator works to encourage transparency and reporting, identifies opportunities for process improvement, acts as a liaison with hospital partners and other hospital departments, develops standards, and assesses ongoing reliability of changes made. In addition, the PS coordinator assists OB/GYN researchers in the collection and use of PS data for research purposes.

Steps to Improve PS/QI

The important steps are to determine how to identify cases of adverse events, report and discuss these cases, identify any action to take, disseminate the feedback, and, finally, educate the care providers to diminish the chance of future similar events. While there are many possible approaches to improving the safety and quality of care, we will describe some of the approaches used at the Washington University School of Medicine in St. Louis (WUSM).

Identify cases

One simple way to identify cases in which PS/QI was inadequate would be to use the already established ACOG clinical indicators.[4] Though not all-inclusive, these indicators include both maternal and neonatal criteria and can be adapted to fit any

☐ 1. Maternal Mortality

☐ 2. Maternal cardiopulmonary arrest

☐ 3. Excessive maternal blood loss (roughly >1500 mL)
Uterine artery laceration? ☐ Yes ☐ No

☐ 4. Postpartum hemorrhage (>1000 mL)

☐ 5. Stillbirth of a baby admitted alive (excluding
extreme prematurity or lethal anomalies)

☐ 6. Cord pH <7.00

☐ 7. Eclampsia

☐ 8. Evidence of unanticipated neonatal depression

☐ 9. Evidence of neonatal trauma

☐ 10. Missed or delayed diagnosis

☐ 11. Delayed or incorrect therapy

☐ 12. Unplanned postpartum return
to delivery room or OR for management

☐ 13. Delivery unattended by the "responsible
physician" (other than precipitous deliveries)

☐ 14. Base excess <−12.0

☐ 15. 5 minute apgar <3

☐ 16. Unplanned maternal
readmission within 14 days

☐ 17. Shoulder dystocia

☐ 18. Cord prolapse

☐ 19. Elective or un-indicated delivery
<39 0/7 gestational weeks

☐ 20. Other_____

(Adapted from the WUSM OB Peer Review Form.)

Figure 20-2. Triggers for review.

particular OB setting. Department leadership and the PS/QI team need to encourage ongoing reporting of cases that meet agreed-upon ACOG PS and quality criteria. This can be through the chief resident managing labor and delivery in an academic setting, through the PS coordinator, or through the team leader. Figure 20-2 lists triggers for case review in obstetrics utilized at the Washington University School of Medicine in St. Louis (WUSM).

Report and discuss cases
As part of establishing criteria for reporting, attention must be paid to creating a culture that supports reporting. Cases may be reported by attendings, residents, nursing staff, and, sometimes, managers. At many hospitals, residents, faculty, and staff can report any case voluntarily through online Event Reporting Systems (ERS). The ERS is kept confidential and reviewed within the department. The case may be brought to the team members for discussion. Input can also be from hospital partners and other hospital departments. Should the hospital or other department see a PS or process issue, it may be brought to the attention of the PS/QI team within the department. Transparency and reporting should be encouraged to identify opportunities to improve processes and communication with other hospital partners and departments.

If a case meets the agreed-upon criteria, then the identified QI leadership or the department leadership will determine the venue in which it will be discussed. Options include M&M, section/divisional meetings, and root cause analysis meetings. Some groups establish a multidisciplinary committee to conduct a weekly case review. This includes input and discussion from maternal–fetal medicine attendings, OB attendings, neonatal intensive care unit (NICU) attendings, OB anesthesiology attendings, PS, and nursing leadership.

The PS/QI team provides ongoing support and encouragement for disclosure and increased transparency. Joint Commission requires that patients be made aware of any unanticipated adverse event that may have taken place while they are under the care of an MD.[5] Thus, MDs have an ethical obligation to communicate in an open and honest way. Studies have shown that when something unexpected happens, patients expect and want to know about it, and they want someone to take responsibility for what happened to them. Much support is available for MDs to seek help in communication of adverse events. Disclosure will only help to increase the transparency of a department and encourage ongoing PS/QI.

Identify actions to take

During case review, all involved are able to make suggestions to improve PS. This review focuses on the department rather than the individual. Although the feedback might be directed to an individual, all are able to learn what might be done differently the next time.

Often, there will be a need to refer a case review to other areas. This can mean referring to another division within our own department, another department that may have participated in the care of the patient, or even to our hospital partners. Each referral that is sent is meant to encourage ongoing teamwork with all those involved in the care of the patient and to increase the transparency across the organization. Referrals are meant to be nonaccusatory, instead helping to bridge a connection between departments across the care continuum. Referrals are sent with the expectation of ongoing dialogue and conversation between all those involved. Oftentimes, the response that is received will require further information/clarification or lead to additional problem solving.

Disseminate feedback

Most health care errors occur as a result of a system, not just one individual.[6] Thus, outputs from case review and discussion need to be clear and concise to encourage ongoing, uninhibited, and unobstructed reporting as well as education and process improvement. Several approaches may be used to ensure that those who actually participate in the day-to-day care of the patients on the inpatient unit learn the information covered in the case review sessions.

Patient Safety Alerts

Patient safety alerts send information to all residents, attendings, and nursing staff. These alerts, delivered via e-mail, are simple, short, and not provider-specific. They convey a simple message such as a reminder about an existing protocol or a clinical technique. In this way, all can learn from the case.

Direct Communication to the MD Involved in the Care of a Particular Patient

Direct communication to the MD involved in the care of a particular patient should come directly from the MD responsible for being the team leader. This communication should be nonconfrontational, not accusatory, and meant to serve as a teaching point going forward. If the team leader thinks there is an issue with an individual MD, it should be referred directly to the chairman.

Educational Lectures or Continuing Education Conferences

Educational lectures or continuing education conferences are good ways to disseminate information to caretakers. For example, if a new process is being implemented for triage of patients in the emergency department, all attendings, residents, and nursing staff in each department will need to know about it. This may require more than one occasion for education and include more than one department. For instance, a presentation can be made at departmental grand rounds or at resident teaching conference. Importantly, information must be conveyed consistently to as many caregivers as possible. The education is meant to focus on the process change and implementation and to allow those that will be working the process to have a voice in the implementation; this may happen with just one encounter or may need ongoing feedback for success. The challenge continues to be how information that is presented at a certain time and place is passed along to those residents who are working through the levels.

Ongoing education

Educational opportunities must be identified to help raise the baseline of the PS literacy of the department. The more that physicians and staff understand the overall climate of the department and the motivation behind the case review and discussion, the easier it will be to create a more open and accepting culture for PS/QI. The goal should be to create an atmosphere of transparency without fear of shame or blame, make the reporting of adverse events an easy process, and convey the commitment to learning and continuous improvement.[4] A transparent process will help create a culture that supports reporting and discussion of cases; this will create an environment that is safer for both patients and caretakers.

Joint Commission has stated that most perinatal adverse outcomes usually result from lack of teamwork and effective communication. They recommend team training to help staff work together and communicate more effectively.[7] One form of education that has demonstrated improvement in maternal and neonatal outcomes is simulation of routine and emergency situations. Simulations can both address clinical education and improve the level of PS learning in a department. These simulations can provide both the technical skills that the residents need and the communication skills that are often necessary in situations that arise in obstetrics. There are many options for simulation programs to best fit the department, and they can be designed to meet the previously identified needs and levels of medical education.[8] Typically, simulations will include all members of the OB care team—OB, Neonatology, Anesthesiology, and Nursing—working together to solve the clinical problem that arises. These simulations focus not just on the clinical aspect of care but also on the essential communication and teamwork.

KEY POINTS
- By encouraging a culture of PS, the environment can change and improve the health and outcomes of women in the obstetric setting.
- By working toward the reduction and identification of errors, we are making a safer environment for our patients.
- By improving communication among the health care team, we can make our environment safer for patients and providers.
- By establishing a PS program in obstetrics, the department will create a culture that is looking out for the safety and well-being of both patients and the health care team.

ONLINE RESOURCES
1. Child Health USA 2011: http://mchb.hrsa.gov/chusa11/hstat/hsi/pages/208mm.html
2. World Health Organization: http://www.who.int/en/
3. American College of Obstetrics and Gynecology: http://www.acog.org
4. Preeclampsia Foundation: http://www.preeclampsi.org

REFERENCES

1. Collaboration between Obstetricians and Neonatologist. Perinatal safety programs and improved clinical outcomes. *Clin Perinatol.* 2010;37:179–88.
2. American College of Obstetrics and Gynecology. Patient safety in obstetrics and gynecology. ACOG committee opinion No. 447. *Obstet Gynecol.* 2009;114:1424–7.
3. American College of Obstetricians and Gynecologists, issuing body. *Hypertension, Pregnancy-Induced—Practice Guideline.* Author.
4. The American College of Obstetrics and Gynecology, Women's Health Care Physicians. *Quality and Safety in Women's Health Care. Committee on Patient Safety and Quality Improvement.* 2nd ed. Washington, DC: American College of Obstetrics and Gynecology; 2010.
5. American College of Obstetrics and Gynecology. Disclosure and discussion of adverse events. ACOG committee opinion. *Obstet Gynecol.* 2012;119(3):686–9.
6. Mulligan MA, Nechodom P. Errors and analysis of errors. *Clin Obstet Gynecol.* 2008;51(4): 656–65.
7. The Joint Commission. *Preventing Infant Death and Injury during Delivery. Sentinel Event Alert Issue No. 30.* Oakbrook Terrace, IL: JC; 2004. http://www.jointcommission.org/sentinel_event_alert_issue_30_preventing_infant_death_and_injury_during_delivery/. Retrieved February 6, 2014.
8. Birsner ML, Satin AJ. Developing a program, a curriculum, a scenario. *Sem Perinatol.* 2013;37:175–8.

21 Patient Safety and Quality Improvement in Anesthesia

Andrea Vannucci, Laura F. Cavallone, and Ivan Kangrga

CLINICAL VIGNETTE

Mr. P was a 75-year-old gentleman with a history of smoking, hypertension, and coronary artery disease who came to the hospital for a left neck dissection. A few months earlier, he had undergone a resection of the floor of the mouth and right neck dissection because of oral cancer. That operation was followed by radiation therapy that couldn't stop the progression of the disease.

On the day of this second surgery, Dr. A, the anesthesiologist, observed the patient to have limited mouth opening and neck rigidity, likely secondary to fibrosis of soft tissues caused by the radiation treatment. Concerned by the possibility of difficult mask ventilation and laryngoscopy, Dr. A decided to proceed with a fiberoptic intubation while maintaining the spontaneous ventilation of the patient. The intubation was performed successfully and without complications.

Before the end of the surgery, a junior anesthesiologist, Dr. Z, took over the case from Dr. A. Dr. Z was informed that the intubation went "smoothly," although, in the handoff, there was no mention of the fiberoptic approach. Reassured by the report of uncomplicated intubation, at the request of the senior surgeon, Dr. Z agreed to extubate the patient "deep." This was meant to avoid "coughing and bucking" at emergence, which could cause bleeding from the surgical site. After assessing full reversal of neuromuscular blockade, Dr. Z inserted a lubricated airway into the left nose hoping that this device would help the patient maintain the patency of the upper airways after extubation. Then, Dr. Z removed the endotracheal tube from the other nostril. This maneuver caused profuse nasal bleeding, and the partially obtunded patient aspirated blood in the airway. Immediately thereafter, Mr. P became unable to ventilate and his oxygen saturation dropped. Dr. Z's attempts of mask ventilation and reintubation under direct laryngoscopy failed because of the ongoing bleeding and patient's very limited mouth opening. The patient had a hypoxic cardiocirculatory arrest, and the surgeon was then forced to perform an emergent cricothyrotomy that was challenging because of the extensive neck fibrosis. Mr. P's oxygenation remained inadequate for more than 10 minutes, resulting in hypoxic brain injury and myocardial ischemia. The patient was resuscitated and then admitted to an intensive care unit (ICU). One week later, Mr. P had not regained consciousness and the ICU physicians, after consulting with Mr. P's family, decided to withdraw care.

INTRODUCTION

The vignette illustrates several crucial elements of a safe anesthetic management: a thorough and updated preoperative assessment, an anesthetic plan that takes into consideration the individual characteristics of patients and surgical procedures, competence in using advanced equipment to manage difficult airways both at induction and at emergence from anesthesia, and the ability to maintain situation awareness and effective communication with all team members.

What steps of the anesthetic management could have helped in preventing the unfolding of the adverse events illustrated in the vignette?

Patient Assessment and Plan

Reviewing the patient's treatment history and physical signs, such as his limited mouth opening, properly alerted the first anesthesiologist of possible difficulties both with intubation and face mask ventilation. This recognition prompted a fiberoptic intubation while the patient's spontaneous ventilation was maintained. In fact, the two main factors contributing to difficult airway management following head and neck radiation therapy are intense neck rigidity due to fibrosis and the presence of chronic airway edema.

Advanced Airway Management

Had Dr. Z fully realized the challenges posed by the airway, he could have planned a staged extubation using an airway exchange catheter (AEC). The AEC is a thin, hollow rubber tube that can be used in an emergency situation either to deliver oxygen via a Luer Lock connector or to attempt some form of ventilation through an Ambu bag with a standard endotracheal tube adapter. The AEC can also be used as a guide to reintubate the patient. In this case, the AEC should be inserted in the endotracheal tube before extubation. The endotracheal tube would then be removed while leaving the AEC in the airway. This is generally well tolerated even by awake, spontaneously breathing patients and can be left in place safely for hours. Extubation of the difficult airway is a very challenging, but often neglected, step of the anesthesia care.[1]

Communication and Situation Awareness

Unfortunately, Dr. A forgot to explain his reasoning in using the flexible bronchoscope to his junior colleague. Consequently, Dr. Z did not take in adequate consideration the perils of a "deep" extubation in a patient with abnormal airway anatomy. In addition, it is very likely that the hierarchy gradient between Dr. Z and the senior surgeon may have played a role in this unfortunate outcome. The "senior" surgeon requested a "deep extubation" for good reasons: "bucking" and "fighting" the ventilator may have indeed increased the risk of bleeding from a neck surgical site. Still, a senior anesthesiologist would have likely anticipated the complications that may have followed a deep extubation in a patient with difficult airways and would have been confident enough to remind the surgeon that a "deep" extubation is safe only in patients with "easy" airways. On the contrary, "junior" anesthesiologists may be reluctant to object to the requests of senior surgeons for the fear of appearing inadequate or lacking self-confidence. This type of communication issue is widely recognized, and the accepted remedy is the development of an organizational culture where all members of the team, regardless of their hierarchical status, feel safe to speak up if they perceive that a dangerous situation is emerging.

The goal of this chapter is to review how anesthesiologists have come to identify threats to patient safety in their field of activities and have been able to develop effective strategies to prevent or mitigate patient harm (Table 21-1). In addition, we will

TABLE 21-1	Technical and Organizational Improvements Supporting Patient Safety in Anesthesia Practice

Category	Items
Medication safety	• Syringe labeling and color coding • Prefilled syringes • Standardization of drug concentration • Infusion pumps with IV medication error prevention software that alerts operators when a pump setting is programmed outside of preconfigured limits • Drug antagonists: naloxone, flumazenil, and sugammadex
Equipment	• Pin Index Safety System (cylinder) and Diameter Index Safety System (pipelines) gas connections to prevent gas crossovers and substitution • Color coding of oxygen and other medical gases • Oxygen pressure failure devices to prevent delivering hypoxic gas mixtures • Oxygen and other gas analyzers
Monitors	• Pulse oximetry • Capnography • Nerve stimulators to monitor neuromuscular block
Devices to assist with difficult airways	• Fiberscope, laryngeal masks, and video laryngoscopes • AECs
Development and implementation of clinical and administrative standards	• Clinical guidelines and practice parameters by ASA and other professional societies
Advanced practices	• Locoregional anesthesia in obstetrics • Transesophageal echocardiography (TEE) in cardiac surgery • Ultrasound-guided locoregional anesthesia • Ultrasound-guided vascular access • Clinical simulation
Cognitive aids	• World Health Organization Surgical Checklist • Guidelines for preanesthesia checkout • Malignant hyperthermia treatment protocol • Anesthesia information management systems with decision support
Ongoing developments	• Large database collection and analysis • Bar code scanner technology with read-back capacity for drugs and blood product administration • Nontechnical skills training

discuss emerging patient safety concerns for those undergoing anesthesia in this era characterized by increased medical knowledge and enhanced technologies but also by the necessity of containing health care costs.

PATIENT SAFETY IN ANESTHESIA

For the purposes of this chapter, patient safety in anesthesia can be defined as the prevention of unnecessary patient harm resulting from anesthesia care.

Historically, the field of anesthesia has pioneered patient safety and quality in health care. The fact that anesthesia is risky and not inherently therapeutic has been recognized by caregivers for a long time.[2] From the very beginning of the specialty this awareness has led the anesthesiology community to focus their clinical attention and research efforts toward prevention of anesthesia-related mortality and complications. Interestingly, anesthesiologists most likely contributed to the field the very term "patient safety." A PubMed search reveals that the two words appear joined for the first time in the title of an article published in 1960 by Dr. Kreul, a leading anesthesiologist from Wisconsin, who was arguing in favor of using locoregional instead of general anesthesia for obstetric procedures.[3] In 1978, Cooper published a seminal paper examining human error and equipment failure in anesthesia practice. He discovered that 82% of preventable adverse events were due to human error.[4] The errors were often due to issues with equipment and supplies, providers' overall inexperience, unfamiliarity with the equipment/device, haste, inattention, fatigue, poor communication, and inadequate training. This early work set the groundwork for future innovation in anesthesia safety and quality. The initial focus was mainly on mortality; then, the interest extended to a progressively larger and articulated category of adverse events, such as central and peripheral nervous system injuries, acute liver failure, perioperative myocardial ischemia and cardiac arrest, respiratory failure, and allergic reactions.

This clinical and research effort was nurtured and structured by the establishment of the American Society of Anesthesiology Closed Claim Project in 1984 and of the Anesthesia Patient Safety Foundation (APSF) in 1985. The goals of the Closed Claims Project have been to identify "major areas of loss, patterns of injury, and strategies for prevention" through an in-depth investigation of closed anesthesia malpractice claims.[5] The APSF's mission is to continually improve the safety of anesthesia by promoting research, education, and patient safety campaigns.[6] Its main communication tool is a newsletter distributed quarterly online and in paper copies. Both organizations have supported acquisition and dissemination of knowledge in patient safety and its translation into everyday clinical practice.

Adverse Outcomes in Anesthesia

Cases of anesthesia-related death have been reported since 1847, only a few months after William Morton, a dentist in Boston, first demonstrated the possibility of inducing general anesthesia with diethyl ether in surgical patients.[7] This event is considered by most historians as the starting date of the modern practice of anesthesia, even if it is now established that ether had already been used since 1842 by two other physicians, William E. Clarke and Crawford W. Long, who missed to timely report their experiences with this inhalational agent. In those early times of the specialty, most fatalities were related to the use of ether, chloroform (discovered in 1847 by the Scottish obstetrician James Young Simpson), and other inhalational agents. In the years following World War II, Beecher and Todd performed the first systematic investigation of anesthesia-related mortality. Their study showed that in highly respected American academic institutions, anesthesia mortality was 64 deaths for 100,000 procedures and that patients receiving curare would die at the much higher rate of 1:370 versus 1:2100 in those who were not paralyzed.[2] Since then, improved understanding of cardiovascular and respiratory physiology; development of safer anesthetic agents, equipment, and monitors; and standardization of clinical care have produced a steady decline in perioperative and anesthetic-related mortality (Table 21-1).

According to a recent review, anesthetic mortality decreased in developed countries from 36 deaths every 100,000 procedures before the 1970s to 34 deaths per 100,000 procedures in the 1990s–2000s and, in developing countries, from 1 death every 100 procedure to 1 death every 1000 procedures over the same time interval, notwithstanding the larger number of surgeries performed on more compromised patients.[7]

Still, when data related to 30- or 60-day outcomes are available (allowing to account for anesthesia risk, but even more for surgical and medical risk), it appears that postoperative mortality is still a very significant burden. A recent study conducted in Europe[8] showed that up to 4% of patients die within 60 days from their initial surgery, and similar results were reported in the US.[9] Interestingly, in the above mentioned European study, even after adjustment for confounding variables, crude mortality rates varied widely between countries (from 1.2% for Iceland to 21.5% for Latvia). This large discrepancy in the observed perioperative mortality[8] suggests that models of hospital care, staffing, and overall national medical practices of health care delivery may have a role in determining patient outcomes. This interpretation of the results of the study calls for the implementation of improvement projects to impact directly on the most important perioperative outcomes: patient morbidity and mortality.

Along with mortality, anesthesia can be associated with multiple complications. In anesthesiology, airway and respiratory issues, cardiovascular complications, drug-related events, and neurologic injuries account for the most severe adverse outcomes, together with procedure-related complications and equipment failure.[10,11] Patients at particular risk of severe anesthesia-related complications are those with significant comorbidities (as captured by the American Society of Anesthesiology physical status score), those in the extremes of age, pregnant women, patients undergoing monitored anesthesia care in remote locations, and patients receiving procedures for chronic pain.[10–12] More recently, new issues have been taken under growing consideration including long-term cardiac morbidity and mortality, delirium, postoperative cognitive dysfunction, awareness, chronic pain after surgery, patient satisfaction with the perioperative experience, and other parameters assessing patient outcomes.[13]

Emerging research is focusing on the possibility of long-term unfavorable outcomes secondary to the administration of anesthesia and to perioperative management. Ongoing developments in this area may have a significant impact on the way patient safety in anesthesia will be approached in the near future.

Over the last few years, the attention of researchers and of the general public has been directed toward the possibility that general anesthesia may cause brain damage. One concern is that, in young children, anesthesia-related neurotoxicity may cause neuroapoptosis and impairment of developmental processes such as neurogenesis and synaptogenesis possibly leading to long-lasting behavioral and learning deficits, severe enough to impair future achievements throughout the entire course of life.[14] In senior patients, serious consequences may be delirium and postoperative cognitive dysfunction. Both delirium and postoperative cognitive dysfunction may be secondary to the inflammatory response induced by major surgical procedures and are associated with longer hospital stay and increased mortality.

Besides cognitive issues, the concept that anesthesia care may influence patient outcome far beyond hospital discharge is recurring in other clinical areas: In 1996, Mangano[15] reported that in-hospital administration of atenolol was associated with decreased overall and cardiac mortality after noncardiac surgery for up to two years. Today, the results of that study (as well as the optimal perioperative use of β-blockers) are considered quite controversial, but the hypothesis that perioperative management may have an impact on long-term outcomes still appears plausible. Also debated are the hypotheses that intraoperative blood transfusions may increase cancer recurrence rate and that the use of locoregional anesthesia may instead have a preventive effect on the development of tumor metastases.[16,17]

Ongoing Safety Issues in Anesthesia: Equipment Failures and Drug Errors

Another current concern is that safety issues with anesthesia equipment and drug administration are still prevalent, notwithstanding the many technologic improvements that have been obtained in these areas. Actually, some of the present problems with anesthesia machines are the "flip side" of the evolution of the technology. Closed-circuit anesthesia machines and ventilators have grown more powerful but also more complex, because of the many components and the computer-driven controls. It is of essence that anesthesia providers gain familiarity with all anesthesia machines in their practice, as they may differ in specific preuse checkout, modality of use, and maintenance. The American Society of Anesthesiology has made available a very useful library of machine-specific preuse checklists.[18]

External infusion pumps have also been involved in patient safety events. These medical devices deliver fluids and drugs to patients at a controlled rate, thereby reducing medication errors and improving patient care. Unfortunately, because of either mechanical or software issues, problems of over- or underinfusion are common, leading to erroneous, missed, or delayed treatments.[19] The U.S. Food and Drug Administration has recently noticed an increasing number and severity of recalls involving infusion pumps. Recognizing that currently none of the available devices is completely safe, the Food and Drug Administration is promoting strategies to help reduce pump-related risk due to design deficiencies or software errors and supporting the development of effective premarket tests for these devices.

Medication errors are a recognized and relatively common cause of anesthetic morbidity and mortality. The rate of drug administration errors is estimated around 1 case for every 133 anesthetics.[20] The most reported errors are incorrect doses and drug substitutions. These errors are so prevalent because anesthesia providers commonly prescribe, draw, and administer drugs directly to patients without additional controls or intermediate steps that may help to catch errors. As suggested in 2010 by APSF, preventative strategies should be multimodal and include standardization. In particular, the following strategies have been proposed and are increasingly adopted: standardization of drugs' concentration, administration through infusion devices containing a drug library with preset dose ranges (although, as discussed above, there may be issues with diffusion devices as well; therefore, vigilance is always imperative), use of labels including standardized abbreviations and tall man lettering (e.g., writing part of a drug's name in uppercase letters to highlight the dissimilar letters in two soundalike, look-alike drugs, thereby helping providers to distinguish between the two), adoption of advanced technology (bar code readers with read-back capability), pharmacy/prefilled/premixed drugs, standardization of anesthesia carts within institutions, and safety culture (reporting, cooperation).[21]

Finally, over the last few years, drug shortages have emerged as a new and significant problem affecting patient safety in the perioperative environment. Medication shortages are defined as "the lack of available supply that results in a change in the way the medication is prepared by the pharmacy, or as the need to change patient management, requiring prescribers to select a therapeutic alternative."[22] Medication shortage often involves intravenous drugs; as a result, the way anesthesia is practiced is frequently affected, and hundreds of errors attributed to medication shortages are reported annually despite the fact that hospital pharmacists have developed increasing experience and competence in managing these situations. The American Society of Health-Systems Pharmacists website[23] provides a web page where it is possible to find a list of current and resolved drug shortages, as well as policies and best practices to deal with these challenges when they occur.

QUALITY IMPROVEMENT IN ANESTHESIA

In the practice of anesthesia, while patient safety and quality of care are closely related, it is difficult to find major outcome measures that are sensitive enough to the quality of care delivery.[24,25] For example, mortality is currently so rare that it has become a poor quality indicator. Even medical complications are not linearly related to quality of anesthesia care, as these unwanted perioperative outcomes are frequently secondary to patient and surgical factors.

In the US, the Centers for Medicare and Medicaid Services (CMS), in an effort to assess and monitor quality of care, has launched the Physician Quality Reporting System (PQRS), a reporting program that uses a combination of incentive payments and payment adjustments to encourage health care professionals to report on specific quality measures.[26]

In 2015, most anesthesia eligible providers (EPs) are required by CMS to report nine measures related to three National Quality Strategy domains. These domains include Patient and Family Engagement, Patient Safety, Care Coordination, Population and Public Health, Efficient Use of Health Care Resources, and Clinical Processes/Effectiveness.

While most EPs can identify and report quality measures specific of their practice settings, "traditional" measures for physician anesthesiologists include the following: preoperative β-blocker in patients with isolated coronary artery bypass graft surgery; prevention of catheter-related bloodstream infections; and perioperative temperature management.

The Anesthesia Quality Institute has recently proposed the definition and the adoption of comprehensive and specific sets of indicators to assess intraoperative, postoperative, and postrecovery patient safety and quality of care outcomes (Figs. 21-1 to 21-3) and is developing a process to systematically collect comprehensive data at a national level.

The goal of this initiative is to overcome two of the historical difficulties that have so far prevented consistent and accurate measurements of the risk of anesthesia and of the impact of complications on patient outcomes: the absence of (1) unequivocal definitions of anesthesia-related mortality and morbidity and (2) adequate and reliable population data.

In fact, until recently, comprehensive national data have not been systematically collected in most countries, with the possible exception of Australia and New Zealand. Most of the currently accepted knowledge on the safety of anesthesia is based

Anesthesia Quality Improvement Intra-Operative

Case Info		Anesthesia type	
Date		Provider ID	
MR #		CRNA ID	
ASA Class		Additional provider	

NO UNTOWARD EVENT		Death (Excludes ASA 6 patients presenting for harvesting)	

Case Cancelled		Unplanned ICU Admission		Operation on incorrect site	
Case Delayed		Unplanned admission of outpatient		Operation on incorrect patient	
Incorrect procedure					

Pulmonary Edema		Cardiac Arrest		Bronchospasm req treatment	
Hypotension requiring unanticipated therapy with a continuous infusion or pressor agents		New PVC's, bradycardia, atrial fibrillation, or other dysrhythmias requiring unanticipated therapy		Myocardial ischemia, indicated by ST segment changes or echocardiography	

Unanticipated difficult airway		Unplanned reintubation		Aspiration	
Inability to secure an airway		Unplanned respiratory arrest		Laryngospasm	

Anaphylaxis		Transfusion Reaction		Delayed emergence	
Other unanticipated adverse reaction to medication		Use of sedation/narcotic reversal agents		Inability to reverse neuromuscular blockade	
Malignant Hyperthermia		Medication error			

High spinal		Failed regional anesthetic		Unintended dural puncture	
Vascular access complication - vessel injury		Vascular access complication - pneumothorax		Local anesthesia systemic toxicity	

Seizure		Surgical fire		Position injury	
Equipment failure		Burn injury		Fall from OR table	
Equipment unavailability		Unanticipated transfusion >10 units of any blood products		Activation of Code Call/Stat Page /Rapid Response Team	

PQRS/SCIP Documentation					
Antibiotics		Central Line Bundle		β-blocker continuation	
Normothermia				DVT prophylaxis	
If other, please describe:					

Figure 21-1. Anesthesia Quality Indicators Capture Sheet (Intraoperative). (From National Quality Institute. Quality Measurements Tools. Available at: http://www.aqihq.org/files/AQI_Clincical_Outcomes_Data_Capture_Sheet_Intraop.docx. Accessibility verified December 5, 2015.)

on the extrapolation of results of investigations performed on relatively small numbers of patients, with data frequently collected over limited periods of time, and in specific geographic locations, thus limiting an exact understanding of incidence and mechanisms of complications. In the near future, more information and insight will be provided by large registries of anesthesia cases.

Table 21-2 provides a recent illustration of the relevant information on complications and anesthesia-related deaths that is currently collected almost in real time and analyzed by the Anesthesia Quality Institute. Since its inception in 2010, the National Anesthesia Clinical Outcomes Registry (NACOR) has collected information about administration and outcome of anesthesia care for more than 32 million of cases (and currently captures 25% of all anesthesia cases performed in the US).

Anesthesia Quality Improvement PACU Discharge

Case Info		Anesthesia type	
Date		Provider ID	
MR #		CRNA ID	
ASA Class		Additional provider	

	Yes	No
Patient is awake and able to contribute to assessment		

Patient Physical Exam:	Yes	No	Pain Score (10-point VAS scale):		
Mental Status at baseline (Y/N)			on PACU admission		
Vital Signs at baseline (Y/N)			Highest pain score		
Airway patency at baseline (Y/N)			Pain score at time of assessment		
Nausea or vomiting requiring treatment			Any occurrence of vomiting		

Did the patient experience an unexpected event during perioperative care?	Yes	No		Yes	No
Unplanned ICU admission			Anaphylaxis		
Unplanned hospital admission			Other medication reaction		
Intraoperative awareness			Delayed emergence		
Epidural hematoma			Respiratory arrest		
Peripheral neurologic deficit			Reintubation		
Corneal abrasion			Dental trauma		
Agitation requiring treatment			Aspiration		
Seizure			Cardiac arrest		
Uncontrolled blood sugar (high or low)			Hypotension requiring treatment		
Subcutaneous emphysema			Unplanned transfusion		
Vascular access complication			Unplanned return to OR		
Pulmonary Edema			Death		
Prolonged PACU stay - patient condition			Prolonged PACU stay - unrelated to patient condition		
New PVC's, bradycardia, arterial fibrillation, or other dysrhythmias requiring treatment			Use of sedation/narcotic reversal agent		
If other, please specify:					

Figure 21-2. Anesthesia Quality Indicators Capture Sheet (PACU Discharge). (From National Quality Institute. Quality Measurements Tools. Available at: http://www.aqihq.org/files/AQI_Clincical_Outcomes_Data_Capture_Sheet_PACU_Discharge.docx. Accessibility verified December 5, 2015.)

This unprecedented and capillary acquisition of electronic information is made possible by the connection with billing systems, quality management systems, and hospital and anesthesia health records[26] of many institutions and anesthesia practices. A current limitation is that the system is not yet set to collect 30-day or 1-year outcomes, thereby missing the opportunity to gain insight on longer-term clinical consequences of anesthesia.

A meaningful example of the unique information that researchers and administrators can gain from the exploration of large databases is provided by the two following studies.

In 2009, Kheterpal reviewed the electronic record of more than 50,000 anesthesia records and was able to estimate that the rate of impossible mask ventilation following induction of anesthesia is 0.15%. This situation poses a significant threat to anesthetized patients, when they have lost the capacity to ventilate following the administration of induction drugs and the anesthesia provider is unable to ventilate

Anesthesia Post-PACU patient assessment

Case Info			Anesthesia type	
Date			Provider ID	
MR #			CRNA ID	
ASA Class			Additional provider	

	QUALITY RATING					
	Strongly Positive	Somewhat	Neutral	Somewhat Negative	Strongly Negative	Don't Know
How satisfied were you with your anesthetic care?						
How likely are you to recommend the facility, personnel and anesthetic technique that you just underwent?						
After you left the recovery room or returned home...						
Did you experience nausea?	Yes	No				
Did you vomit at any time?	Yes	No				
How would you rate your pain on a scale of 1-10? (1 – no pain at all, 10 – worst pain ever						
Has your pain medicine been effective	Yes	No				
Did you experience any unexpected events related to your procedure or the anesthetic?	Yes	No				
If so, please explain...						

Figure 21-3. Patient Satisfaction Capture Sheet (Postrecovery). (From National Quality Institute. Quality Measurements Tools. Available at: http://www.aqihq.org/files/AQI_Clincical_Outcomes_Data_Capture_Sheet_PACU_Discharge.docx. Accessibility verified 12/5/15.)

TABLE 21-2	National Anesthesia Clinical Outcomes Registry		
Category	**Subcategory**	**N**	**%***
Major	Anaphylaxis	127	0.0103
	Awareness	134	0.0097
	Central nervous system (CNS) injury	282	0.0183
	Hemodynamic instability	1414	0.0769
	Infection	48	0.0205
	Malignant hyperthermia	11	0.0015
	Medication error	29,060	2.4622
			(Continued)

| TABLE 21-2 | National Anesthesia Clinical Outcomes Registry (Continued) |

Category	Subcategory	N	%*
	Patient wrong, site, fall, burn	58	0.0053
	Peripheral nerve injury	175	0.0151
	Respiratory	2134	0.1176
	Resuscitation	2198	0.263
	Spinal/epidural/nerve block	75	0.0058
	Upgrade of care	4554	0.2756
	Vascular access	227	0.0159
	Visual loss	10	0.004
	Total events	40,507	3.3017
Minor	Airway/intubation	4493	0.286
	Any postoperative nausea and vomiting	144,141	9.6597
	Blood—vascular	154	0.0358
	Central line/IV problem	196	0.0315
	Dental/oral/tooth/mouth	790	0.0428
	Dural/wet/headache	580	0.0373
	Equipment/monitor	471	0.0537
	Eye/ocular/corneal	2291	0.1331
	Hemodynamic instability	53,499	3.7004
	Inadequate postoperative pain control	52,142	5.8053
	Neuro—any	570	0.0671
	Regional anesthesia problem	342	0.0352
	Respiratory—pulmonary	809	0.0729
	Reversal narcotics	262	0.065
	Reversal neuromuscular blocking agents	806	0.1288
	Unanticipated upgrade of care	1658	0.1287
	Total events	263,204	20.2833
Mortality	Mortality	577	0.033

This table was kindly provided by the Anesthesia Quality Institute and is based on the data available on August 26, 2013. "The data presented are rough aggregates of what is collected in NACOR, based on a minimum number of practices which report that outcome. Definitions vary from practice to practice, especially in the 'minor' category.*Not all practices report all outcomes. This creates varying denominators for rate calculations. Consequently, some outcomes might have a higher count (N) but a lower rate (%) as compared to others."

them by mask and bag valve mask resuscitator (e.g., Ambu bag). In the setting of a difficult or impossible intubation, the inability to provide oxygenation to a patient who is not breathing spontaneously may lead to severe consequences, such as hypoxic brain damage or death. This study was the first to reliably assess the incidence of impossible mask ventilation in anesthetized subjects.

In addition, the investigators identified and validated several predictors of impossible mask ventilation, such as previous radiation treatment of the neck, male sex, sleep apnea, Mallampati III or IV, and presence of beard. These clinical predictors can all be easily assessed during the preoperative evaluation of surgical candidates, allowing anesthesia providers to customize the anesthetic management on the characteristics of the patient and possibly improving the safety of anesthesia induction.[27]

In 2013, Bateman, by reviewing a data set of more than 140,000 surgical and obstetric patients collected by the Multicenter Perioperative Outcomes Group, was able to estimate an incidence of epidural hematomas requiring surgical evacuation following epidural catheterization ranging between 1 event per 4300 and 1 event per 22,000 epidural catheter placement.[28] Such information is valuable both in guiding anesthetic management and promoting shared decision making with the patient.

Patient experience is an increasingly important component of the quality of anesthesia: it encompasses the full spectrum of anesthesia care, from the preoperative assessment to the discharge process. At present, there are numerous valid questionnaires to measure patient satisfaction with anesthesia care that can be applied to different clinical settings and patient populations[29]; those metrics can provide adequate information to conduct and assess the outcomes of improvement initiatives, if used systematically.

To make sense of collected quality data and drive improvement efforts, a rigorous statistical approach is needed. Statistical process control is the method of quality control applied to these purposes. In addition, statistical methods to recognize "outlier" providers or performances are also increasingly pursued.[30] Of note, it is recognized that feeding-back information concerning performance data to providers is paramount to increase the understanding of their practice and to promote the acceptance of changes aiming at improving quality of care.[24]

Finally, quality of anesthesia care is based on the systematic application of minimum clinical standards, evidence-based guidelines, and recommendations promoted by professional societies. In the US, the American Society of Anesthesiologists publishes and periodically updates practice parameters to guide clinicians toward high-quality clinical behaviors. In 2007, the European Society of Anaesthesiology published their "Guidelines for safety and quality in anaesthesia practice in the European Union."[31] The two societies have very similar perspectives and goals. They both support the following concepts:

• All anesthesiologic medical work should be led and personally supervised by a physician anesthesiologist.
• Patients should be assessed and optimized preoperatively; equipment should be available and be consistent with minimum standards or guidelines.
• Syringes containing drugs should be color coded.
• Clinical and administrative documentation should be complete and intelligible.

Of note, the European guidelines place a greater focus on the fact that anesthesia providers have an obligation to minimize fatigue in the context in which they are working while employers have an obligation to optimize rosters and working/resting conditions to minimize the risk of fatigued anesthetists. These principles were also received in a European Working Hour Directive.[31] In the US, the Joint Commission

TABLE 21-3	Choosing Wisely Campaign: The American Society of Anesthesiology Has Proposed the Following Five Recommendations

1. Don't obtain baseline laboratory studies in patients without significant systemic disease (ASA I or II) undergoing low-risk surgery—specifically complete blood count, basic or comprehensive metabolic panel, coagulation studies when blood loss (or fluid shifts) is expected to be minimal.
2. Don't obtain baseline diagnostic cardiac testing (transthoracic/esophageal echocardiography—TTE/TEE) or cardiac stress testing in asymptomatic stable patients with known cardiac disease (e.g., coronary artery disease, valvular disease) undergoing low- or moderate-risk noncardiac surgery.
3. Don't use pulmonary artery catheters (PACs) routinely for cardiac surgery in patients with a low risk of hemodynamic complications (especially with the concomitant use of alternative diagnostic tools [e.g., TEE]).
4. Don't administer packed red blood cells (PRBCs) in a young healthy patient without ongoing blood loss and hemoglobin of ≥6 g/dL unless symptomatic or hemodynamically unstable.
5. Don't routinely administer colloid (dextrans, hydroxylethyl starches, albumin) for volume resuscitation without appropriate indications.

(http://www.choosingwisely.org/doctor-patient-lists/american-society-of-anesthesiologists/)

has acknowledged the link between fatigue, patient safety events, and quality of care (sentinel event alert 48 and Ref.[32]), but no working hour limitations have been enforced by the specialty governing bodies, with the exception of the Accreditation Council for Graduate Medical Education that restricted working hours for residents of all specialties.

Finally, the American Society of Anesthesiology has recently joined the "Choosing Wisely" campaign,[33] an initiative of the American Board of Internal Medicine Foundation, whose focus is to encourage "physicians, patients and other health care stakeholders to think and talk about medical tests and procedures that may be unnecessary, and in some instances can cause harm." The five measures identified by the American Society of Anesthesiology (ASA) are reported in Table 21-3.

PROMOTING PATIENT SAFETY IN THE PRACTICE OF ANESTHESIA

The science of complexity has clarified that accidents and adverse outcomes are likely in complex systems where multiple agents perform several simultaneous tasks generating nonlinear and, therefore, largely unpredictable interactions and outcomes.[33]

The clinical work of anesthesia providers is certainly complex because it involves dealing with patients that are vulnerable due to age and/or comorbidities, surgical procedures that alter normal physiology, emergency conditions, and time pressure, all the while striving for efficiency, multitasking, and cooperating with many surgeons and consultants with different priorities and mind-sets.

In this context, the goal of preventing patient harm should be based on principles derived from cognitive psychology, human factors, and system thinking. Therefore, the leadership of every anesthesia practice or academic department should be engaged in building and sustaining a resilient and highly reliable system, capable of minimizing the chances of errors of clinicians and mitigating the adverse consequences of medical mistakes on patient outcomes.

A first important step in this direction is to design and implement an organized pathway for patient flow across all of the different phases of the perioperative period, from the preoperative assessment to the discharge from the hospital, to assure an effective and efficient patient management and to prevent fragmentation of care. In addition, the scheduling of elective and emergent cases should guarantee adequate first-line personnel and supervision and help minimizing providers' fatigue.

The leadership should support and assess providers' performance. Providers' skills can be promoted through training, in-services, and maintenance of competences sessions. Furthermore, there is currently a strong consensus that good communication and teamwork are essential to promote patient safety. An interesting development in this area consists in adopting medical simulation for maintaining clinical competences and promoting nontechnical skills.[33] Similar to aviation, simulation has become a standard approach used to teach nontechnical skills (situation awareness, communication, teamwork, leadership, etc.) to health care providers.[32] Of note, assessing providers' performance is requested and regulated by the Joint Commission for accreditation purposes (ongoing and focused provider performance evaluation).

An additional and essential safety and quality measure in clinical practice consists in standardizing care according to evidence-based clinical protocols. Furthermore, the systematic adoption and implementation of surgery checklists, such as the one proposed by World Health Organization, have been effective in decreasing perioperative complications and mortality.[29] It is currently acknowledged that checklists are more effective when "adjusted" to local realities, and the whole health care team participates in their execution, with "active voice" and "reading back." Importantly, a "routine debriefing" at the end of the procedure is a very effective tool to generate a shared understanding of "what went well and what went wrong," to establish next clinical priorities and to plan the next steps of patient management.

Another critical component of delivering state-of-the-art anesthesia care is the availability of adequate monitors and equipment (anesthesia machines, difficult airways cart, ultrasound for vascular access and regional anesthesia, rapid infusion systems, infusion pumps with drugs library and limits). Anesthesia information management systems can support safe practices when they are configured to deploy electronic reminders (e.g., for the administration of antibiotics), to provide decision support (for instance, operating room crisis checklists), and to facilitate reporting adverse events and near misses. It is likely that in the near future, the integration and analysis of physiologic signals coming from different monitors will allow clinicians to timely recognize patterns of situations at risk of adverse outcome,[33] thereby triggering appropriate interventions.

While information technology can be a major tool in supporting patient safety and quality efforts, it is crucial to maintain a balanced and realistic perspective on its current limitations. In particular, information technology that does not take into consideration clinicians' workflow may be distracting and represent an additional burden on clinical performance and patient safety.[31]

A final necessary step to promote patient safety is to establish a consistent process for reporting adverse events and near misses. Such an effort should include dedicating enough personnel and resources to collect and analyze performance data and to review complicated cases (under the umbrella of peer-review or morbidity and mortality conferences). To make sure that the "lessons learned" are not forgotten, the understanding gained in the review process should ultimately be translated into system improvements and increased providers' knowledge.

It is also imperative to assure that, in case of patient complications, adverse events are properly disclosed to patient and family members. Disclosure is often more effective if performed in collaboration with other services involved in the care of the patient. In the field of anesthesia, the development and implementation of effective system improvements frequently depend on the anesthesiologists' capacity to cooperate with other hospital services involved in the perioperative care of patients.

In conclusion, it is the interest of our society to make medicine more effective and safer, but also affordable and accessible to all. To this goal, it is vital to eliminate waste in health care and to "bend the health care cost curve."[35] It is a present challenge to guarantee that anesthesia clinical processes are safe and effective and, at the same time, economically sustainable. The approach that every single institution will adopt to match this financial priority will have an impact on the way anesthesia care is delivered and influence the distribution of roles and responsibilities among the members of the anesthesia team: physicians, nurse anesthetists, and anesthesia assistants.

SUMMARY

- Anesthesiologists have contributed to create the discipline of patient safety and have emerged as leaders and innovators in this field.
- Perioperative outcomes have improved due to the development of standards of care, enhanced providers' training, and technical and organizational progresses.
- New concerns are emerging of a possible negative long-term impact of anesthesia on neurologic patient outcomes such as postoperative cognitive dysfunction in elderly patients and acquired learning disability in young children.
- Data acquisition from large electronic databases and analysis is providing increasing opportunities to understand predictors and measure outcomes of anesthesia-related adverse events.
- Ongoing developments of anesthesia management information systems including decision support and adverse event reporting capabilities may play a major role in supporting patient safety and quality of care at the front line.
- Promotion of situation awareness, decision making, and communication skills may enhance clinical performance of frontline workers.

REFERENCES

1. Cavallone LF, Vannucci A. Extubation of the difficult airway and extubation failure. *Anesth Analg.* 2013;116(2):368–83.
2. Beecher HK, Todd DP. A study of the deaths associated with anesthesia and surgery: based on a study of 599, 548 anesthesias in ten institutions 1948-1952, inclusive. *Ann Surg.* 1954;140(1):2–35.
3. Kreul W. Regional anesthesia for increasing obstetrical patient safety. *Wis Med J.* 1960;59: 370–3.
4. Cooper JB, et al. Preventable anesthesia mishaps: a study of human factors. *Anesthesiology.* 1978;49(6):399–406.
5. Closed Claim Project and U.M. Center. *Closed Claims Project and Its Registries.* December 5, 2015. http://depts.washington.edu/asaccp/
6. Mission Statement of the Anesthesia Patient Safety Foundation. December 5, 2015. http://apsf.org/about.php
7. Bainbridge D, et al. Perioperative and anaesthetic-related mortality in developed and developing countries: a systematic review and meta-analysis. *Lancet.* 2012;380(9847):1075–81.
8. Pearse RM, et al. Mortality after surgery in Europe: a 7 day cohort study. *Lancet.* 2012;380(9847):1059–65.
9. Sigakis MJ, Bittner EA, Wanderer JP. Validation of a risk stratification index and risk quantification index for predicting patient outcomes: in-hospital mortality, 30-day mortality, 1-year mortality, and length-of-stay. *Anesthesiology.* 2013;119(3):525–40.

10. McNicol L, Mackay P. Anaesthesia-related morbidity in Victoria: a report from 1990 to 2005. *Anaesth Intensive Care.* 2010;38(5):837–48.
11. Metzner J, et al. Closed claims' analysis. *Best Pract Res Clin Anaesthesiol.* 2011;25(2):263–76.
12. Haller G, Laroche T, Clergue F. Morbidity in anaesthesia: today and tomorrow. *Best Pract Res Clin Anaesthesiol.* 2011;25(2):123–32.
13. Anesthesia Quality Institute. Outcomes of anesthesia. December 5, 2015. http://www.aqihq.org/files/Outcomes_of_Anesthesia_Summer_2013.pdf
14. IARS. *Smart Tots.* December 5, 2015. http://smarttots.org/
15. Mangano DT, et al. Effect of atenolol on mortality and cardiovascular morbidity after non-cardiac surgery. Multicenter Study of Perioperative Ischemia Research Group. *N Engl J Med.* 1996;335(23):1713–20.
16. Kavanagh T, Buggy DJ. Can anaesthetic technique effect postoperative outcome? *Curr Opin Anaesthesiol.* 2012;25(2):185-90.
17. Snyder GL, Greenberg S. Effect of anaesthetic technique and other perioperative factors on cancer recurrence. *Br J Anaesth.* 2010;105(2):106–15.
18. American Society of Anesthesiology. ASA recommendations for pre-anesthesia check-out: sample procedures. [cited December 5, 2015]. https://www.asahq.org/resources/clinical-information/2008-asa-recommendations-for-pre-anesthesia-checkout
19. US Food and Drug Administration. Medical devices—infusion pumps. December 5, 2015. http://www.fda.gov/MedicalDevices/ProductsandMedicalProcedures/GeneralHospitalDevicesandSupplies/InfusionPumps/default.htm
20. Webster CS, et al. The frequency and nature of drug administration error during anaesthesia. *Anaesth Intensive Care.* 2001;29(5):494–500.
21. Merry AF, et al. Multimodal system designed to reduce errors in recording and administration of drugs in anaesthesia: prospective randomised clinical evaluation. *BMJ.* 2011;343:d5543.
22. De Oliveira GS, Jr., Theilken LS, McCarthy RJ. Shortage of perioperative drugs: implications for anesthesia practice and patient safety. *Anesth Analg.* 2011;113(6):1429–35.
23. American Society of Health-System Pharmacists. Drug shortages: current drugs. December 5, 2015. http://www.ashp.org/DrugShortages/Current/
24. Benn J, et al. Using quality indicators in anaesthesia: feeding back data to improve care. *Br J Anaesth.* 2012;109(1):80–91.
25. Haller G, et al. Quality and safety indicators in anesthesia: a systematic review. *Anesthesiology.* 2009;110(5):1158–75.
26. Dutton RP, Dukatz A. Quality improvement using automated data sources: the anesthesia quality institute. *Anesthesiol Clin.* 2011;29(3):439–54.
27. Kheterpal S, et al. Prediction and outcomes of impossible mask ventilation: a review of 50,000 anesthetics. *Anesthesiology.* 2009;110(4):891–7.
28. Bateman BT, et al. The risk and outcomes of epidural hematomas after perioperative and obstetric epidural catheterization: a report from the Multicenter Perioperative Outcomes Group Research Consortium. *Anesth Analg.* 2013;116(6):1380–5.
29. Barnett SF, et al. Patient-satisfaction measures in anesthesia: qualitative systematic review. *Anesthesiology.* 2013;119(2):452–78.
30. Jones HS, Spiegelhalter DJ. The identification of "unusual" health-care providers from a hierarchical model. *Am Statistician.* 2011;65(3):154–63.
31. Eur-Lex. Access to European law. December 5, 2015. http://eur-lex.europa.eu/LexUriServ/LexUriServ.do?uri=CELEX:32003L0088:EN:NOT
32. Sinha A, Singh A, Tewari A. The fatigued anesthesiologist: A threat to patient safety? *J Anaesthesiol Clin Pharmacol.* 2013;29(2):151–9.
33. ABIM Foundation Choosing Wisely. December 5, 2015. http://www.choosingwisely.org/
34. Sessler DI, et al. Hospital stay and mortality are increased in patients having a "triple low" of low blood pressure, low bispectral index, and low minimum alveolar concentration of volatile anesthesia. *Anesthesiology.* 2012;116(6):1195–203.
35. Berwick DM, Hackbarth AD. Eliminating waste in US health care. *JAMA.* 2012;307(14):1513–6.

22 Intensive Care

Charl de Wet, Douglas J. E. Schuerer,
and Michael H. Wall

CLINICAL VIGNETTE

A 35-year-old 180-kg man with a history of obstructive sleep apnea and hypertension undergoes an uneventful laparoscopic gastric banding. He is discharged from the recovery room to the observation unit with morphine patient-controlled analgesia (PCA) for postoperative analgesia and will be monitored with intermittent pulse oximetry. At 02:00, he is found unconscious and unresponsive in pulseless electrical activity (PEA) arrest. He is successfully resuscitated but has a devastating neurologic injury and care is withdrawn 10 days later.

• Could telemonitoring or tele-intensive care unit (ICU) have prevented this complication?
• What is the role for a rapid response team (RRT) in decompensating patients?
• How could bundles or protocols be used to prevent complications or near misses?

INTRODUCTION

Critical care units, by their nature, care for the sickest patients in any hospital, and most patients have one or more organ failures being supported at once. Patients are often completely dependent on pharmacologic or mechanical support, have numerous continuous and intermittent monitors of physiologic function, and have ongoing testing and evaluation. These patients are also cared for by an extensive team consisting of intensivists, consultants, nurses, clinical pharmacists, physical therapists, and occupational therapists. Because of the complex nature of the patients, the disease, and the care team, patient safety and quality improvement activities are an absolute necessity in the ICU. This chapter will briefly review the role of telemonitoring or tele-ICU, trigger tools and RRTs, and the use of bundles and protocols in the ICU.

TELEMONITORING/TELE-ICU

Telemonitoring or tele-ICU means many different things to many different people.[1] It could be as simple as a cardiac telemetry technician monitoring a cardiac telemetry floor in a hospital or as complex as a remote monitoring location staffed with a team of teleintensivists and tele-ICU nurses continuously monitoring more than 100 patients in many ICUs at several hospitals with the use of real-time, continuous two-way audio/video robotic communication and complex computerized clinical decision support tools.

This section will focus on the more comprehensive (and expensive) tele-ICU model. In 2010, it was estimated that tele-ICU programs were in use in more than 40 US health care systems covering more than 4900 adult ICU beds in several hundred hospitals. A hospital's tele-ICU system typically consists of a monitoring location, which may be remote or on site and staffed by teleintensivists and nurses with the ability for real-time two-way audio and video communications. Typically, each intensivist can oversee up to 150 patients, and each tele-ICU nurse can observe 30–45 patients.[2] Several studies have evaluated the effectiveness of telemedicine. It should be noted that all of these studies are before-versus-after studies that are subject to bias. Lilly et al. reported the results of implementation of a tele-ICU system at a single academic institution in 7 ICUs with over 6000 patients over 17 months. They found that after implementation, there were significant decreases in adjusted mortality (13.6% vs. 11.8%, adjusted odds ratio [OR] 0.4, 95% confidence interval [CI] 0.31–0.52), ventilator-associated pneumonia (VAP) (13% vs. 1.6%, OR 0.15, 95% CI 0.09–0.23), catheter-related infection, and hospital stay. They also showed improved compliance with best practice and protocol adherence.[3] Willmitch et al. examined the before-versus-after results in 10 adult ICUs in a 5-hospital community health system over a 4-year period involving more than 24,000 patients. They showed that the tele-ICU was associated with a 23% decrease in the relative risk of adjusted mortality (95% CI 0.69–0.87; $p < 0.001$) and a 14% decrease severity-adjusted hospital length of stay (LOS) ($p < 0.001$) and a 13% decrease in ICU LOS ($p < 0.001$).[4] Young et al. performed a systematic review and meta-analysis on the impact of tele-ICU on patient outcomes. They included 13 studies from 35 ICUs involving more than 41,000 patients. Tele-ICU was associated with a decrease in ICU mortality (OR 0.8, 95% CI 0.66–0.097; $p = 0.02$) and ICU LOS (-1.2 days, 95% CI -7.21 to -0.03; $p = 0.01$). However, there was no difference in hospital mortality (OR 0.82, 95% CI 0.65–1.03; $p = 0.08$) or hospital LOS (mean reduction of 0.64 days; 95% CI -1.52 to 0.25; $p = 0.16$).[5] The authors commented on several serious limitations in tele-ICU studies to date including the huge differences in tele-ICU models and implementation, before-versus-after study design, and the fact that most studies have been funded by the vendors of these systems.

These systems are expensive. Start-up costs are in the range of $2 to $5 million per ICU, and annual operating costs may be $1 million per year per ICU.[6] Franzini et al. evaluated the costs and cost-effectiveness of a tele-ICU system from more than 4000 patients in 6 ICUs in a five-hospital system. They showed that tele-ICU increased hospital daily cost ($4302 to $5340), hospital cost per case ($21,967 to $31,318), and cost per patient ($20,231 to $25,846). This study showed that in patients with a simplified acute physiology score (SAPS II), the tele-ICU did not change hospital mortality, and they were not cost-effective. On the other hand, in patients with a SAPS II >50, mortality decreased from 30.7% to 19.3% and tele-ICU was cost-effective. Kumar performed a systematic review and analysis on eight studies and from a network of seven Veteran's Health Administration (VHA) hospitals. They found the implementation and first-year costs to be $50,000 to $100,000 per bed. Hospital costs were even more difficult to predict and ranged from a reduction to $3000 per patient to an increase of $5600. The authors point out several limitations of these data including the lack of outcome and cost-effectiveness data, the different methods of depreciation calculations, and difficulties in obtaining actual implementation costs.[7]

In conclusion, definitive studies showing the outcome and cost-effectiveness of tele-ICUs have not been done. However, as Marcin et al. commented in a recent review of a pediatric tele-ICU, "tele-medicine, in and of itself, will not result in improved care. Rather, tele-medicine is a technologic tool that can enable providers to provide better care."[8]

TRIGGER TOOLS

Patient safety has become a top priority in health care. Many changes and new protocols to improve patient safety have been suggested and implemented since the original report on deaths resulting from preventable medical errors from the Institute of Medicine (IOM) in 1999. It has been suggested that the tracking of adverse events (AEs), or harm to patients, can be used to evaluate the success or failure of safety processes.

There are several ways to track AEs. Voluntary reporting by health care providers is often incomplete. The Agency for Healthcare Research and Quality defined patient safety indicators (PSIs) using ICD-9 diagnosis codes from administrative discharge data, literature review, clinical panels, and empirical analysis, whereas the Institute of Healthcare Improvement (IHI) uses a list of triggers with a systematic chart review process (http://www.qualityindicators.ahrq.gov/modules/psi_resources.aspx. Accessed 12/10/15). According to the IHI, the use of "triggers," or clues, to identify AEs is an effective method for measuring the overall level of harm from medical care in a health care organization. The focus of these trigger tools is somewhat different in that they are designed to find harm related to medical care whether or not it was the result of an error.[9]

Harm is classified in categories according to the National Coordinating Council for Medication Error Reporting and Prevention (NCC MERP). For a full list of the NCC MERP error reporting classifications, see Chapter 13, Event Analysis.

A. Temporary harm that required intervention
B. Temporary harm that required ICU readmission or prolonged hospitalization
C. Permanent harm
D. Intervention required to sustain life
E. Patient death (not related to medical care)

Traditional efforts to detect AEs have focused on voluntary reporting and tracking errors. However, only 10–20% of all errors are reported, and of those, 90–95% cause no harm to patients. The ICU AE trigger tool is based on IHI's global trigger tool (GTT). There are various trigger tools available at IHI.org for use in different settings: the GTT for measuring AEs, trigger tools for measuring adverse drug events in general or in specific settings, such as in a children's hospital, a mental health setting, or nursing homes. Trigger tools are also available for use in specific populations or during specific periods such as in the perioperative surgical population, during the perinatal period, or for use in the neonatal ICU.

According to the IHI, these trigger tools provide an easy-to-use method for accurately identifying AEs and measuring the rate of AEs over time. The process is standardized: charts are randomly selected by trained reviewers throughout the year, and to maximize efficiency, time is limited to 20 minutes per chart. Rather than a page-by-page review of the chart, the trigger tool uses a predefined checklist of triggers. Specific areas of the charts are queried to look for the trigger, and if the trigger is found, then further relevant information is searched for in the chart in order to make an informed judgment as to whether the trigger resulted in an AE. The trigger "positive blood culture" will lead the reviewer to search in the summary section for microbiology, whereas naloxone administration will be searched for in the medication administration record (MAR). Electronic records provide the ability to improve efficiency of the searching process, some of which can be automated.

The ICU AE trigger tool is designed to identify harmful events in the ICU and uses records of patients who have been in the ICU for at least 2 days. The trigger tool does not track errors that do not lead to harm. The GTT has a very high detection rate. However, since the medical record is not searched from front to back and since there is no gold standard for detecting AEs, the true sensitivity and specificity of these tools remain unknown.

There is currently little published data on the utility and validity of these tools. Landrigan et al. used the GTT during their retrospective study of a stratified random sample of 10 hospitals in North Carolina and found that during the period of January 2002 through December 2007, there was no significant change in overall rate of harm. When using the GTT, they showed very good internal interrater reliability but very poor agreement by external reviewers.[10] Mattsson et al. used the GTT in a high-volume oncology service in Denmark. The two review teams identified mean AEs of 32–37 per 1000 admission days. They concluded that different review teams identified different AEs and reached different conclusions on the safety process. They showed that only 31% of all AEs were identified by both teams with only moderate interrater agreement ($\kappa = 0.45$) between teams. This gave rise to different conclusions on the safety process. Another concern is that there is poor agreement among teams in the categorization of identified AEs especially when related to temporary harm. They also pointed out that mean values of harm rates were within the measurement error of the GTT. Therefore, making changes in the harm rate is almost impossible to track unless AEs doubled.[11]

It is clear that different detection methods identify different AEs. Some suggest combining these different methodologies to measure patient safety for internal quality improvement (Table 22-1).

TABLE 22-1	Rationale for Triggers in ICU Patients
ICU Trigger	**Rationale for Trigger/Possible Mechanisms**
Positive blood cultures	Measure of quality, frequently iatrogenic; associated with poor outcome
Abrupt drop in Hgb > 4 g/dL	Clue to possible surgical bleed/complication or anticoagulant problems
Clostridium difficile positive	Antibiotic usage or inappropriate coverage/duration
aPTT > 100 s	Anticoagulant related, test sampling error, disseminated intravascular coagulation (DIC)
International normalized ratio (INR) > 6	Anticoagulant related (very common)
Glucose < 50 mg/dL	Related to insulin/tube feeding interruption
↑BUN and/or Creatinine to 2× baseline	Possibly related to drugs (IV contrast dye, antibiotics, etc.)
Radiologic tests for emboli or clot	Immobility in ICU/inadequate or lack of DVT prophylaxis

(Continued)

TABLE 22-1	Rationale for Triggers in ICU Patients (*Continued*)
ICU Trigger	Rationale for Trigger/Possible Mechanisms
Benadryl	Allergic reaction/used as sleeping aid (possible delirium)
Vitamin K	Coumadin reversal in over anticoagulation/bleeding
Flumazenil	Sedative reversal. Often related to lethargy/hypotension
Naloxone	Analgesia-related complications/respiratory depression
Antidiarrheals/Laxatives	Can signal a Clostridium difficile infection or constipation
Antiemetics	Often due to over use of narcotics
Sodium polystyrene (Kayexalate)	Hyperkalemia related to drugs or renal failure
Code	Review carefully. Not all codes are related to harm caused
Pneumonia onset in unit	Nocosomial pneumonias are adverse events and a measure of quality
Readmission to ICU	Premature discharge or unrecognized problem in ICU
New-onset dialysis	Possible perioperative surgical problems or ICU events
In unit procedures	Evaluate reason for procedure: e.g., arterial line for hypotension/sepsis. Chest tube for iatrogenic pneumothorax
Intubation/reintubation	Frequently related to AEs
Abrupt medication stop	Often because of drug side effects/complications
Oversedation/lethargy/hypotension	Often related to medication AEs
Other	Uncovered event that does not fit any of the above categories

(Adapted from the Institute for Healthcare Improvement ICU Adverse Event Trigger Tool. © VHA/Institute for Healthcare Improvement, January 2002. Available on www.IHI.org)

It is clear that the incidence of AEs remains very high. AEs are often unrecognized or not reported. While multiple safety initiatives have been proposed and implemented since the landmark report by the Institute of Medicine (IOM), evidence of any dramatic beneficial effect on improving outcomes in patient safety is still lacking. Some of these patient safety initiatives may not go far enough or may have unintended or unrecognized negative effects. Press et al. examined the impact of resident duty hour reform on hospital readmission rates, as well as death during the admission or within 30 days of discharge, and found no changes associated with resident duty hour reform.[12]

RAPID RESPONSE TEAMS FOR DECOMPENSATING PATIENTS

Survival to discharge after inhospital cardiopulmonary resuscitation by so-called code teams remains only 7–26%.[13] This failure to rescue patients, and evidence to suggest that most serious AEs are preceded by clinically observable warning signs, has led to the development of the rapid response team (RRT). RRT is a multidisciplinary group of hospital personnel that respond promptly to acutely deteriorating patients outside of the ICU. The rapid response system uses various terms and definitions such as RRT (led by a nurse, with or without physician consultation available), medical emergency team, a medical emergency response team (physician leads the team), or critical care outreach teams (ICU-based teams that follow general ward patients).[14] There is considerable heterogeneity in the application of these terms. For the purposes of this discussion, we will use the term RRT.[15]

RRTs were widely implemented following publication of five single center studies that made before-and-after comparisons. These studies showed a reduction in the rate of cardiac arrests and more care provided to patients by the RRT. The effectiveness of the RRT however remains somewhat controversial.[15] The large multicenter cluster-randomized controlled trial called the Medical Early Response Intervention and Therapy (MERIT) study failed to demonstrate any direct benefit.[16] Even though RRTs have been shown to reduce cardiopulmonary arrests outside of the ICU, subsequent meta-analyses also have failed to demonstrate a significant reduction in hospital-wide mortality in adult patients after RRT implementation. Beitler et al. were one of the first to show a benefit. In a long-term cohort study from 2003 to 2008, following more than 150,000 patients admitted to a tertiary facility, they showed that RRTs were associated with a significant reduction in unadjusted hospital-wide mortality, out-of-ICU mortality, and out-of-ICU cardiopulmonary arrest codes. The reduction in hospital-wide mortality remained statistically significant even after adjusting for inpatient mortality trend over time.[17]

RRTs were widely introduced without level 1 evidence showing effectiveness. Clinicians need to understand the controversies surrounding them. While they have many potential benefits as "rescue" therapy, the primary goal should still focus at preventing these events in the first place and fostering a culture of patient safety.

USE OF BUNDLES AND PROTOCOLS TO IMPROVE CARE

Bundles, protocols, and guidelines are all important in the care of the ICU patient and to standardize care to improve quality and outcomes. Nomenclature of these items is often confusing and overlapping. For the purpose of this review, guidelines are evidence-based statements on how to provide optimal care of a particular patient condition, such as what antibiotics should be routinely used for undifferentiated ventilator associated pneumonia (VAP). Protocols are then an extension of those guidelines, particularly centered on patient care flow or how to "operationalize" a guideline based on the structure of one's own ICU. In many organizations, the terms "protocol" and "guidelines" are used more or less interchangeably, likely due to perceived legal ramifications of using certain terms over others. An ICU bundle is a set of treatment goals (usually three to seven) that, when grouped and achieved together over a finite time span, are believed to promote optimal outcomes.[18]

Initially, care bundles were promulgated by the Institute for Healthcare Improvement.[19] Bundle-driven care is grounded in evidence-based medicine. The various components of the bundle have been shown in various studies to be effective, although all components of individual bundles may not have the backing of level-one evidence, namely, two or more randomized controlled trials. Bundles exist for many disease patterns, such as VAP, preventing surgical site infections, or treatment of sepsis. Figure 22-1 shows a typical sepsis bundle. Multiple studies have shown that bundles can improve outcomes.[20–22] Unfortunately, most of those trials have been retrospective in nature and based on historical controls. Bundles likely help most by promoting consistency in the care of clinical conditions.[23] Critics of bundles point to the fact that the data are lacking in randomized trials, some items of a successful bundle may in fact not contribute to positive outcomes and may even be harmful, "cookbook" medicine is not for individual patients, and regulators and payers may use bundle adherence as an incorrect measure of quality.[24]

Protocols have much more prospective data with good information on everything from weaning mechanical ventilation to ensuring compliance to one's own list of best practices.[25,26] Protocols are usually developed at the institution or unit level, in response either to a safety event or to standardize care based on new research or evidence-based guidelines. In the past, in spite of good evidence, guidelines have not always taken hold in bedside care. Protocols develop a pathway so that such evidence-based care is consistently applied to the correct patient scenario, and compliance with the protocols can be easily measured as a marker of quality. By standardizing care, they may also decrease costs by improving outcomes and decreasing variability. Decreasing variability has been shown to decrease the amount of testing, such as eliminating standard daily labs, thereby decreasing cost.

SURVIVING SEPSIS CAMPAIGN CARE BUNDLES

TO BE COMPLETED WITHIN 3 HOURS:

1) Measure lactate level
2) Obtain blood cultures prior to administration of antibiotics
3) Administer broad spectrum antibiotics
4) Administer 30 mL/kg crystalloid for hypotension or lactate ≥4 mmol/L

TO BE COMPLETED WITHIN 6 HOURS:

5) Apply vasopressors (for hypotension that does not respond to initial fluid resuscitation) to maintain a mean arterial pressure (MAP) ≥65 mm Hg
6) In the event of persistent arterial hypotension despite volume resuscitation (septic shock) or initial lactate ≥4 mmol/L (36 mg/dL):
    - Measure central venous pressure (CVP)*
    - Measure central venous oxygen saturation (ScvO2)*
7) Remeasure lactate if initial lactate was elevated*

*Targets for quantitative resuscitation included in the guidelines are CVP of ≥8 mm Hg, ScvO2 of ≥ 70%, and normalization of lactate.

Figure 22-1. Surviving sepsis campaign care bundles. (From Dellinger RP, Levy M, Rhodes A, et al. Surviving sepsis campaign: international guidelines for management of severe sepsis and septic shock, 2012. *Intensive Care Med.* 2013;39(2):165–228.)

In practice, all of these tools must be used while understanding their benefits and shortcomings. We know that not every patient can have all of his or her care directed by protocol, but there is a large component of everyday care that can be governed by information from well-validated studies. The practicing ICU physician should be a part of the team that develops ICU and organizational protocols based on evidence-based guidelines and local practice patterns. When there are several of these that relate to a single disease process, they can be included in a care bundle. These practices will provide consistency and reduce variability in those patients, allow data collection and elucidate change if the protocol proves ineffective. The practitioner must also recognize either when a patient does not fit a given protocol or when such prescribed care is not effective. In those cases, the true art of medicine, including experience and judgment, must come above standardized care. In other words, we should use these tools to make sure we apply well-proven elements of care, leaving our time for the truly difficult dilemmas that we encounter in the ICU on a daily basis. In the clinical vignette, it is likely that a protocol to recognize potential sleep apnea patients and a bundle that included continuous central monitoring and limiting narcotics (all recommended guidelines) could have prevented such a devastating event.

KEY POINTS

* Telemedicine is a tool that may allow clinicians to provide better care.
* Studies of telemedicine are limited by before-versus-after study design, heterogeneity, and potential bias.
* Telemedicine is expensive, and cost-effectiveness studies are limited.
* Trigger tools have been developed to provide an easy-to-use method for accurately identifying AEs related to medical care. Currently, there is little published data on the utility and validity of these trigger tools.
* Multidisciplinary RRTs were developed to respond promptly to acutely deteriorating inpatients outside the ICU. Statistically, their effectiveness remains somewhat controversial.
* Bundles are a set of treatment goals that are grouped together to provide optimal patient care.
* Protocols are extensions of evidenced-based guidelines that promote consistency and aid in quality data collection.
* Bundles and protocols are not perfect, need to evolve, and should never replace clinical decision making.

REFERENCES

1. Lilly CM, Fisher KA, Ries M, et al. A national ICU telemedicine survey: validation and results. *CHEST J.* 2012;142(1):40–7.
2. Ward NS, Afessa B, Kleinpell R, et al. Intensivist/patient ratios in closed ICUs: a statement from the society of critical care medicine taskforce on ICU staffing. *Crit Care Med.* 2013;41(2):638–45.
3. Lilly CM, Cody S, Zhao H, et al. Hospital mortality, length of stay, and preventable complications among critically ill patients before and after tele-ICU reengineering of critical care processes. *JAMA.* 2011;305(21):2175–83.

4. Willmitch B, Golembeski S, Kim SS, et al. Clinical outcomes after telemedicine intensive care unit implementation. *Crit Care Med.* 2012;40(2):450–4.
5. Young L, Chan PS, Lu X, et al. Impact of telemedicine intensive care unit coverage on patient outcomes: a systematic review and meta-analysis. *Arch Intern Med.* 2011;171(6):498–506.
6. Franzini L, Sail KR, Thomas EJ, et al. Costs and cost-effectiveness of a telemedicine intensive care unit program in 6 intensive care units in a large health care system. *J Crit Care.* 2011;26(3):329.
7. Kumar G, Falk DM, Bonello RS, et al. The costs of critical care telemedicine programs: a systematic review and analysis. *CHEST J.* 2013;143(1):19–29.
8. Marcin JP. Telemedicine in the pediatric intensive care unit. *Pediatric Clin North Am.* 2013;60(3):581–92.
9. Griffin FA, Resar RK. *IHI Global Trigger Tool for Measuring Adverse Events.* 2nd ed. Cambridge, MA: Institute for Healthcare Improvement; 2009.
10. Landrigan CP, Parry GJ, Bones CB, et al. Temporal trends in rates of patient harm resulting from medical care. *N Eng J Med.* 2010;363(22):2124–34.
11. Mattsson TO, Knudsen JL, Lauritsen J, et al. Assessment of the global trigger tool to measure, monitor and evaluate patient safety in cancer patients: reliability concerns are raised. *BMJ Qual Saf.* 2013;22(7):571–9.
12. Press M, Silber J, Rosen A, et al. The impact of resident duty hour reform on hospital readmission rates among medicare beneficiaries. *J Gen Intern Med.* 2011;26(4):405–11.
13. Ehlenbach WJ, Barnato AE, Curtis JR, et al. Epidemiologic study of in-hospital cardiopulmonary resuscitation in the elderly. *N Eng J Med.* 2009;361(1):22–31.
14. DeVita MA, Bellomo R, Hillman K, et al. Findings of the first consensus conference on medical emergency teams. *Crit Care Med.* 2006;34(9):2463–78.
15. Jones DA, DeVita MA, Bellomo R. Rapid-response teams. *N Eng J Med.* 2001;365(2):139–46.
16. Hillman K, Chen J, Cretikos M, et al.; MERIT Study Investigators. Introduction of the medical emergency team (MET) system: a cluster-randomised controlled trial. *Lancet.* study date: 2005;365(9477):2091–7.
17. Beitler LN, Bails DB, et al. Reduction in hospital-wide mortality after implementation of a rapid response team: a long-term cohort study. *Crit Care Med.* 2011;15:R269.
18. Dellinger RP, Townsend SR. Point: are the best patient outcomes achieved when ICU bundles are rigorously adhered to? yes. *CHEST J.* 2013;144(2):372–4.
19. Resar R, Griffin FA, Haraden C, Nolan TW. Using care bundles to improve health care quality. *IHI Innovation Series White Paper.* 2012. http://www.ihi.org/knowledge/Pages/IHIWhitePapers/UsingCareBundles.aspx. Accessed 10/1/13.
20. Pronovost P, Needham D, Berenholtz S, et al. An intervention to decrease catheter-related bloodstream infections in the ICU. *N Eng J Med.* 2006;355(26):2725–32.
21. Hasibeder WR. Does standardization of critical care work? *Curr Opin Crit Care.* 2010;16(5):493–8.
22. Levy MM, Dellinger RP, Townsend SR, et al. The surviving sepsis campaign: results of an international guideline-based performance improvement program targeting severe sepsis. *Crit Care Med.* 2010;38(2):367–74.
23. Levy MM, Pronovost PJ, Dellinger RP, et al. Sepsis change bundles: converting guidelines into meaningful change in behavior and clinical outcome. *Crit Care Med.* 2004;32(11): S595–7.
24. Marik PE, Raghunathan K, Bloomstone J. Counterpoint: are the best patient outcomes achieved when ICU bundles are rigorously adhered to? no. *CHEST J.* 2013;144(2):374–8.
25. Kress JP, Pohlman AS, O'Connor MF, et al. Daily interruption of sedative infusions in critically ill patients undergoing mechanical ventilation. *N Eng J Med.* 2000;342(20):1471–7.
26. Byrnes MC, Schuerer DJE, Schallom ME, et al. Implementation of a mandatory checklist of protocols and objectives improves compliance with a wide range of evidence-based intensive care unit practices. *Crit Care Med.* 2009;37(10):2775–8.
27. Dellinger RP, Levy M, Rhodes A, et al. Surviving sepsis campaign: international guidelines for management of severe sepsis and septic shock, 2012. *Intensive Care Med.* 2013;39(2): 165–228.

23 Patient Safety in the Emergency Department

Richard T. Griffey, Ryan Schneider, and Robert F. Poirier

CLINICAL VIGNETTE

Mrs. Stevens has been in hallway bed 7 of the emergency department (ED) for 20 hours. During the third handoff in her care, oncoming providers are told that she has pneumonia and is admitted and waiting for a bed. The trauma pager goes off and a nurse asks the off-going doctor for a prescription for a patient being discharged. Sign-out ends quickly, and as the team finishes responding to the trauma, a nurse says "I need your help. Mrs. Stevens in hallway 7 is hypotensive, tachycardic, and short of breath." Review of her record reveals that she has missed a dose of antibiotics and that she never received a third liter of fluid resuscitation. Now she is septic and will require intubation, resuscitation, and admission to an intensive care unit (ICU).

* What system issues contributed to this and similar common scenarios?
* What measures can prevent such cases?

INTRODUCTION: THE ED MINEFIELD

The ED is a unique and dynamic setting with the principal mission of the acute stabilization and disposition of patients, sometimes described as managing chaos. The ED now accounts for nearly one-third of the 354 million annual acute care visits in the United States, practically all acute care provided after hours and on weekends, more acute care for the uninsured than in all other settings combined, and nearly 50% of hospital admissions in the US. The ED is increasingly the site of care of last resort for the most vulnerable and underresourced patients.[1,2] Many features of work in the ED (illustrated in Table 23-1) combine to make this an area fraught with potential for error.

Attention to the organization of work, leadership in advocating for patients and staff in the ED, and open lines of communication in collaborating with other services are needed to ensure a successful environment for emergency care. While principles of patient safety discussed in other sections of this manual apply to the ED, in this chapter, we discuss some areas of patient safety that are of particular importance to the ED.

CROWDING, BOARDING, AND ITS EFFECTS

If you were to ask emergency physicians to identify the single biggest threat to patient safety in the ED, most will tell you that boarding of inpatients and consequent crowding is by far the biggest concern. In many ways, the ED is the canary in the coal mine,

TABLE 23-1	Features contributing to error in the ED setting

- Increasing patient complexity and volume
- Mandate never to miss high-risk conditions
- High decision density and production pressures
- Continuous 24/7/365 function
- Lack of control of arrival or egress of patients
- Coordination of care with many other providers
- Frequent interruptions
- Fatigue
- Inadequate health information system support
- Numerous shift changes and handoffs
- Social disasters and failures of the outpatient network
- Unfunded mandates and accounting systems that reinforces consideration among health system administrators of the ED as a loss leader

where problems in the health system first manifest. One of the biggest challenges and patient safety problems in the ED is lack of patient flow. For admitted patients, patient flow means the forward progression of patients from ED presentation and initial evaluation, to egress from the ED after initial evaluation, management, and stabilization to a hospital bed. Decreased flow leads to decreased capacity, ED over-crowding, and numerous patient safety concerns. Figures 23-1 and 23-2 show typical ED arrival pattern by time of the day and by day of the week. As patients are evaluated as to the severity of their complaints and conditions, those who have been sorted or "differentiated" and have had treatment initiated are often less worrisome than the undifferentiated patient sitting in the waiting room with an occult emergency. Emergency physicians must necessarily be on the lookout for the next disaster walking through the door and often lack the time, training, and expertise to perform ongoing inpatient care simultaneously in the ED. Though boarding of admitted patients in

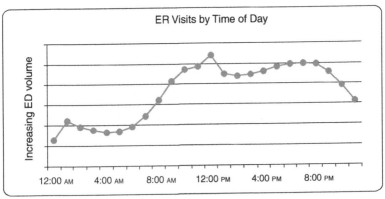

Figure 23-1. This graph shows a typical plot of ED volume increasing in the morning arriving at a peak level around noon. Volume then often remains steady or continues to increase from noon until around 10 PM. (From Washington State Hospital Association. Emergency Room Use. October, 2010. http://www.wsha.org/files/127/ERreport.pdf. Accessed 6/19/15.)

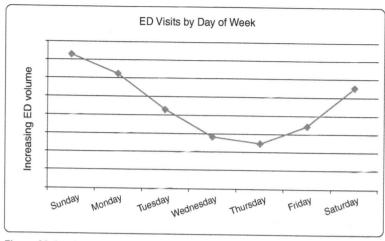

Figure 23-2. This graph displays a typical ED arrival pattern by day of the week. Volume increases on Friday and tends to peak on Sunday or Monday evenings. Volume tends to nadir on Thursday morning. (From Washington State Hospital Association. Emergency Room Use. October, 2010. http://www.wsha.org/files/127/ERreport.pdf. Accessed 6/19/15.)

the ED and consequent crowding have garnered national attention over the past two decades, there has been little improvement in conditions.[3] The American College of Emergency Physicians (ACEP) defines a boarding patient as one "who remains in the ED after they have been admitted to a facility, but has not transferred to that inpatient unit." Studies have shown that boarding ED patients results in poor pain control and decreased patient satisfaction; delays antibiotic administration; increases waiting times and the number of patients who leave the ED (from the triage waiting area) prior to being seen by a provider; increases the frequency of medical errors, the number of sentinel events, patient mortality, and malpractice claims; and has severe financial consequences.[4-7] While policies related to crowding seem to assume that the ED has unlimited capacity to expand, the reality is that emergency physicians must always focus on the undifferentiated patients in the waiting room who may have occult life-threatening conditions, and so a hall bed in the treatment area can become a very unsafe place for patients who require admission, as they may receive suboptimal care. ED physicians and nurses are specifically trained in their given specialty, and this does not include long-term care of the ICU or medical/surgical patient. Missed timing of medication doses and laboratory testing and longer hospital lengths of stay are associated with boarding in the ED.[6,8]

Successful strategies used by hospitals to address boarding include moving admitted patients from ED hall spots to inpatient hall spots until beds are available when the boarding burden hits certain thresholds. Though this practice has been shown to be safe, resulting in increased turnover of beds and improved patient satisfaction, and to make financial sense, it is often underutilized as this is perceived by the hospital and nursing administration to be unsafe, unacceptable, or unprofitable.[3,9] This is often one of the highest-level interventions that is part of hospital surge protocols that consist of tiered, transparent, actionable responses tied to specific levels of ED's crowding. Other strategies have included reorganizing work to a more patient-centered approach, matching patient demand with availability of services, including scheduling of elective surgical cases to smooth out the spikes in bed requirements following surgery to avoid those days where high surges are predictable and over which a hospital has less control.[3]

A common response to crowding and boarding has been to increase capacity by building more beds. Unless processes are improved, however, increasing the footprint of an ED or the number of beds has been shown to result in a temporary improvement followed by an even bigger boarding problem.[10] Boarding and overcrowding in the ED can cause a significant strain to its physical capacity and resources and to personnel time. While improving flow is the ultimate goal, the focus should not be on working faster. Instead, efforts need to be on smarter and more efficient functioning of the hospital and health care systems as a whole. Adequate ED flow is a precondition for safe and high-quality patient care.

TIME-CRITICAL DIAGNOSES

Care for time-critical conditions is a core mission of emergency medicine. This task requires a high level of coordination of services to rapidly muster and intensely apply resources for diagnosis and therapeutic interventions. Conditions and burdens that threaten the ability to accomplish these tasks, such as ED crowding, or incentives that distract time-dependent resources impair this core mission.

In 2005, the Centers for Medicare and Medicaid Services (CMS) began publically reporting hospital "core" process of care measures focused on heart failure, heart attack, pneumonia, and surgical care. Many of these measures were focused on time-critical diagnoses and treatment. Examples for acute myocardial infarction (MI) care include aspirin at arrival, thrombolytics administered within 30 minutes of arrival, or PCI within 90 minutes of arrival. Examples for pneumonia include timing of antibiotics from arrival and correct choice of antibiotics. An early pneumonia measure requiring administration of antibiotics within 4 hours of arrival reveals the potential for perverse incentives in quality measurement. When physicians and hospitals felt they were being penalized for delayed diagnosis of pneumonia among patients with vague symptoms diagnosed only after extensive evaluations, administrators were incentivized to "uptriage" these patients, potentially at the expense of sicker patients, to administer antibiotics to patients who did not require them, or to take other actions to game the system. The unintended consequences of these measures based on tenuous evidence led to a sustained uproar from the medical community, and the measures were subsequently modified and ultimately removed.[11,12]

Other recognized time-critical conditions include severe trauma where a "golden hour" after injury for successful resuscitation has long been recognized. More recently, data suggesting benefit of thrombolysis in the treatment of stroke for patients presenting in the first 3 hours has driven discussions of regionalization of care and prioritization of these patients on presentation to achieve the best care and fastest time possible for reperfusion of brain tissue.

DIAGNOSTIC ERROR

Since the Institute of Medicine (IOM) report, areas such as medication error and surgical safety have enjoyed increased attention. Though thought to be one of the largest areas leading to adverse events and waste in the form of underutilization and overutilization of services, diagnostic error remains a black box, tending to be much more difficult to identify and prevent than other areas of patient safety. Consequently, diagnostic error has been a largely neglected area of patient safety and is considered "the next frontier of patient safety."[13] Though it is not truly the mission of the ED to make final diagnoses, but rather to exclude life- and limb-threatening illness, there are some diagnoses, especially those with time-critical elements, that should not be missed. Missed diagnoses of fractures and myocardial infarction are historically among the most common and the most costly diagnostic errors in emergency medicine, respectively. Many of the aforementioned conditions conspire to lead to decision making that is susceptible to common cognitive biases. Though the effectiveness of doing so remains to be explored, training in emergency medicine includes focus on debiasing techniques to help avoid common diagnostic errors. These include routine education about classic mimics for common complaints including MI masquerading as gastroenteritis, abdominal aortic aneurysm presenting as flank pain, hip fracture presenting as knee pain, etc. Education also focuses on avoiding overreliance on viewing test results as a yes/no binary means to rule out disease but rather viewing these in a Bayesian framework as increasing or decreasing the probability of disease.

PROCEDURAL SAFETY

The ED is increasingly the setting for many procedures that may have previously been performed in other settings. This includes procedures such as placement of central venous catheters, drainage of abscesses, reduction of fractures and dislocations, aspiration of fluid from joints and cavities, and IV procedural sedation to facilitate patient comfort and safety. Though, historically, procedural safety has primarily focused on the operating room, the volume of bedside procedures bears increased attention to safety in areas like the ED. While the literature on procedural safety in the ED is limited, several conceptual models and recommendations have been made in recent years in other clinical areas, such as in the operating room. Some of those principles and practices may at least partially apply to an ED setting.

There are a number of differences between ED-based procedures and those taking place in the OR. Most procedures taking place in the ED are on awake, alert patients (if not sedated) with obvious external pathology. While this may make certain risks, such as wrong-sided procedures, less likely, other factors, such as patient acuity, suboptimal environmental conditions, time pressures, and provider variability, increase procedural risk.[14] Some examples include life- or limb-threatening situations, availability of needed equipment, physical layout, change of shifts for nursing or physician staff, and the need to perform procedures on patients with potentially full stomachs.

Many routine ED procedures are low risk in nature (i.e., IV insertion, laceration repair). However, emergency care requires that providers train to be proficient in performing infrequent high-risk procedures, such as cricothyrotomy, thoracotomy, and pericardiocentesis. The age-old teaching method of "see one, do one, teach one" is no longer an acceptable approach. Instead, training now should include simulation and clinical competence in the use of advanced technologies like bedside ultrasound before providers are allowed to independently perform high-risk procedures. In addition, the Joint Commission now requires all bedside procedures to use the same Universal Protocol that is required in the operating room. Specific suggested interventions that may increase PS in the ED setting include adoption of clinical protocols and procedural checklists, use of evolving technology, and team training.[14]

Unfortunately, there is no "one-size-fits-all" application that has been specifically designed and can be used for procedural safety in the ED. Therefore, procedural safety in the ED needs to incorporate a hybrid model that encompasses specific elements from the World Health Organization (WHO) Surgical Safety Checklist, the Joint Commission Universal Protocol, and current conceptual models and recommendations.

STAFF SAFETY

Violence against health care providers in the US continues to escalate each year. It is reported that 53% of hospital assaults occur in the ED. Recent studies have shown that 80% of ED staff know at least one staff member injured by a violent patient in the past 5 years, while 43% reported physical attacks on staff occur at least once a month in their ED. Over 10% of hospitals in a recent survey reported weapon threats against staff occurring each month. Health care workers experience violent workplace assaults four times higher than the average in other industries. Seventy-five percent of emergency physicians report being threatened in the past year, and 28% have reported being assaulted on the job in the past. Despite these figures, it is well known that ED violence remains significantly underreported. Some believe that health care workers have come to accept that workplace violence is just part of the job.

Visits to the ED by patients with behavioral health issues and/or drug- and alcohol-related illness continue to increase. Violence against health care workers is more prevalent in environments that see higher-level mental health and substance abuse illness. Numerous negative effects impact health care workers who have experienced workplace assaults. These include posttraumatic stress, fear of their workplace, feelings of helplessness and guilt, depression, and decreased productivity.

Improving safety begins with education/training, awareness, and increased hospital support for health care workers. Panic alarms, metal detectors, and 24-hour security have reduced violence in high-risk health care settings. Recognizing the signs of impending violence and having the training/skills to de-escalate the situation are essential. Highly coordinated rapid teamwork by physicians, nurses, and security has been shown to make the workplace safer. Aggressive reporting of workplace violence events along with guidelines on reporting to police and state prosecutors helps establish a culture of zero tolerance for violence. These measures reduce the helplessness some health care workers feel in their environment. Unfortunately, only half the states in the US have strict penalties for assaults against health care workers.

Workplace violence prevention programs are successful when there is employee involvement and hospital management commitment. Comprehensive programs that include security and health care personnel safety training along with incident debriefing are important components. Environments where health care workers feel safe and protected promote higher quality of care provided to patients, improved morale, and increased productivity.

TEAMS AND TEAMWORK

When the terms team and teamwork come to mind, most people think about their favorite baseball or football organization. In the complex environment of health care, teams and teamwork are essential to providing safe and optimal patient care. Applying teamwork to clinical practice can prove to be quite challenging and is still a relatively new concept. And despite it being a challenge, the health care arena is an excellent venue to form teams as it already consists of groups of individuals.

How can teams impact ED performance? One must first focus on the difference between a group and a team. A group can be thought of as a number of people without a shared focus on certain values, while a team usually consists of people who have a shared purpose. For the team to be successful, they have to have a shared understanding of intended goals and be aware of each team member's roles and responsibilities.[15] A typical team in the ED may consist of the bedside RN, patient care tech, emergency physician, social worker, case coordinator, and consulting physicians.

While having a team leader is important in the functioning of a team, the ability to flatten hierarchy is essential for success and to avoid hazards.[16] Empowering front-line staff to speak up when they have a safety concern can make the difference between high performance and failure. This kind of culture change can be difficult and requires having all the staff on board. Data demonstrate that workplaces with higher levels of teamwork outperform those with lower levels.[17,18] Overall, high-functioning medical teams consist of individuals who have a shared goal and mental model and work fluidly to provide safe and effective health care.

COMMUNICATION

It may come as no surprise that a significant portion of adverse events and outcomes in the ED is the direct result of poor communication practices. This is particularly evident in communication that occurs across transitions of patient care (i.e., shift changes, admitted patients, speaking with consultants). Emergency medicine providers are faced with daily challenges such as frequent interruptions, increased production pressures, and high-impact decision making that all contribute to challenging communication. Therefore, it is essential that emergency medicine providers incorporate communication strategies into their daily practice. Some examples of communication strategies include using a standardized handoff tool, protocol, or read back technique.[19] Patient safety in the ED can only improve once an overall awareness of the importance of effective communication is appreciated.

COORDINATION OF CARE

It is recognized that a minority of superusers drive a disproportionate amount of costs and resource utilization in health care. According to the Center for Medicaid and Children's Health Insurance Program (CHIP) Services, 5% of Medicaid beneficiaries account for 54% of the program's total expenditures and 1% account for 25% of the total.[20] A report funded by the Agency for Healthcare Research and Quality found that 5% of the population accounts for 49% of health care spending.[21] In addition, among Medicare patients admitted to the hospital, nearly 20% are readmitted within 30 days of being discharged, and nearly three-quarters of those admissions may be preventable.[22] Combined with an increasing elderly population, the prevalence of limited health literacy, a threadbare primary care network, and a high proportion of uninsured patients, it is more important than ever that the health system make unprecedented efforts to coordinate care for patients trying to navigate the fragmented health care system. This is essential to get patients the right care and timely care and to keep them out of the hospital and out of the ED. This will involve participation of hospital departments, third-party payers, community providers, and patients in sharing information in a community care network. Recently, a number of initiatives have focused on confirming readiness for discharge from the hospital, setting up follow-up appointments and home health and transportation services. A number of EDs have instituted nurse follow-up call programs, appointment scheduling, and other interventions to help optimize coordination of care. Providing alternatives for unscheduled acute care visits including services such as extended primary care physician office hours, urgent care appointments and home infusion services are important for helping keep patients healthy and out of the hospital.

DISCHARGING PATIENTS SAFELY FROM THE ED

Discharge from the ED is increasingly recognized as a high-risk transition of care with the potential for loss of important information. The prevalence of limited health literacy among ED patients is high, and print materials for patients are often written at a higher reading level than that possessed by many patients. Though providers believe in the effectiveness of techniques to improve communication, they rarely use them,[23] and few verify confirmation of discharge instructions.[24] It is recommended that patients receive written and verbal communication about their ED visit that explains in plain language their diagnosis, information about tests and treatment rendered, home care, medication, follow-up instructions, and reasons to return to the ED. Comprehension of discharge instructions should be confirmed asking the patient to repeat back their instructions and receive clarifying feedback.[19] Nearly all patients being discharged from the ED should be given instructions to make a follow-up appointment with a primary care provider. Unfortunately, many patients do not have primary care providers, or follow-up appointments cannot be scheduled for weeks later. Coordination of care including primary care and unscheduled acute care options outside the ED are components of the health care safety net that are badly needed. Lack of outpatient options can lead to worse outcomes and return ED visits.

KEY POINTS

In summary, emergency medicine is an exciting and mission-critical area of patient care, but the ED can also be a dangerous place for patients if structure and processes are not in place to ensure timely, reliable systems that address problems that arise. This includes:

- Attention to the safety and organization of work
- Leadership in addressing issues such as boarding and crowding
- Clear communication and teamwork in caring for patients with time-critical diagnoses

When the ED functions well within the health care system, this leads to more coordinated care and better outcomes for patients.

REFERENCES

1. Schuur JD, Venkatesh AK. The growing role of emergency departments in hospital admissions. *N Engl J Med*. 2012;367:391–3.
2. Pitts SR, Carrier ER, Rich EC, Kellermann AL. Where Americans get acute care: increasingly, it's not at their doctor's office. *Health Aff (Millwood)*. 2010;29:1620–9.
3. Rabin E, Kocher K, McClelland M, et al. Solutions to emergency department 'boarding' and crowding are underused and may need to be legislated. *Health Aff (Millwood)*. 2012;31:1757–66.

4. Hollander JE, Pines JM. The emergency department crowding paradox: the longer you stay, the less care you get. *Ann Emerg Med.* 2007;50:497–9.
5. Walsh P, Cortez V, Bhakta H. Patients would prefer ward to emergency department boarding while awaiting an inpatient bed. *J Emerg Med.* 2008;34:221–5.
6. Liu SW, Thomas SH, Gordon JA, et al. A pilot study examining undesirable events among emergency department-boarded patients awaiting inpatient beds. *Ann Emerg Med.* 2009;54:381–5.
7. Forster AJ, Stiell I, Wells G, et al. The effect of hospital occupancy on emergency department length of stay and patient disposition. *Acad Emerg Med.* 2003;10:127–33.
8. Liu SW, Chang YC, Weissman JS, et al. An empirical assessment of boarding and quality of care: delays in care among chest pain, pneumonia, and cellulitis patients. *Acad Emerg Med.* 2011;18:1339–48.
9. Viccellio A, Santora C, Singer AJ, et al. The association between transfer of emergency department boarders to inpatient hallways and mortality: a 4-year experience. *Ann Emerg Med.* 2009;54:487–91.
10. McHugh M, VanDyke K, McClelland M, et al. Improving Patient Flow and Reducing Emergency Department Crowding. Rockville, MD: AHRQ; 2011. Report No.: 11(12)-0094.
11. Fee C, Weber EJ, Sharpe BA, et al. When is a scarlet letter really a red badge of courage? the paradox of percentage of pneumonia patients receiving antibiotics within 4 hours in accordance with JCAHO and CMS core measures. *Ann Emerg Med.* 2007;50:205–6.
12. Walls RM, Resnick J. The joint commission on accreditation of healthcare organizations and center for medicare and medicaid services community-acquired pneumonia initiative: what went wrong? *Ann Emerg Med.* 2005;46:409–11.
13. Wachter RM. Why diagnostic errors don't get any respect—and what can be done about them. *Health Aff (Millwood).* 2010;29:1605–10.
14. Pines JM, Kelly JJ, Meisl H, et al. Procedural safety in emergency care: a conceptual model and recommendations. *Jt Comm J Qual Patient Saf.* 2012;38:516–26.
15. Croskerry P, Cosby KS, Schenkel SM, et al. *Patient Safety in Emergency Medicine.* Philadelphia, PA: Wolters Kluwer Health; 2009.
16. Wachter RM. *Understanding Patient Safety.* 2nd ed. New York, NY: McGraw Hill Medical; 2012.
17. Makary MA, Sexton JB, Freischlag JA, et al. Operating room teamwork among physicians and nurses: teamwork in the eye of the beholder. *J Am Coll Surg.* 2006;202:746–52.
18. Pronovost PJ, Berenholtz SM, Goeschel C, et al. Improving patient safety in intensive care units in Michigan. *J Crit Care.* 2008;23:207–21.
19. DeWalt DA, Callahan LF, Hawk VH, et al. *Health Literacy Universal Precautions Toolkit.* Rockville, MD: Agency for Healthcare Research and Quality; 2010.
20. CMCS Informational Bulletin. In: Services: DoHaH ed. Baltimore, MD: CMCS Informational Bulletin. 2013:1–39.
21. Conwell LJ, Cohen JW. Characteristics of people with high medical expenses in the U.S. civilian noninstitutionalized population, 2002. In: Quality AfHRa, ed. Rockville, MD: Quality AfHRa; 2005.
22. MPAC (MEDPAC). Payment Policy for Readmissions Report to the Congress: Promoting Greater Efficiency in Medicare. Washington, DC: MEDPAC; 2007:103–20.
23. McCarthy DM, Cameron KA, Courtney DM, et al. Self-reported use of communication techniques in the emergency department. *J Emerg Med.* 2012;43:E355–E61.
24. Vashi A, Rhodes KV. "Sign right here and you're good to go": a content analysis of audio-taped emergency department discharge instructions. *Ann Emerg Med.* 2010;57:315–22 e1.

24

Patient Safety in Pediatrics

Ahmed S. Said, Kara Kniska, Matthew I. Goldsmith, and Nikoleta S. Kolovos

CLINICAL VIGNETTE

MT is a 12-year-old boy (weighing 60 kg and 156 cm in length) whose past medical history is significant for relapsed acute lymphocytic leukemia (ALL). He was admitted to the pediatric intensive care unit (PICU) with profound septic shock secondary to *Escherichia coli* colitis. His ICU course was complicated by the development of abdominal compartment syndrome, renal failure, and respiratory failure requiring extended mechanical ventilation. As he recovered, he was successfully extubated but, due to narcotic habituation, required initiation of a hydromorphone infusion delivered by a computerized ambulatory drug delivery (CADD) pump. On the evening of the event, he was exhibiting signs of agitation and discomfort. An order was entered in the computer to administer a 0.016 mg/kg bolus of intravenous hydromorphone; he was inadvertently given a 0.16 mg/kg dose. Thirty minutes later, the dosing error was recognized when he was noted to be hypopneic, with pinpoint pupils and increasing lethargy. He was treated with naloxone with subsequent improvement in his symptomatology, and the hydromorphone infusion was restarted 3 hours later without incident. The dosing error was disclosed to the family who expressed their understanding of the circumstances and the plan. The order was reviewed and was written correctly in the computerized order entry system.

Questions

• Utilization of smart pumps has demonstrated a reduction in PICU medication errors.
   a. True
   b. False

   True. Larsen et al. reported a 73% reduction in medication-related errors after implementation of standard devices and drug concentrations.

Larsen GY, Parker HB, Cash J, et al. Standard drug concentrations and smart-pump technology reduce continuous-medication-infusion errors in pediatric patients. *Pediatrics.* 2005;116(1):e-21–5.[1]

- Full disclosure of medical errors results in increased lawsuits.
  a. True
  b. False

  False. Boothman and Hoyler demonstrated a reduction in lawsuits following the development of an early disclosure program.

Boothman R, Hoyler MM. The University of Michigan's early disclosure and offer program. *Bull Am Coll Surg.* 2013;98(3):21–5.[2]

INTRODUCTION

Children are not little adults. This fact poses unique challenges regarding patient safety and quality in pediatrics. Rates of medical errors are similar in adults and children, but the potential for adverse drug events within the pediatric inpatient population is approximately three times higher than in hospitalized adults.[3]

UNIQUE SAFETY ISSUES IN PEDIATRICS

The increased vulnerability of children in the health care setting has been attributed to several factors.[4]

- Many health care settings are structured for the care of adult patients and lack trained staff oriented to pediatric care, protocols and safeguards, and up-to-date and easily accessible pediatric equipment and reference materials such as drug dosing manuals, vital sign ranges, and textbooks of common physical findings. Emergency departments may be particularly risk-prone environments for children.[5]
- Younger children are less capable of communicating adverse effects they may be experiencing.
- Children have less mature hepatic, renal, and immune systems and are more prone to experience the physiologic adverse effects of medication errors.
- Most commercially available medications are prepared and packaged for adults. These medications often then have to be prepared in different volumes and concentrations prior to administration to pediatric patients. The need to alter the original medication formulation and/or dose requires a series of pediatric-specific calculations and tasks, each significantly increasing the possibility of error.

TECHNOLOGY IN PEDIATRICS

In response to the 1999 Institute of Medicine Report and leading health care initiatives, many hospitals began implementing various available technologies to improve patient safety. These technologies included innovations such as computerized order entry, "smart" infusion pumps, and bar coding devices. While all designed to minimize errors, each had potential to introduce unanticipated outcomes. For example, the introduction of computerized order entry at a major children's hospital was designed to decrease errors related to dosing and illegible handwriting but was paradoxically associated with an increase in mortality.[6] Smart infusion pumps have been shown to decrease the number of errors in the pediatric population[1]; however, the incidence of serious medication events was unchanged with the use of that same technology in another study.[7] Bar coding and positive patient identification also has promise in the prevention of wrong-patient medication administration and laboratory sampling; however, research has demonstrated conflicting results as to its effectiveness. In neonates, a 47% reduction in adverse drug events has been demonstrated,[8] although these data have not been replicated in children or adults.

Of particular concern with all technology is the "work-around" phenomenon as these devices may increase a provider's workload. For example, "charting by exception" is a shortcut whereby a bedside provider transfers prior chart values in a time-saving maneuver. Caregivers may also find ways to decrease the time it takes to enter medications, for example, by removing identifying labels, combining them, and scanning them at one time. If work-arounds are discovered, a key component of improving the culture of safety is to listen to the frontline providers as to why such actions were necessary. Resources such as unit safety committees and hospital quality oversight committees can be useful in commissioning debriefing events and analyses to identify practical solutions that improve care delivery.

While technology is important in enhancing systems, programs designed to hone assessment skills are also important in the care of the child, particularly those who are unable to communicate secondary to either developmental milestones or medical fragility. Pediatric Early Warning Systems have been developed and validated, which use objective criteria from a patient's neurobehavioral status, cardiovascular system, and respiratory parameters to generate a score that indicates a need for increased monitoring or escalation of care.[9,10] The Institute of Healthcare Improvement has also advocated rapid response teams; data in both children and adults have been inconclusive as to improved outcomes. However, rapid response teams represent good clinical practice and promote a culture of safety, particularly among trainees and personnel with less experience.

COMMUNICATION WITH PARENTS AND FAMILIES

Family-Centered Care

Children are frequently unable to speak for themselves, and as such, their parents and caregivers are acting not only as advocates but also as decision makers. Parents (and guardians, including grandparents) provide unique understanding to a child; for children who are in frequent interaction with the health care environment, this information is essential. The American Academy of Pediatrics has established guidelines and recommendations regarding the concept of family-centered care. Familial presence at bedside rounds should be considered standard practice, and parents should be offered the opportunity to be present during procedures.[11] A typical concern is the impact such a structure has on both families and trainees. When studied, most parents responded that attendance at rounds reduced their concerns and increased their confidence in the health care team; medical trainees were less likely to support this and believed that care and learning opportunities were blunted when families were present.[12]

Consent, Permission, and Assent

A key aspect in the care of children is the relationship between physicians, patients, and families in the decision-making process, not only in medical care but also in the research arena. The concepts of parental permission and patient assent are adjuncts to the tenet of informed consent. The responsibility for *informed consent* in children is frequently assumed by a parent or guardian, which, although rare, may prove problematic when the adult's beliefs are incongruent with the best interest of the child. *Parental permission* is the notion that decisions regarding the care of a young child involve a common responsibility between practitioners and families. *Patient assent* involves the concept that children who have reached an age of understanding should be included in the discussions surrounding care or research protocols.[13]

MEDICATION SAFETY

Medication errors are one of the most frequent adverse events that occur in health care settings. Pediatric patients are at higher risk of error as compared to adults, with increased potential for harm.[14] The true incidence of medication errors is unknown as this is dependent upon accurate reporting; using a trigger tool, there was an average of 11.1% rate of adverse drug events in pediatric patients.[15] A study published in 2003 aimed at characterizing medication errors in pediatrics concluded that the majority of errors occurred at the ordering stage. Potentially harmful errors were more likely to involve errors in dosing, allergies, or frequency.[16] A recent study in an academic, university-affiliated hospital found that 10-fold medication errors were a significant source of risk to pediatric patients. Morphine was the most frequently error-reported medication, and opioids were the most frequently reported drug class. Intravenous formulations, paper ordering, and drug delivery pumps were frequent error enablers. Errors of dose calculation, documentation of decimal points, and confusion with zeroes were frequent contributing causes to 10-fold medication errors.[17]

There are numerous reasons that the pediatric patient is more susceptible to medication errors. In contrast to most medications used in adults, pediatric dosages are calculated based upon their weight, introducing an extra step where an error may occur. Additionally, pediatric doses are calculated in the metric system; most parents and patients in the US are familiar with body weight measured in pounds, not kilograms. Depending upon the size of the patient, doses may contain decimal points, which predisposes a patient to a potential dosing error by a factor of 10. To minimize this risk, the Joint Commission recommends using a leading zero in front of the decimal point and never using a trailing zero after the decimal point.[14] Another source of dosing errors in pediatrics is a failure to recognize the adult dose of a medication. Many pediatricians and pediatric trainees know the weight-based dose for specific medications; however, for an older child or adolescent patient, this dose may be higher than the adult dose.

Another pediatric medication challenge is the commercially available dosage preparation. Solid oral dosage forms, such as tablets and capsules, are not typically the correct dose needed for a child. Even if the dose is correct, infants, toddlers, and children cannot swallow tablets and capsules. Availability of liquid preparations may be limited, particularly in remote areas, compounding pharmacies face challenges in maintaining stability of liquid preparations, and data on how to prepare the compounds may be unavailable. In addition, intravenous medications are not packaged with the pediatric patient in mind. Frequently, available concentrations are often not conducive for use in the pediatrics, and the drugs must first be diluted to obtain the correct dose. Also, manufacturers may recommend that the adult dose be place into a certain volume (i.e., 100 mL) for administration. In neonates and children with congenital or acquired heart disease, this volume could lead to fluid overload. It is recommended that medications for pediatric patients be made as a standard concentration to reduce the likelihood of a dilution or calculation error and with as few concentrations as possible.[4]

TABLE 24-1   Medication Administration Process Measure for Error Reduction

- Establish a pediatric formulary system for drug evaluation, selection, and use.[18]
- Standardize timing of orders (e.g., day 0 or day 1).
- Limit the number of concentrations of high-alert medications to a minimum.
- Standardize the volume and concentration of compounded oral medications and total parenteral nutrition for both inpatient and home use.
- Use standardized syringes for oral medications.

A final challenge in the safe use of medications in the pediatric patient is the lack of drug studies in this population. Most medications are developed, tested, and approved for adult use. Once the drug is approved, the medication can be used off-label for other indications, including use in pediatric patients. Along with the challenge of the dosing formulations already discussed, if the medication is thought to be beneficial in a pediatric patient, determining the correct dose can be problematic. Depending upon the age of the patient, children have different pharmacokinetic parameters as compared to adults. This may affect the volume of distribution, metabolism, clearance, and overall exposure to the medication. This also changes throughout the stages of development; therefore, there is a need to study the medications in all pediatric age ranges. The development of "gray baby syndrome" with chloramphenicol and kernicterus with sulfa medications are examples of adverse drug reactions, which can occur in neonates, due to their age-related pharmacokinetic differences. New medications need to be studied in the pediatric patient to determine safety and efficacy; caution should be used when initiating a medication that has not been thoroughly studied in pediatrics.

A summary of recommendations to minimize pediatric medication errors is highlighted in Tables 24-1 through 24-3.

TABLE 24-2   Recommendations for Pharmacy Management

- A practitioner trained in pediatrics should be assigned to committees responsible for oversight of medication management.
- Immediate access to current pediatric-specific information for all hospital staff should be available, including drug reference materials, pediatric growth charts, normal vital sign ranges, emergency dosage calculations, and research study data.
- New pharmacy staff should be oriented to specialized neonatal/pediatric pharmacy services available in each institution.[19]
- Preparation of dosage calculation sheet for patients in intensive care settings[20] including both emergency and commonly used medications.[19]
- Development of preprinted medication order forms and clinical protocols to reflect a standardized approach to medication ordering, preparation, and administration.
- Ensure available information about monitoring parameters.
- Pediatric satellite pharmacies or pediatric-trained pharmacists and technicians should be present on newborn/pediatric intensive care and oncology units.[3,19]
- Pediatric medications should be stored and prepared in areas separate from those where adult medications are stored and prepared.

TABLE 24-3	Practical and Procedural Management to Reduce Medication Errors

- Ensure ability to accurately measure the additives for intravenous solutions, including total parenteral nutrition.
- Ensure availability of dose range checking software in hospital or pharmacy information systems enabled to provide alerts for potentially incorrect doses.
- Medications in automated dispensing cabinets should be limited to those needed for emergency use or to those medications under the control of licensed independent prescribers.
- Education for providers who interact with infusion/smart pumps.
- Use consistent physiologic monitoring, including pulse oximetry, while children receiving procedural sedation.[21]
- Health care facilities are encouraged to develop bar coding technology with pediatric capability, including the ability to provide readable code for small-volume, pediatric-specific dose labels.

KEY POINTS

- Many health care settings are designed for the adult patient, putting children at risk.
- Most commercially available medications are prepared, packaged, and dosed for adults.
- Technologic innovation may have unintended consequences in children for whom the technology may not be optimized.
- Health care organizations that care for children are encouraged to develop technology with pediatric capability.
- Basic physical assessment skills are paramount in the care of a child.
- Parents and caregivers are an essential component of the pediatric health care team.
- Clear communication among the members of the health care team is essential to devise plans and clarify changes for patients who may not be able to speak for themselves.

ONLINE RESOURCES[22]

1. Safer Health Care for Kids: www.aap.org/saferhealthcare
2. Children's Hospital Association: www.childrenshospitals.org
3. Institute for Safe Medication Practices: www.ismp.org
4. National Initiative for Children's Healthcare Quality: www.nichq.org

REFERENCES

1. Larsen GY, Parker HB, Cash J, et al. Standard drug concentrations and smart-pump technology reduce continuous-medication-infusion errors in pediatric patients. *Pediatrics.* 2005;116(1):e-21–5.
2. Boothman R, Hoyler MM. The University of Michigan's early disclosure and offer program. *Bull Am Coll Surg.* 2013;98(3):21–5.
3. Kaushal R, Bates DW, Landrigan C, et al. Medication errors and adverse drug events in pediatric inpatients. *JAMA.* 2001;285(16):2114–20.

4. The Joint Commission. Preventing pediatric medication errors. *Sentinel Event Alert.* Issue 39, April 11, 2008.
5. Institute of Medicine. *Emergency Care for Children: Growing Pains.* Washington, DC: National Academies Press; 2007.
6. Han YY, Carcillo JA, Venkataraman ST, et al. Unexpected increased mortality after implementation of a commercially sold computerized physician order entry system. *Pediatrics.* 2005;116(6):1506–12.
7. Rothschild JM, Keohane CA, Cook EF, et al. A controlled trial of smart infusion pumps to improve medication safety in critically ill patients. *Crit Care Med.* 2005;33(3):533–40.
8. Morriss FH, Jr., Abramowitz PW, Nelson SP, et al. Effectiveness of a barcode medication administration system in reducing preventable adverse drug events in a neonatal intensive care unit: a prospective cohort study. *J Pediatr.* 2009;154(3):363–8.
9. Egdell P, Finlay L, Pedley DK. The PAWS score: validation of an early warning system for the initial assessment of children in the emergency department. *Emerg Med J.* 2008;25(11):745–9.
10. Parshuram CS, Duncan HP, Joffe AR, et al. Multicentre validation of the bedside paediatric early warning system score: a severity of illness score to detect evolving critical illness in hospitalised children. *Crit Care.* 2011;15(4):R184.
11. Committee on Hospital Care, American Academy of Pediatrics. Family-centered care and the pediatrician's role. *Pediatrics.* 2003;112(3):691–6
12. Grzyb MJ, Coo H, Ruhland L, et al. Views of parents and health care providers regarding parental presence at bedside rounds in a neonatal intensive care unit. *J Perinatol.* 2014;34(2):143–8.
13. Committee on Bioethics, American Academy of Pediatrics. Informed consent, parental permission, and assent in pediatric practice. *Pediatrics.* 1995;95(2):314–7.
14. The Joint Commission. Facts about the official "do not use list." June 18, 2013.
15. Takata GS, Mason W, Taketomo C, et al. Development, testing, and findings of a pediatric-focused trigger tool to identify medication-related harm in US children's hospitals. *Pediatrics.* 2008;121(4):e927–35.
16. Fortescue EB, Kaushal R, Landrigan CP, et al. Prioritizing strategies for preventing medication errors and adverse drug events in pediatric inpatients. *Pediatrics.* 2003;111(4):722–9.
17. Doherty C, McDonnell C. Tenfold medication errors: 5 years' experience at a university-affiliated pediatric hospital. *Pediatrics.* 2012;129(5):916–24.
18. Committee on Drugs and Committee on Hospital Care, American Academy of Pediatrics. Policy statement—prevention of medication errors in the pediatric inpatient setting. *Pediatrics.* 2003;112(2):431–6.
19. Levine SL, Cohen MR. Preventing medication errors in pediatric and neonatal patients. In Cohen MR, ed. *Medication Errors.* 2nd ed. Washington, DC: American Pharmacists Association; 2007:469–92.
20. Hazinski MF. Reducing calculation errors in drug dosages: the pediatric critical information sheet. *Pediatr Nurs.* 1986;12(2):138–40.
21. Cote CJ. Sedation disasters in pediatrics and concerns for office based practice. *Can J Anesth.* 2002;49(90001):R10.
22. Steering Committee on Quality Improvement and Management and Committee on Hospital Care, American Academy of Pediatrics. Principles of pediatric patient safety: reducing harm due to medical care. *Pediatrics.* 2011;127:1199–210.

Medical Imaging

James R. Duncan and Andrew Bierhals

CLINICAL VIGNETTE

A portable chest radiograph was obtained to assess causes for poor oxygenation in a patient admitted to an intensive care unit (ICU). The image was reversed when loading it into the hospital's picture archiving and communication system (PACS). Distorted anatomy allowed the error to escape detection during the initial image interpretation. As a result, the patient's new pneumothorax was interpreted as being on the left instead of the right. The ICU team was promptly notified of a new left pneumothorax, and the error was not detected until after a chest tube had been placed.

INTRODUCTION

Imaging has become an indispensable tool for modern health care since it frequently supplements the medical history and laboratory evaluation. Imaging not only has reduced the need for invasive procedure but also is being used to guide an increasing number of minimally invasive procedures. These advances have led to faster diagnosis, treatment, and recovery. The drawback is a complex and segmented system where key steps such as selection of the most appropriate imaging study, image acquisition, study interpretation, and treatment decisions are distributed across different individuals and teams.[1] Such complexity and segmentation can degrade system performance unless reliability concepts such as checks, redundancies, and error recovery strategies are added. High-reliability organizations recognize that errors can and will occur at any step.[2] Ensuring safe, high-quality medical imaging requires a systematic assessment of multiple processes.

SYSTEMATIC APPROACH TO MEDICAL IMAGING

The steps necessary for imaging to add value have been compared to the Five Rights of Medication Administration. The ideal imaging system includes five steps: Right Study, Right Order, Right Way, Right Report, and Right Action. This process starts with a clinical question. Data are collected and analyzed to answer the question. The results are then used to drive treatment decisions. In this process, information is also available from other sources such as history, physical examination, laboratory evaluation, and prior encounters. The information from these sources can assist with choosing the most appropriate imaging study or focusing on the most likely diagnosis. In some cases, information from these sources can completely obviate the need for an imaging study. Given the risks, delays, and costs of gathering data, the ideal system will only collect enough data to answer the question at hand.[3] One should avoid situations where data are collected to satisfy one's curiosity or confirm an established diagnosis. In this ideal system, data-gathering activities are tightly linked to treatment decisions.

The Right Study

Choosing the right study begins with determining if imaging is the best source of the information and ends with choosing a particular imaging study. Regrettably, evidence-based decision guidelines for imaging have only been developed a few scenarios.[4] Observation versus head CT for children with minor head trauma is a well-studied example. A recent large study confirmed that when certain criteria are met, the pretest probability of discovering a clinically important finding with head CT is extremely low.[5] Unless continued observation over the next few hours reveals new information, the child's parents should be informed that the available data set predicts a complete recovery. From the perspective of information theory,[6] the additional data provided by the head CT are redundant. Still, many anxious parents will often ask about getting a head CT "just to be sure." However, in settings where the pretest probability of a serious injury is extremely low, the risks of the ionizing radiation as well as risks of falsely positive or negative studies should be part of the decision-making process.[1] Any result other than "normal" undermines the reassurance that parents experience when hearing the results. In addition, the benefit of any abnormal diagnostic study is linked to the health system's ability to act on the result and promote recovery. Indeed, some have suggested that not knowing about a potentially serious condition such as prostate cancer has benefits because the treatment can be worse than the disease.[7] Failure modes for selecting the right study are found in Table 25-1.

This Bayesian approach to medical decision making requires frontline teams to look for patterns in the available data before determining whether an imaging study will add value to the existing data set. In many cases, time and energy spent collecting additional history, prior imaging exams, and laboratory results will better address diagnostic uncertainty and guide therapeutic interventions than an additional imaging study. The importance of obtaining and reviewing prior imaging exams cannot be overemphasized. "The Right Study" is often the one that was performed last week in a physician's office or an hour ago in the outside hospital. While most of the data embedded in electronic medical records cannot be shared between facilities, medical imaging utilizes a standardized format (DICOM) that allows gigabytes of information to be quickly and reliably conveyed to the point of care. Information systems

TABLE 25-1	Right Study	
Subtask	Failure Mode	Example
Patient assessment	Inadequate evaluation	Imaging study ordered prior to patient evaluation
Choose an imaging study rather than a better alternative	Alternative provides equivalent benefit with less risk	Observation instead of head CT for children with minor head trauma

can clearly improve their ability to support frontline teams by leveraging the ever-increasing amount of data captured in electronic formats.

Once the decision is made that a new imaging study is needed to guide care, the question becomes, which study among the numerous imaging choices is "the Right Study"? This problem can be compared to a common navigation problem. One typically relies on personal experience when navigating from point A to B, but when personal experience is lacking, navigation aids become critical. Imaging professionals often serve as guides who plot a course using their knowledge of the terrain and the traveler's desired destination. The decision-making algorithms used by these guides are increasingly being incorporated into computerized systems. In the same way that GPS navigation systems not only help plot the route but also update the guidance information as the trip unfolds, clinical decision support systems can use information about the patient's current condition and goals of therapy to update their recommendations. The ever-increasing array of diagnostic studies such as ultrasound, CT, magnetic resonance imaging (MRI), and positron emission tomography (PET) can be considered different waypoints along a route that leads to treatment and recovery. While consultation with an imaging expert may still be needed to discern the best path through a unique clinical situation, the 80/20 rule suggests that the 80% of imaging decisions follow a relatively limited number of paths. Automated decision support tools promise to help frontline teams find these optimal paths in common situations with 24/7 availability.

The Right Order

Orders for imaging studies frequently fail to convey the necessary information (Table 25-2). These orders should receive the same diligence that is being used to ensure accuracy with medication orders. Although no reasonable provider would submit an order of "antibiotic for pneumonia," vague orders for imaging studies such as "brain scan to rule out pathology" remain all too common. As orders for imaging studies become more specific, imaging departments work to reconcile the study order with the most appropriate study. A common example is chest CT where studies are frequently ordered without and with intravenous contrast. Such dual or combination studies are very rarely needed, but there is a natural human tendency to believe that "more is better."

TABLE 25-2	Right Order	
Subtask	Failure Mode	Examples
Order exam	Vague order	Order reads "brain scan"
	Incorrect order	Foot radiographs requested for patient with ankle trauma
	Over order	Chest CT ordered as without and with IV contrast for suspected pulmonary embolism
Provide history	Inadequate history	History reads "R/O pathology"

Choosing the most appropriate exam includes communicating the site and nature of the clinical concern. Foot radiographs are often ordered for evaluation of ankle injuries, and the site of maximal tenderness is often absent from the request. While these errors are often corrected by the technologist performing the exam, it requires additional work to contact the ordering provider, cancel the existing exam, and order the correct study.

Multiple exams are often concurrently requested to address the same clinical question. A more reasonable strategy would be to select the most appropriate study first and evaluate that result before proceeding to the next study. While the shotgun approach might occasionally seem more efficient, it is akin to prescribing multiple drugs for same symptom in hope that one is effective. Although some may contend that multiple antibiotics are often given concurrently when the organism causing a serious infection is uncertain, the difference is that while multiple antibiotics can be given concurrently, it is usually not possible to simultaneously perform multiple imaging studies. Thus, one must decide upon a sequence of imaging studies, typically balancing diagnostic yield versus access, invasiveness, and cost.

The Right Way

The imaging department typically controls whether the study is performed in "the Right Way," and selected failure modes are found in Table 25-3. Choices start with selecting the "right" equipment and settings to maximize the probability of answering the clinical question while minimizing risk. While the details of this optimization process are beyond the scope of this chapter, one good example occurs when imaging children.

TABLE 25-3	Right Way	
Subtask	Failure Mode	Example
Selection of imaging equipment	Inappropriate equipment	Fluoroscope lacking dose monitoring equipment is used to perform a complex procedure[8]
Select imaging protocol	Appropriate protocol is not available	Facility lacks size-specific pediatric protocols
	Appropriate protocol is not selected	Pediatric protocol is available but it is not used
Image according to protocol	Variation from protocol	Scanned volume during a CT exam extends above or below the specified region (Z-axis overscanning)

TABLE 25-3	Right Way (Continued)	
Subtask	Failure Mode	Example
Imaging data are processed for review	Mislabeled images	Left marker is placed on an image of the right arm
Check for diagnostic images	Failure to check that exam includes the entire volume of interest	Abdominal radiographs obtained for potential intraoperative foreign body fail to include all recesses of the peritoneal cavity
	Check leads to unneeded additional images	Patient moved during a portion of a CT exam. Rather than just repeating selected images, the entire study is repeated
Imaging data are stored	Not properly stored	Key images not sent to PACS

Most imaging equipment has been designed to serve the much larger adult market. As a result, the imaging equipment even in pediatric specialty centers is identical or nearly identical to that used to image adults. However, the marked differences in patient size between newborns, toddlers, and teenagers have prompted pediatric specialty centers to develop size-specific imaging protocols.[9] In the same way that doses of medications are adjusted for the child's weight, machine settings for pediatric imaging should be adjusted for the patient's size. This is particular important for CT scans and radiographs since x-ray penetration drops geometrically as body part diameter increases. The amount of ionizing radiation needed to adequately image a 15-cm thick abdomen is typically one-tenth that needed to image a 30-cm thick abdomen.

The "right way" for imaging studies includes making the most informative images accessible to everyone treating the patient. While it might seem ideal to make the entire study immediately available, network bandwidth issues arise when trying to share imaging studies that exceed a gigabyte. Further, locating the key images within studies that consist of several hundred images takes time. To preserve bandwidth, decrease storage costs, and improve physician workflow, a subset of the entire study is often uploaded to the picture archiving and communication system (PACS). PACS is also used to identify prior studies and make them available for comparison.

The Right Report

Radiologists play a central role in the acquisition and interpretation of most imaging studies. They review large amounts of imaging data and summarize the key findings in a report that ideally concludes by addressing the clinical question. Image interpretation can be considered a type of data compression where gigabytes of imaging data are distilled into kilobytes of text. High levels of compression occur when imaging data can be succinctly described as "normal" or "unchanged from the prior study." Abnormalities and interval changes in the imaging data can usually be summarized by referring to the responsible pathophysiology and pertinent details, for example, "5.0-cm diverticular abscess in the left lower quadrant." Multiple failure modes undermine efforts to generate the Right Report (Table 25-4).

TABLE 25-4 Right Report		
Subtask	Failure Mode	Example
Prior studies reviewed	Prior studies not reviewed	Although a study is being used to assess treatment response, current exam is not compared to prior studies because the prior studies are not available or failure to perform the comparison
Key findings detected	Key finding not detected	Finding is below the reviewer's perceptual threshold Multiple findings lead to premature termination of search
Findings are used to formulate a differential diagnosis	Finding is misinterpreted, and as a result, the correct diagnosis is not included Qualifying statements lead to an excessively long differential diagnosis	Finding is believed to reflect normal variant rather than pathology "Likely normal variant but cannot rule out neoplastic process"
Important result called to provider	Result not perceived as requiring immediate notification Notification delayed because provider is unknown or unavailable	Indeterminate pulmonary nodule No contact information for ordering physician or he/she does not answer call
Report generated	Reporting errors	Reporter says "left" when he/she means "right"
Report available for distribution	Errors not corrected when checking report Delay in report distribution	Left versus right error is not corrected Report is not available until after treatment decision is made

Images from prior studies should be reviewed as part of interpreting the current exam. Pathophysiology is a dynamic process and often the question is not whether disease is present but whether it is responding to treatment. Such assessments are impossible without prior studies. Prior studies from the same institution are readily retrieved from an institution's PACS. Subspecialty care and second opinions are increasingly prompting patients to bring their prior imaging studies on compact discs. Many sites now load these outside studies into their PACS so that they can be compared to prior or subsequent studies. More advanced solutions are being developed to facilitate rapid transfer of imaging information across great distances.[10]

Image interpretation begins with focusing visual attention. Both attention and the subsequent perception of patterns are heavily influenced by expectations at the conscious and subconscious levels. The common adage is that "you only see what you know." When multiple abnormalities are present, the detection of each depends on completing an exhaustive search. The satisfaction of search phenomena describes premature termination of the search since finding several abnormalities early in the search pattern can cause attention to shift to interpretation rather than completing the search.[11]

Once patterns are detected, image interpretation then progresses to pattern characterization. Findings are categorized as normal or abnormal although normal variants and incidental findings create substantial latitude for categorization. Pattern analysis leads to a differential diagnosis. Decisions are then made regarding where each possibility is placed in this list. Ideally, the most likely entity is placed at the top of the list, and the list only contains reasonable possibilities. Generating exhaustive lists of ten or more possible diagnoses might improve diagnostic sensitivity but at the expense of specificity.

Time-sensitive, critical findings warrant immediate attention and trigger notification of the primary team. Unfortunately, notification of critical findings is impeded by multiple failure modes. The image interpreter and primary team might have different definitions of what constitutes a "time-sensitive, critical finding." While all might agree that tension pneumothorax and ruptured abdominal aortic aneurysm warrant immediate notification, disagreements occur with pulmonary nodules and similar abnormalities. Deciding whether the abnormality is clinically important requires insight into the mental model of the primary team.[12] Again, the radiologist must try to balance sensitivity and specificity. An overly sensitive trigger might lead to contacting the primary team for every abnormality. Conversely, setting the trigger threshold too high will almost certainly lead to complaints such as "I should have been called about this report." While critical notification of lab results is triggered by comparing results to an objective threshold, the process is far more subjective for imaging studies.

The ideal radiology report is accurate, timely, succinct, complete, and easily to comprehend and includes ancillary information such as technique, radiation exposure, and notes as to who was notified and when notification occurred. The report might also include annotated copies of key images. The report is distributed to requesting teams and a copy is archived.

The Right Action

The final step in this sequence is using the imaging information to impact patient care. The Right Action means that the care provider receives the information, reviews it, understands it, and takes appropriate action in a timely manner. Numerous failure modes can undermine this step (Table 25-5). Many patients have multiple physicians,

TABLE 25-5	Right Action	
Subtask	Failure Mode	Example
Report sent to provider	Report sent to wrong provider	Biopsy result sent to consulting rather than primary physician
Report received	Failure to review report	Key result is included in report, but providers believe they will be called about any key result
Report understood	Report misunderstood	Report of *superficial* femoral vein thrombosis does not trigger standard treatment for deep venous thrombosis
Appropriate action	Report understood but no action is taken	Outpatient CT scan demonstrates hydronephrosis and primary team attempts to call the patient. The line is busy and the call is forgotten because another urgent matter arose before a second call was made
	Report understood but wrong action is taken	CT head shows a right subdural hematoma. Despite an accurate report and plans for the correct therapy, a lapse leads to surgery on the left side

and it is not uncommon that some but not all of the patient's physicians receive a copy of the report. Even with electronic systems where all reports are available, the signal can be lost due to alert fatigue or lack of clarity as to which physician is responsible for reviewing the results and taking action. Indeed, one unintended consequence of critical result notification is that some teams have developed the expectation that they will be called about any important result.

Communication breakdowns can cause a failure to understand the implications of the radiology report. A common example is the lack of a shared mental model for both the message's sender and receiver. The report might describe severe pancreatitis with lack of enhancement in the pancreatic body and tail, but the primary team might not recognize this as a description of necrotizing pancreatitis or fully understand the implications of that diagnosis.

Even in cases where the diagnosis is understood, failure to take appropriate action occurs. This includes meaning to act but being interrupted during the process and then forgetting to resume a planned sequence. It also occurs when a slip or lapse occurs during an intended action.

Quality and Safety Issues in Radiology

Exposing Patients to Ionizing Radiation

With exception of ultrasound and MRI studies, medical imaging requires exposing patients to ionizing radiation (Table 25-6). Ionizing radiation is in the form of x-rays for radiographs, CT exams, and fluoroscopic procedures. For nuclear medicine studies, the ionizing radiation includes γ rays and emission of charged particles. Ionizing radiation damages biologic tissue predominantly by causing double-strand breaks in

TABLE 25-6	Estimated Radiation Dose for Common Procedures[a]
Procedure	Effective Dose (mSv)
Bone densitometry	0.001
Dental intraoral x-ray	0.005
Knee series	0.005
Chest x-ray (1 view)	0.02
Mammogram (4 views)	0.4
Abdominal x-ray	0.7
Lumbar spine series	1.5
CT of the head without contrast	2
Endoscopic retrograde cholangiopancreatography	4
Barium swallow	6
Bone scan (Tc-99, MDP)	6
CT of the chest without contrast	7
Coronary angiography (diagnostic)	7
Cardiac rest–stress test (Tc-99, sestamibi)	9
Abdominal angiography (diagnostic)	12
PET/CT (F-18 FDG)	14
CT of the abdomen and pelvis with contrast	14
CT of the liver (triple phase)	15
Coronary intervention (angioplasty, stent, or radiofrequency ablation)	15
Transjugular intrahepatic portosystemic shunt placement (TIPS)	70

[a]The effective doses will vary widely between patients and institutions.[13] Even greater variation occurs with fluoroscopic procedures such as coronary angiography and TIPS.

DNA molecules.[14] In some cases, the DNA damage leads to immediate cell death, but in others, it induces a mutation, which is passed to the cell's progeny. Since cancer induction is linked to DNA mutations, ionizing radiation is classified as a carcinogen.[15] Ionizing radiation should be viewed as a drug with a narrow therapeutic window. Underuse of radiation increases the likelihood of a treatment failure due to a paucity of diagnostic information. Overuse of radiation does not improve diagnostic accuracy but does increase the probability of side effects such as skin injury and future neoplasms.

The linkage between ionizing radiation exposure and cancer induction is well accepted with high-level exposures, but there is considerable controversy about the risks of low-level exposure. The best available evidence points to a linear no-threshold model where the future cancer risk attributable to radiation exposure increases equally with each increment in exposure (Fig. 25-1). The current models also predict that risks do not dissipate with time.

Different units are used to express radiation exposure and its relative risks. Exposure is expressed using milligray (mGy) where the mGy is measure of how much energy was deposited in tissue. Given that different tissues vary in their likelihood of developing cancer, a different unit, the millisievert (mSv) is used to estimate the probability of cancer induction. Stated another way, exposure to ionizing radiation is measured in mGy and the result used to estimate the probability of a biologic impact using mSv. As shown in Figure 25-2, for any given exposure, the probability of future cancer induction is substantially higher in neonates than their grandparents.

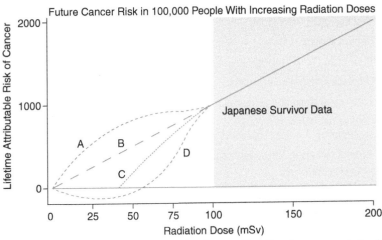

Figure 25-1. Risk models for radiation-induced cancer. Data from Japanese atomic bomb survivors are indicated by *solid line* and the *gray box*. Below 100 mSv, the data are less clear, and while the linear no-threshold model (*B, long dashed line*) is currently favored by the National Academy of Sciences,[14] at least three other models (*A*, *C*, and *D*) have been proposed. In model *A*, low doses are considered more carcinogenic. In model *C*, a threshold is proposed. In model *D*, low doses are considered protective since they trigger upregulation of DNA repair mechanisms. Essentially, all diagnostic procedures and almost all interventional procedures have doses <100 mSv.

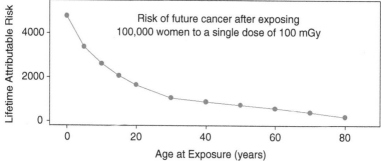

Figure 25-2. Children are a particularly vulnerable population because they are far more sensitive to the detrimental effects of ionizing radiation. The risks of developing cancer after exposure to ionizing radiation have been repeatedly estimated. The most recent report by the National Academy of Sciences Committee to Assess Health Risks from Exposure to Low Levels of Ionizing Radiation provided these estimates.[14] The risks of germline mutations that are passed to future generations and the risks of radiation-induced organ dysfunction are in addition to these estimated cancer risks.

The risk of future cancer induction is generally estimated as 1 in 1000 for a 10-mSv exposure, and the delay between radiation exposure and cancer induction is measured in decades. The assessment of these long-delayed risks is further compounded by the inability to differentiate between cancers caused by radiation exposure and any other cause. The risks of medical exposure to ionizing radiation must be considered in the context of radiation exposure from natural sources and the baseline lifetime probability of developing cancer. We are exposed to natural sources of ionizing radiation every day of our lives. A large portion of the exposure results from decay of naturally occurring isotopes such as radon and potassium. Exposure to cosmic radiation varies depending on altitude. The result is a baseline annual exposure of approximately 3 mSv from natural sources. While low radiation exposure is ubiquitous, cancer is also prevalent. The lifetime risk of developing cancer is estimated at 30% or more. While medical imaging has led to a rapid and sizable increase in per capita exposure (Fig. 25-3), any small increase in cancer rate will be difficult to detect.

MRI Safety

The high magnetic field used for MRI creates a hazardous environment. The magnetic field is present even when the scanner is not acquiring imaging. It can interfere with pacemakers, IV pumps, and other electronic devices. It can also transform metallic objects into projectiles. Patients and personnel must be screened before they can safely enter this environment. Resuscitation events (codes) are a particularly dangerous situation since unscreened personnel often rush into the room in an attempt to rescue the patient. The resulting tragedies prompted the Joint Commission to recommend that resuscitation never be attempted in the MRI room.[17]

The strong radiofrequency gradients needed for MRI can also induce currents in electrical cables and metal objects. In some cases, the resulting heating has caused skin burns. The liquid nitrogen and helium used to cool magnets to low temperatures needed for superconductivity are another hazard. Serious injuries have occurred because inadequate ventilation led to accumulation and suffocation due to displacement of oxygen.

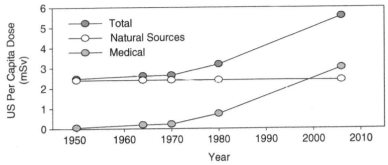

Figure 25-3. Trends in US per capita exposure to ionizing radiation. Before 1970, the predominant source of ionizing radiation was from natural sources, but since then, there has been a rapid increase in medical imaging that has doubled the per capita exposure. CT is the largest contributor due to the marked increase in the number of CT studies and the substantial radiation dose needed to create the 10–300 images in a typical CT study. Increases in nuclear medicine studies and fluoroscopic interventions have also played a role. (Adapted from Mettler FA Jr, Bhargavan M, Faulkner K, et al. Radiologic and nuclear medicine studies in the United States and worldwide: frequency, radiation dose, and comparison with other radiation sources—1950–2007. *Radiology.* 2009;253(2):520–31, Ref. 16.)

Image-Guided Procedures

Imaging is being used to perform an increasing number of procedures. This includes ultrasound-guided procedures, such as central venous access, CT-guided biopsies, and fluoroscopic procedures, such as vascular interventions. In each case, images are being used to help the operator guide long, slender tools (needles and/or catheters) toward specific targets while avoiding obstacles. The visual information creates a feedback loop where course and distance to target and location of intervening obstacles are transmitted back to the operator.

Fluoroscopic procedures provide a clear example of how low-quality images contain sufficient information to guide intraprocedural decisions. While each fluoroscopy frame is typically acquired with 20- to 100-fold less radiation than its corresponding diagnostic x-ray image, the human visual system is still able to process these low signal-to-noise images and recognize key patterns (Fig. 25-4).

The ionizing radiation used for fluoroscopic procedures creates a situation where the operators have a vested interest in patient safety. Their radiation dose is linked to patient exposure. This linkage prompts the operator to continually strive to minimize the amount of fluoroscopic information needed to successfully complete the procedure. Since these procedures frequently occur outside of radiology, steps, which can reduce patient and operator dose, are briefly reviewed here.

The simplest method of reducing dose is to reduce the number of images. For dynamic procedures, this typically means reducing the frame rate. While fluoroscopy frame rates of 30 frames per second may be needed in situations with rapid motion, many fluoroscopy units are capable of pulsed fluoroscopy at 7.5 frames per second or less. This reduction in temporal resolution provides a fourfold reduction in operator and patient dose.

Multiple methods will reduce the dose per image. Images can be acquired with lower signal-to-noise ratios (Fig. 25-4). Operators should strive to reduce the distance

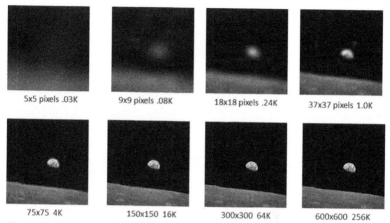

| 5x5 pixels .03K | 9x9 pixels .08K | 18x18 pixels .24K | 37x37 pixels 1.0K |
| 75x75 4K | 150x150 16K | 300x300 64K | 600x600 256K |

Figure 25-4. Demonstration of the sigmoidal relationship between diagnostic accuracy and image resolution.[3] At low resolutions, few observers would correctly recognize the image as the earth appearing above the lunar surface. While highest resolution images may be more visually appealing, once above a certain level, additional data do not improve diagnostic accuracy.

between the patient and the image detector (Fig. 25-5). Since attenuation increases geometrically with object diameter, the oblique and lateral images of the abdomen tend to have doses/images 2- to 10-fold higher than anteroposterior images (Fig. 25-5).

The teams performing these procedures can reduce their exposure by increasing the distance between them and the patient. The operator's dose primarily results from photons, which are scattered from the patient, and the highest dose is usually found on the same side as the x-ray generator (inferior to the table in Fig. 25-5A).

Complex fluoroscopic procedure in the thicker portions of large patients can lead to substantial skin doses. Skin injuries ranging from transient erythema to full-thickness necrosis occur but are largely preventable through a combination of awareness and dose management.[18,19] Since the x-ray beam is attenuated as it passes through tissue, these injuries occur on the skin closest to the x-ray generator and typically have a shape (circular or rectangular) that matches the field of view.

RADIOLOGY CONSULTATION

Advances in imaging techniques have made the ordering of imaging studies a complex process, as studies are commonly tailored to answer a specific clinical question. For example, the settings used to perform a CT scan of the chest vary depending on whether the region of interest is the coronary arteries, great vessels, tracheobronchial tree, or pulmonary parenchyma. Requesting a "CT scan of the chest" is akin to referring the patient to a specialist with a history of "chest problem." Ideally, radiology should be viewed as any other consultant service, where the consultant is asked to evaluate the patient and is supplied with the pertinent data. For radiology, this includes formal requests for consultation that are entered into the medical record or calls/visits to the reading room.

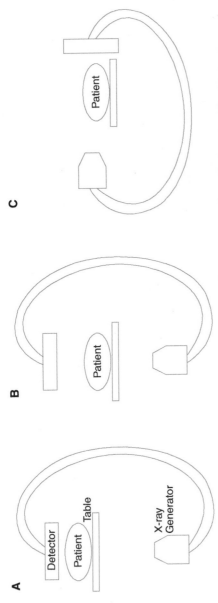

Figure 25-5. Dose considerations for different C-arm geometries during fluoroscopic procedures. Configuration (A) minimizes dose to the patient and the team performing the procedure. In this configuration, the scatter is highest below the table. In (B), the distance between the patient and the detector leads to a higher dose. In (C), the dose increases because it must penetrate more tissue before reaching the detector.

KEY POINTS

1. Imaging is a complex, multistep process. Numerous factors can degrade system performance.

2. The ionizing radiation used for CT scans, radiographs, fluoroscopic procedures, and nuclear medicine studies carries risks of cancer induction and skin injuries. In most cases, the benefits of these imaging studies greatly exceed their risks. However, radiation should be viewed as a high-hazard medication with a narrow therapeutic window.

3. While MRI avoids the risks associated with ionizing radiation, the strong magnetic fields and radiofrequency energy needed to create these images create a hazardous environment. Patients and personnel must be screened for metallic implants, pacemakers, and other items not suited to high magnetic fields before entering this environment.

ONLINE RESOURCES

1. Choosing Wisely: http://www.choosingwisely.org/
2. Image Gently: http://www.pedrad.org/associations/5364/ig/
3. Image Wisely: http://www.imagewisely.org/
4. ACR Appropriateness criteria: http://www.acr.org/Quality-Safety/Appropriateness-Criteria

REFERENCES

1. National Academies of Sciences, Engineering, and Medicine. *Improving Diagnosis in Health Care*. Washington, DC: The National Academies Press; 2015.
2. Ebeling CE. *An Introduction to Reliability and Maintainability Engineering*. New York, NY: McGraw Hill; 1997.
3. Duncan JR, Evens RG. Using information to optimize medical outcomes. *JAMA.* 2009;301(22):2383–5.
4. American College of Radiology. Appropriateness Criteria. 2013. http://www.acr.org/Quality-Safety/Appropriateness-Criteria. Accessed 11/6/13.
5. Kuppermann N, Holmes JF, Dayan PS, et al. Identification of children at very low risk of clinically-important brain injuries after head trauma: a prospective cohort study. *Lancet.* 2009;374(9696):1160–70.
6. Pierce JR. *An Introduction to Information Theory: Symbols, Signals & Noise*. 2nd rev. ed. New York, NY: Dover Publications; 1980.
7. Welch HG, Schwartz L, Woloshin S. *Overdiagnosed: Making People Sick in the Pursuit of Health*. Boston, MA: Beacon Press; 2011.
8. National Council on Radiation Protection and Measurements. *Radiation Dose Management for Fluoroscopically Guided Interventional Medical Procedures*. Bethesda, MD: National Council on Radiation Protection and Measurements; 2011.
9. Strauss KJ, Goske MJ, Kaste SC, et al. Image gently: ten steps you can take to optimize image quality and lower CT dose for pediatric patients. *AJR Am J Roentgenol.* 2010;194(4):868–73.
10. Radiological Society of North America. Image share. 2013. http://www.rsna.org/Image_Share.aspx. Accessed 11/6/13.
11. Berbaum KS, Franken EA Jr. Satisfaction of search in radiographic modalities. *Radiology.* 2011;261(3):1000–1001; author reply 1001–2.
12. Senge PM. *The Fifth Discipline: The Art and Practice of the Learning Organization*. Rev. and Updated ed. New York, NY: Doubleday/Currency; 2006.

13. Smith-Bindman R, Lipson J, Marcus R, et al. Radiation dose associated with common computed tomography examinations and the associated lifetime attributable risk of cancer. *Arch Intern Med.* 2009;169(22):2078–86.

14. National Research Council (U.S.), Committee to Assess Health Risks from Exposure to Low Level of Ionizing Radiation. *Health Risks from Exposure to Low Levels of Ionizing Radiation: BEIR VII Phase 2.* Washington, DC: National Academies Press; 2006.

15. World Health Organization. Medical radiation exposure. 2013. http://www.who.int/ionizing_radiation/about/med_exposure/en/index.html. Accessed 11/6/13.

16. Mettler FA Jr, Bhargavan M, Faulkner K, et al. Radiologic and nuclear medicine studies in the United States and worldwide: frequency, radiation dose, and comparison with other radiation sources—1950–2007. *Radiology.* 2009;253(2):520–31.

17. The Joint Commission. Preventing accidents and injuries in the MRI suite. 2008. http://www.jointcommission.org/assets/1/18/SEA_38.PDF. Accessed 11/6/13.

18. Stecker MS, Balter S, Towbin RB, et al. Guidelines for patient radiation dose management. *J Vasc Interv Radiol.* 2009;20(7 Suppl):S263–73.

19. Balter S, Hopewell JW, Miller DL, et al. Fluoroscopically guided interventional procedures: a review of radiation effects on patients' skin and hair. *Radiology.* 2010;254(2):326–41.

26 Patient Safety and Quality in Ambulatory Care

Emily Fondahn and Michael Lane

CLINICAL VIGNETTE

Ms. R is a 45-year-old woman who presented to her primary care physician (PCP) for her yearly physical examination. She pointed out a new mole on her right arm and on her right thigh to her PCP and was referred to a local dermatologist. At the dermatologist's office, she had a biopsy performed of both moles. After 2 weeks, she called the dermatology office for her test results and was told that the lesion was benign. The following year, she returned to her PCP for her yearly exam. Her PCP shared the same EMR as the dermatologist and discovered that the lesion on her right arm was melanoma and the lesion on her right thigh was benign. Later, it was discovered that the pathology report for the right arm lesion was accidentally misfiled, so the nurse only reported the results of the benign lesion.

- What are some key differences between patient safety for inpatients and outpatients?
- What are the most common types of errors in the outpatient setting?
- What methods are used to decrease the risk for failing to communicate results to patients?

INTRODUCTION

The majority of patient safety and quality research has focused on the inpatient setting, leaving a lack of intervention-based research in patient safety and quality for the ambulatory setting. There were an estimated 1.1 billion ambulatory visits in the US in 2010 with this number expecting to rise due to the shift from inpatient to outpatient care and the aging population.[1] Given these numbers, the potential harm in outpatient medicine is immense. According to the Colorado and Utah Medical Practices Study, an estimated 75,000 hospitalizations per year are due to preventable adverse events in the ambulatory setting. The most common types of ambulatory adverse events were medication events, surgical events, or diagnostic adverse events.[2] Safety and quality principles, such as just culture, infection prevention, event identification and analysis, and communication and medication safety, have been researched for inpatients and can be modified for the outpatient setting. On the other hand, differences between caring for inpatients and outpatients can make other safety methodology less relevant (Table 26-1).

Outpatient care encompasses a wide variety of patients, acuity of care, and health care settings. Outpatient practices can range from a single provider to a

TABLE 26-1	Differences between Inpatient and Outpatient Care
Inpatient	**Outpatient**
Episodic, high-intensity care	Longitudinal care
Technologically complex	Larger volume of patients
One medical record	Multiple medical records frequently with pertinent information
Comprehensive care of patient	Diffuse care settings requiring information exchange
Quality and safety officers employed by the hospital	Fewer resources with more staff multitasking
Services and providers readily available	Offsite laboratories and providers
Medical team arranges care coordination	Patients responsible for care coordination
More regulatory agencies	More diversity of patients

large, multispecialty group, with or without hospital affiliation. Given the variety of outpatient settings, there is likewise a wide range of quality and safety programs and initiatives.

Types of outpatient settings

1. Physician practices and clinics
2. Ambulatory surgery centers
3. Urgent care facilities
4. Emergency departments
5. Dialysis centers
6. Imaging centers
7. Oncology centers
8. Endoscopy centers
9. Rehabilitation centers
10. Sleep centers

Multiple barriers exist for initiation and sustainment of quality and safety programs in the outpatient setting. Within a large medical group, there can be a wide range of management policies, resources, and electronic health record use, especially if the medical group is a merger of multiple smaller, relatively independent practices. Hospital-affiliated centers may have safety and quality resources provided by the hospital. Smaller practices may have more difficulty obtaining and maintaining quality measurements due to financial and personnel constraints.[3] Team members, including the physicians, may not have sufficient training or protected time for safety and quality work. Additionally, with the advent of hospitalists, many primary care providers do not see patients in the inpatient setting resulting in decreased interaction with other providers and increasing isolation. However, given the increasing amount of care provided in the ambulatory setting, these barriers need to be addressed to improve patient care.

In the inpatient setting, medical care is delivered by a multidisciplinary team including physicians, nurses, respiratory therapists, and physical and occupational therapists, allowing for coordination of all care aspects. In the outpatient setting, the individual patients are often responsible for coordinating the majority of their health care without the same level of support; the burden of care is on the patient and his or her outpatient caregivers (family, friends, etc.). Poor patient outcomes and adverse events can occur due to the patient's increased accountability for managing his or her own health and making treatment decisions. For example, patients with congestive heart failure will make numerous decisions to guide their health every day, such as taking their medications as prescribed, eating a low-salt diet, regularly weighing themselves, and calling their health care provider with worsening symptoms. However, if patients do not follow or understand their care instructions, they may be at increased risk for worsening disease and a poor outcome.

PATIENT SAFETY IN AMBULATORY CARE

Outpatient care may also be viewed as safer given the lower acuity of illness in healthier patients. However, patient harm can and still does occur. Errors are frequently not reported in the ambulatory setting. Outpatient visits outnumber hospital discharges by more than 30–1. On average, an individual will have approximately 4 visits to an ambulatory care center each year; however, only approximately 10% of Americans will have an inpatient stay in a given year.[1] Despite the fact that the vast majority of medical care is delivered in the ambulatory setting, only 4.1% of sentinel events reported to the Joint Commission occurred in the ambulatory setting.[4] Error reporting is difficult in the ambulatory setting due to short patient interactions, multiple providers in different settings, lack of consensus about error definitions, and lack of ambulatory error reporting systems.[5] Improved classification of outpatient errors can help create categories for future study.[6] In 2011, the American Medical Association (AMA) published a 10-year review entitled "Research in the Ambulatory Patient Safety," which identified the top six errors made in the ambulatory setting and current gaps in research.[7] The top six errors identified include the following:

- Medication errors
- Diagnostic errors
- Laboratory errors
- Clinical knowledge errors
- Communication errors
- Administrative errors

Understanding these errors helps teach us when to recognize an error when it occurs and prevent future errors. Some of these topics are covered in more detail in other chapters (Medication Safety, Diagnostic Errors).

MEDICATION ERRORS

Medication errors are very common in the outpatient setting. This section highlights some of the unique difficulties with medication safety for the ambulatory setting. In the inpatient setting, physicians can generally assume that the patient is receiving what is listed on the medication list at the correct times and dosages and can monitor closely for adverse events and drug levels. However, given the longer feedback loops in outpatient care, providers lose much of this control and become more reliant on patients to accurately report all medications and dosages they are taking. The number of patients experiencing medication errors in the ambulatory setting is staggering; a report from the Institute of Medicine in 2006 estimated 530,000 Medicare beneficiaries in ambulatory clinics experienced a medication-related error in the year.[8,9]

Medication Reconciliation

Medication reconciliation should occur at every transition of care and patient appointment. However, patients frequently do not know medication names or doses, and time is not available to go through the entire medication list. It has been estimated that a complete medication reconciliation process takes between 15 and 30 minutes.[10] Given the time pressures on clinicians in the ambulatory setting, it is not surprising that medication reconciliation may not routinely be completed. There is significant potential for harm though as on discharge from the hospital, 23% of patients were not taking their discharge medications and 29% had a discrepancy between their discharge medication list and what they were actually taking.[11]

Patient Adherence

Health care providers may fail to recognize the contribution of nonadherence to a patient's health and medical condition. In one study examining 195,000 newly prescribed e-prescriptions, only 72% were filled.[12] Medications for chronic conditions, such as diabetes, hypertension, and hyperlipidemia, were more likely to have noncompliance. Health care providers may overestimate patient's understanding of medications. In one study of 359 adults waiting for an ambulatory appointment, understanding of prescription label instructions ranged from 53% to 89%.[13] Tools to help patients adhere and understand their medications include providing a medication list at every visit, encouraging patients to bring medications to all appointments, providing patients with a pill box, using patient-friendly language on the prescription instructions, and educating patients and caregivers about important side effects and interactions.

Medication Monitoring

Many medications require careful monitoring in the outpatient setting. Outpatient clinicians must create reliable processes to accurately monitor these medications. The most common errors are failure to act on available information, such as signs, symptoms, or laboratory values of drug toxicity (e.g., failure to respond promptly to systems suggestive of digoxin toxicity) and inadequate laboratory monitoring of drug therapies (e.g., checking International normalized ratio [INRs] for patient on warfarin).[9]

Medication Prescribing

Prescribing errors are some of the most common in ambulatory medicine. In one study evaluating 1879 prescriptions, 7.6% had a medication error that was life threatening, serious, or significant.[14] E-prescribing has shown promise to decrease this amount of errors by requiring complete, legible prescriptions, checking interactions, and checking allergies. A small study of 15 providers showed a decrease in error rates from 42/100 prescriptions to 6/100 prescriptions after implementation of an e-prescribing system with clinical decision support including dosing recommendations and checks for drug–drug interactions, patient allergies, and duplicate therapy.[15]

DIAGNOSTIC ERRORS

Diagnostic errors are defined as a delayed, missed, or incorrect diagnosis. Given the brief, episodic nature of ambulatory care, diagnostic errors are a threat to clinicians and patients. In one series of 307 closed malpractice claims, cancer was the most commonly missed diagnosis (24% breast cancer, 7% colorectal cancer, 8% skin cancer), followed by infections (5%), fractures (4%), and myocardial infarctions (4%).[16] These cases led to significant or major physical adverse outcomes in 59% of cases and death in 30% of cases. The breakdown points in the diagnostic process are listed in Table 26-2.

The outpatient setting is prone to diagnostic errors for a wide variety of reasons. The clinician may receive inaccurate or insufficient information from the patient or colleagues and may have inadequate or overwhelming information from the patient's medical record. The busy and rushed nature of ambulatory care lends itself to premature closure and other cognitive bias by the provider. The physicians are often reliant on the patient to follow up with requested laboratory or diagnostic testing to make a diagnosis and to adhere to the treatment plan.

Methods to improve the diagnostic process focus on the provider–patient encounter and the electronic medical record.[17] Web portals that allow patient and physician electronic transmission of laboratory and diagnostic test results, recommendations, and communication are one promising future strategy. Additionally, equipping EMRs with triggers, mnemonics, or checklists is one possibility to help providers fully evaluate a diagnosis. Employing point of care testing whenever possible allows for immediate communication of results and establishment of a plan of care.

TABLE 26-2 Breakdown Points in the Diagnostic Process

Breakdowns in Diagnostic Process	% of Cases
Initial delay by patient to seek care	9
Failure to obtain adequate medical history or physical exam	42
Failure to order appropriate diagnostic or laboratory test	55
Diagnostic or laboratory test ordered but not performed	9
Diagnostic or laboratory test performed incorrectly	8
Incorrect interpretation of diagnostic or laboratory test	67
Responsible provider did not receive diagnostic or laboratory test results	13
Diagnostic or laboratory test results not transmitted to patient	12
Inappropriate or inadequate follow-up plan	45
Failure to refer	26
Failure for requested referral to occur	5
Failure to refer to physician to convey relevant results to referring clinician	2
Patient nonadherence to the follow-up plan	17

COMMUNICATION ERRORS

Numerous studies have shown that lapses in communication contribute to poor quality care and patient safety. As discussed previously, the providers rely on the patients to bring forward concerns, symptoms, and accurate medical histories to help them diagnose problems and identify potential adverse medication errors. However, during the clinical encounter, physicians often lack the information needed. In a survey of 253 clinicians in 32 Colorado practices, important information was missing at the time of the visit in 13.6% of cases.[18] The lack of information was thought to likely lead to delayed care or duplicated care in 59.5% of the cases. The likelihood of missing information increased as the number of active medical problems increased (Fig. 26-1).

Similarly, the patients expect that their providers will provide them with prompt information from study or laboratory results and clear follow-up and treatment plans. Numerous gaps currently exist in the follow-up of laboratory or radiology results. Reasons for errors in laboratory result notification can be as simple as misfiling a paper or not having a chart available. If patients do not hear from their physician, they may incorrectly assume that the results were within normal limits and "no news is good news." Physicians report spending well over an hour per day managing test results (74 minutes/day), but 83% reported that they wished they had reviewed at least one test in the last 2 months earlier.[19] Among surveyed ambulatory medical practices, 52% reported having a system to record tests ordered while only 32% of practices had systems to detect if patients missed tests.

In the outpatient setting, the referral process is prone to breakdowns and errors. Both specialists and primary care providers express frustration about the referral process and communication between providers. The referral process can be difficult due to physician time restraints, lack of clarity regarding reason for referral, patient self-referrals, insurance limitations, different medical record systems, and unclear follow-up plans (Table 26-3).[20] In a survey of 48 primary care providers, 63% reported being dissatisfied with the referral process. Additionally neither the PCP nor the specialist felt like they were receiving the information needed from the other provider. In the

Patient		Provider
• Symptoms • Past medical history • Allergies • Medications		• Laboratory or diagnostic test results • Follow-up plan • Treatment plan

PCP		Specialist
• Reason for referral • Previous laboratory or diagnostic studies • Patient medical problems • Patient medications		• Timely recommendations Results of test and procedures • Plan for future care and role in medical management

Figure 26-1. Ambulatory lapses in communication.

TABLE 26-3	Breakdowns and Errors in the Outpatient Referral Process
Primary Care Providers	**Specialists**
Timeliness of information from specialists	Timeliness of information from PCP
Redundant aspects of current process	Time required for insurance approvals for studies and procedures
Time required to create adequate referral note	Time required for medication management approvals
Difficulty in finding a specialist	Lack of clarity of note content from PCP
Lack of knowledge of role of medical management	Time required to create an adequate note for PCP
Time required for medication management approvals	Redundant aspects of current process

outpatient setting, much of the referral process occurs via notes and letters, rather than conversations between practitioners. This lack of clear communication hinders the utility of many referrals.

LABORATORY ERRORS

Primary care providers order lab tests on an estimated 29–38% of encounters.[21] These laboratory tests can contribute to between 15% and 54% of errors in primary care. Primary care providers review a tremendous amount of test results per week—one report found that a full-time primary care provider will review 930 chemistry/hematology reports and 60 pathology and radiology reports in a week.[22] Given that there is usually a delay between seeing the patient, ordering the test, and obtaining the test result, it is easy to forget about test results. Ambulatory offices lag behind hospitals in developing and implementing systems to prevent errors from occurring. There are multiple steps that occur between ordering a test to acting upon the test results; errors may occur at each of these steps (Fig. 26-2). Types of errors include missed/delayed provider of test results, patient follow-up of test results, patient notification about test result, and laboratory errors such as incorrectly labeling or processing a specimen. Unfortunately, few practices have systems in place to accurately track labs ordered, reporting of results, and patient notification.[23] A survey of primary care providers similarly showed that 37% of providers had seen a patient in the last 2 weeks with a missed test result.[24] The most commonly missed diagnostic studies included imaging (29%), common clinical pathology (22%), anatomic pathology (9%) and other studies (40%). The most common diagnosis that had a delay in care was cancer (34%). In addition to the process steps, errors can occur if the provider orders the wrong test or when the appropriate test is not ordered.[25] Standardization of the test result process is one important tool to decrease errors. Practices should have a standard way to order tests, track results, respond and document test results, and notify patients.[21] Engaging patients to be active participants in their care is one potential strategy for mitigating risk. Although many patients may assume that "no news is good news," encouraging patients to actively seek out their test results may add another layer of

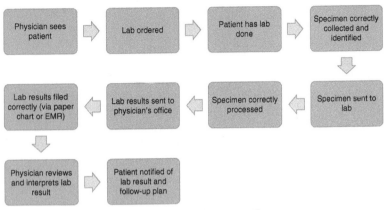

Figure 26-2. Steps in ordering and receiving a laboratory result.

defense against missed test results. Electronic tracking systems and patient portals are promising methods for monitoring test results, but more research is still needed to investigate best practices for ordering and following up on abnormal labs.

ADMINISTRATIVE ERRORS

Currently, there is very little research on administrative errors in the outpatient setting. However, many providers will experience events like a misplaced laboratory result or the front desk forgetting to call a patient to schedule an appointment; all of these common scenarios can lead to adverse events. Creating a culture of safety and designing systems with built-in safeguards are two important principles to mitigate these types of errors. Specific interventions suggested by a study of family physicians included stopping using carbon copy prescription forms, doing urgent lab tests in the office, and using flagging systems.[26] Best practices from the Joint Commission include standardization of:

- Types of files, shapes, colors, and labels.
- Formatting of files.
- Process used for filing such that it becomes habitual.
- Method of sign-off.
- Methodology of nonsoftware filing systems on every person's computer.
- Forced functions built into software systems such that filing something incorrectly will be immediately noticed and intercepted.[5]

Patients often make their first impressions of a practice based on the medical office staff that often function as a gateway to the medical providers. Being on time and accessible are important for patient satisfaction and can signal how an office is functioning. Potential metrics to measure include number of patient "touches," being time, on-time starts, appointment access, and telephone access.[27]

Improving communication among office staff is another potential means to reduce the risk of error. For example, creating an interdisciplinary team (e.g., physician, nurse, office manager, scheduler) to improve the handling of phone messages could be done using PDSA cycles,[27] leading to a collaborative and sustainable solution. Ambulatory practices can benefit from the use of daily briefings and huddles to improve communication among team members.[27]

SAFETY AND QUALITY IN PRIMARY CARE

Primary care providers have a crucial role in following and managing patients. Given the increasing complexity of health care, many people now are receiving care by a variety of clinicians in many different settings and facilities. The PCP is supposed to be the link between all these different providers. However, PCPs are under increased pressure to see more patients, maximize billing, manage transitions of care, and track quality. The agenda in an outpatient visit is jam-packed: addressing patient concerns and medical problems, creating and updating a problem list, reconciling medications, reviewing allergies, documenting a review of systems, completing a physical exam, ordering tests, prescribing new medications, making referrals, coordinating testing logistics, allowing time for questions, and doing this all in a patient-centered manner! The average primary care encounter lasts around 17–20 minutes and covers six topics.[28,29] Unfortunately, there is little time to do all that needs to be done.

A gap exists between recommended care and actual care received by patients. For example, in 2011, between only 58.4% and 65.4% of patients diagnosed with hypertension had adequate control. The breast cancer screening rate varies between 50.4% and 70.5%.[30] Another analysis showed that only 54.9% of the population received recommended preventative care.[31] Common outpatient quality improvement projects often involve preventive and chronic care. The Ambulatory Care Quality Alliance (AQA) was started in 2004 as collaboration between the American Academy of Family Physicians (AAFP), the American College of Physicians (ACP), America's Health Insurance Plans (AHIP), and the Agency for Healthcare Research and Quality (AHRQ) to improve collection and reporting of ambulatory quality measures.

A "starter set" of 26 measures was developed for ambulatory care covering cancer screening, vaccination, tobacco use and cessation, coronary artery disease, heart failure, diabetes, depression, asthma, prenatal care, and antibiotic use.[32] This starter set is one possible framework for practices that wish to begin collecting, analyzing, and improving on ambulatory quality metrics.

The creation of Primary Care Medical Homes (PCMH) is another possible mechanism to improve the quality and safety provided to patients. The AHRQ defines a PCMH as a "mechanism for organizing primary care to provide high-quality care across the full range of an individual's health care needs. It focuses on teams of health care professionals proving coordinated and accessible care to an identifiable group of patients."[33] PCMH aim to create care that is patient centered, comprehensive, coordinated, accessible, and committed to quality and safety. Each patient has an ongoing relationship with a personal physician. The practice works as a team to address the patient's needs, ongoing care, and access to services.[34] A systematic review showed that PCMH has a small positive effect on patient experience and small to moderate positive effect on preventative care.[33] This concept is also expanding to Patient Centered Medical Home Neighbors for specialty and subspecialty practices to improve communication and comanagement between PCPs and consultants.

CREATING AN OUTPATIENT SAFETY AND QUALITY PROGRAM

To date, much of the safety and quality focus has been on the inpatient setting. However, with increasing emphasis on value-based purchasing and public reporting, outpatient medical practices will face increasing pressure to create and maintain quality and safety programs. The EHR incentive program includes clinical quality measures that practices will have to report on. A recommended core set of measures for adults and pediatrics that focuses on high-priority health conditions and best practices has been complied, which includes controlling high blood pressure, tobacco use screening and cessation, and childhood immunization status.[35] Many physicians are being required to perform a self-assessment and quality improvement project for their practice as part of their maintenance of certification through their medical board.

Many practices may feel overwhelmed by quality improvement projects and data reporting. Historically, safety and quality improvement have been a relatively small component in medical education, making it difficult for existing practices to create a safety and quality program that engages the multitude of roles involved in safe medical care. At a minimum, components of an outpatient safety and quality improvement program should include the following:

• Providing training for staff
• Identifying key areas for improvement
• Identifying and removing barriers of improvement
• Creating a tracking system for quality and safety issues
• Developing specific safety and quality goals that are reviewed regularly
• Developing metrics that measure the safety and quality of care
• Assigning of responsibility and accountability to monitor metrics
• Supporting a Just culture and reporting of errors
• Engaging patients[36]

Multiple preexisting frameworks exist for quality improvement programs, and some of these programs will assist with the analysis of data. Many different specialty societies have quality programs with suggested metrics. National organizations have preestablished metrics that can be followed based upon disease, specialty, and patient population. These resources can be beneficial for practices learning about quality improvement.

SUMMARY

Improving patient safety and quality for the ambulatory setting is a much needed next step for the quality movement. As more care is transitioned to outpatients, the potential amount of harm will be increasing. Creating a taxonomy to define errors is a first step, followed by creating a safe culture and error reporting systems, to finally creating system-based solutions to decrease errors. Major areas of interest include communication, medication safety, diagnostic error, laboratory error, and administrative error. While principles learned from the inpatient setting may be useful to improve care, these tools will need to be adapted to the outpatient setting. Despite many of the difficulties, some safety and quality initiatives in the outpatient setting may be more feasible since patients are not as acutely ill, allowing them to be more engaged. Additionally, most outpatient clinics will have a smaller staff, which may make it easier to implement and communicate changes. Therefore, smaller, easier tools or system changes can have large impacts without as much time and money invested when compared to the inpatient setting.[4] Practices need to look at their relationship with consultants, laboratories, hospitals, and home health organizations to ensure that they have methods to track patients and communicate results.

KEY POINTS

- Outpatient safety and quality differs from inpatient care due to the large volume of patients, longitudinal care, and the diffuse care environment.
- The wide variety of outpatient settings and providers can make safety and quality work challenging.
- Outpatient practices need to identify ways to standardize systems, identify errors, and maintain a just culture.
- Causes of errors include medication errors, diagnostic errors, laboratory errors, clinical knowledge errors, communication errors, and administrative errors.

ONLINE RESOURCES

1. Patient Safety Tools for Physician Practices: http://www.mgma.com/pppsahome/
2. The Ambulatory Care Quality Alliance Recommended Starter Set: The Ambulatory Care Quality Alliance. May 2005. Agency for Healthcare Research and Quality, Rockville, MD: http://www.ahrq.gov/professionals/quality-patient-safety/quality-resources/tools/ambulatory-care/starter-set.html
3. Patient Centered Primary Care Collaborative: http://www.pcpcc.org/

REFERENCES

1. *National Ambulatory Medical Care Survey: 2010 Summary Tables.* 2010 [cited 2013 8/18/13]. Available from: http://www.cdc.gov/nchs/data/ahcd/namcs_summary/2010_namcs_web_tables.pdf
2. Woods DM, Thomas EJ, Holl JL, et al. Ambulatory care adverse events and preventable adverse events leading to a hospital admission. *Qual Saf Health Care.* 2007;16(2):127–31.
3. Landon BE, Normand. *National Voluntary Consensus Standards for Ambulatory Care: Measurement Challenges in Small Group Settings.* Washington, DC: National Quality Foundation; 2006.
4. *Summary Data of Sentinel Events Reviewed by the Joint Commission.* 2012. Available from: http://www.jointcommission.org/assets/1/18/2004_4Q_2012_SE_Stats_Summary.pdf
5. The Joint Commission, Fry HM, eds. *A Patient Safety Handbook for Ambulatory Care Providers.* 1st ed. Oakbrook Terrace, IL: Joint Commission Resources; 2009.
6. Pace WD, Fernald DH, Harris DM, et al. Developing a taxonomy for coding ambulatory medical errors: a report from the ASIPS collaborative. In: Henriksen K, Battles JB, Marks ES, et al., eds. *Advances in Patient Safety: From Research to Implementation.* Rockville, MD: Agency for Healthcare Research and Quality; 2005.
7. Lorincz CY, Drazen E, Sokol PE, et al. *Research in Ambulatory Patient Safety 2000–2010: A 10-Year Review.* Chicago, IL: American Medical Association; 2011.
8. Aspden P, Wolcott J, Bootman JL, et al. *Preventing Medication Errors: Committee of Identifying and Preventing Medication Errors.* Washington, DC: Institute of Medicine; 2006.
9. Gurwitz JH, Field TS, Harrold LR, et al. Incidence and preventability of adverse drug events among older persons in the ambulatory setting. *JAMA.* 2003;289(9):1107–16.
10. Gleason KM, Brake H, Agramonte V, et al. *Medications at Transitions and Clinical Handoffs (MATCH) Toolkit for Medication Reconciliation. Prepared by the Island Peer Review Organization, Inc., under Contract No. HHSA2902009000 13C.* Rockville, MD: Agency for Healthcare Research and Quality; 2011.
11. Schnipper JL, Kirwin JL, Cotugno MC, et al. Role of pharmacist counseling in preventing adverse drug events after hospitalization. *Arch Intern Med.* 2006;166(5):565–71.
12. Fischer MA, Stedman MR, Lii J, et al. Primary medication non-adherence: analysis of 195,930 electronic prescriptions. *J Gen Intern Med.* 2010;25(4):284–90.

13. Davis TC, Federman AD, Bass PF III, et al. Improving patient understanding of prescription drug label instructions. *J Gen Intern Med.* 2009;24(1):57–62.
14. Gandhi TK, Weingart SN, Seger AC, et al. Outpatient prescribing errors and the impact of computerized prescribing. *J Gen Intern Med.* 2005;20(9):837–41.
15. Kaushal R, Kern LM, Barrón Y, et al. Electronic prescribing improves medication safety in community-based office practices. *J Gen Intern Med.* 2010;25(6):530–6.
16. Gandhi TK, Kachalia A, Thomas EJ, et al. Missed and delayed diagnoses in the ambulatory setting: a study of closed malpractice claims. *Ann Intern Med.* 2006;145(7):488–96.
17. Singh H, Weingart SN. Diagnostic errors in ambulatory care: dimensions and preventive strategies. *Adv Health Sci Educ Theory Pract.* 2009;14(Suppl 1):57–61.
18. Smith PC, Araya-Guerra R, Bublitz C, et al. Missing clinical information during primary care visits. *JAMA.* 2005;293(5):565–71.
19. Poon EG, Gandhi TK, Sequist TD, et al. "I wish I had seen this test result earlier!": Dissatisfaction with test result management systems in primary care. *Arch Intern Med.* 2004;164(20):2223–8.
20. Gandhi TK, Sittig DF, Franklin M, et al. Communication breakdown in the outpatient referral process. *J Gen Intern Med.* 2000;15(9):626–31.
21. Hickner JM, Fernald DH, Harris DM, et al. Issues and initiatives in the testing process in primary care physician offices. *Jt Comm J Qual Patient Saf.* 2005;31(2):81–9.
22. Poon EG, Wang SJ, Gandhi TK, et al. Design and implementation of a comprehensive outpatient Results Manager. *J Biomed Inform.* 2003;36(1–2):80–91.
23. Smith ML, Raab SS, Fernald DH, et al. Evaluating the connections between primary care practice and clinical laboratory testing: a review of the literature and call for laboratory involvement in the solutions. *Arch Pathol Lab Med.* 2013;137(1):120–5.
24. Wahls TL, Cram PM. The frequency of missed test results and associated treatment delays in a highly computerized health system. *BMC Fam Pract.* 2007;8:32.
25. Dovey SM, Meyers DS, Phillips RL, et al. A preliminary taxonomy of medical errors in family practice. *Qual Saf Health Care.* 2002;11(3):233–8.
26. Dovey SM, Phillips RI, Green LA, et al. Family physicians' solutions to common medical errors. *Am Fam Physician.* 2003;67(6):1168.
27. Webster JS, King HB, Toomey LM, et al. Understanding quality and safety problems in the ambulatory environment: seeking improvement with promising teamwork tools and strategies. In: Henriksen K, Battles JB, Keyes MA, et al., eds. *Advances in Patient Safety: New Directions and Alternative Approaches.* Vol. 3: Performance and Tools. Rockville, MD: Agency for Healthcare Research and Quality (US); 2008:1–15.
28. Tai-Seale M, McGuire TG, Zhang W. Time allocation in primary care office visits. *Health Serv Res.* 2007;42(5):1871–94.
29. Chen LM, Farwell WR, Jha AK. Primary care visit duration and quality: does good care take longer? *Arch Intern Med.* 2009;169(20):1866–72.
30. *Focus on Obesity and on Medicare Plan Improvement; The State of Health Care Quality 2012.* National Committee for Quality Assurance; 2012:1–230.
31. McGlynn EA, Asch SM, Adams J, et al. The quality of health care delivered to adults in the United States. *N Engl J Med.* 2003;348(26):2635–45.
32. Ambulatory Care Quality Alliance. *Ambulatory Care Quality Alliance Recommended Starter Set.* Available from: http://www.ahrq.gov/professionals/quality-patient-safety/quality-resources/tools/ambulatory-care/starter-set.html
33. Jackson GL, Powers BJ, Chatterjee R, et al. The patient-centered medical home a systematic review. *Ann Intern Med.* 2013;158(3):169–78.
34. *Patient-Centered Primary Care Collaborative.* Available from: http://www.pcpcc.org/
35. 2014 Clinical Quality Measures. Available from: https://www.cms.gov/Regulations-and-Guidance/Legislation/EHRIncentivePrograms/2014_ClinicalQualityMeasures.html. Accessed 12/14/15.
36. Guinane C, Davis N. *Improving Quality in Outpatient Services.* Boca Raton, FL: CRC Press; 2011.

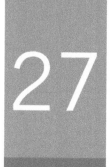

27 Patient Safety Issues Specific to Psychiatry

Anne L. Glowinski

CLINICAL VIGNETTE

Mr. L is a 22-year-old Caucasian male group home resident. His live-in caretakers assist him daily for functional impairment secondary to his intellectual disability. He presents to the emergency department (ED) with 2 days of acute mood and behavior changes. He is eating and sleeping poorly and is uncharacteristically "on and off" grumpy. Mr. L suffers from long-standing generalized epilepsy. No seizures have been observed since he started topiramate 10 days ago. While in the ED, Mr. L alternates between calm and agitated states. A brief physical exam is uninformative. His heart rate fluctuates between 75 and 135. Psychiatry is consulted for "mental status changes." The psychiatry consultant lists "delirium" as the likely diagnosis and recommends identifying and correcting the underlying cause of delirium to avoid a worsening clinical course. He particularly recommends talking to Mr. L's neurologist today about epilepsy management because topiramate is a known deliriogenic agent. The patient, calm for 2 hours, is discharged with a diagnosis of "rule out psychiatric disorder" and a recommendation to arrange follow-up with his neurologist. Mr. L is back in the ED a few hours later. He became agitated again and broke a chair on the head of another group home resident.

- What are the basic steps for diagnosing and treating delirium?
- What might have prevented serious injury to another person?

INTRODUCTION

The interface of Psychiatry and General Hospital Medicine presents significant opportunities to positively impact and improve the quality and safety of patient care. This is because psychiatric and behavioral disorders, with or without other comorbidities, are ubiquitous across health care settings.[1-3]

Large-scale psychiatric epidemiologic studies, such as the National Comorbidity Survey Replication, have demonstrated that many individuals with mental health problems, including severe and chronic disorders, are still unlikely to ever be seen or followed for those problems.[4] Hence, the patient with psychiatric symptoms in acute medical settings will typically not have been assessed previously or longitudinally by a mental health expert. Furthermore, that patient will be under the care of physicians with a relative paucity of knowledge or expertise in the identification and management of psychiatric syndromes. Such a patient will be at risk of harm from both suboptimal management of his or her psychiatric disorders due to provider inexperience and poorer management of medical problems occurring in the context of comorbid psychiatric or behavioral symptoms. How perilous is the latter for patients? It is very serious, as illustrated by several studies documenting that, when compared with other patients, those with psychiatric disorders have notably worse outcomes from their medical problems.[5]

Nevertheless, psychiatric disorders remain relatively underemphasized in medical education, including in residency training for clinical specialties where the psychiatric contribution to patient morbidity and mortality is pervasive. For instance, a general pediatric resident training in 2014 must rotate through 2 months of neonatal critical care and 2 months of pediatric critical care (as per ACGME guidelines) but is not required to rotate through Child and Adolescent Psychiatry.[6] This is but one example of a training curriculum that clashes with reality as suicide is consistently the second or third leading cause of pediatric death in youth 10–18 and the CDC currently reports a 16% incidence of serious suicidal ideation by US high school students in the past 12 months.[7]

Pragmatically addressing this expertise deficit in settings where patients with psychiatric disorders routinely and normatively present is a fundamental task for any group, project, organization, or institution leading efforts to enhance patient safety and quality of medical care.

DELIRIUM

The hallmark of delirium (sometimes also called "acute confusional state" by nonpsychiatrists) is a consciousness disturbance (e.g., decreased attention focus, sustenance, or control), characteristically over brief periods of time (e.g., hours or days). It is characterized by a fluctuating course (e.g., disturbance alternating with periods of normal or less abnormal level of consciousness). Table 27-1 details the Diagnostic and Statistical Manual of Mental Disorders 5th edition (DSM-5) diagnostic criteria for delirium.[8] Not considered to be core criteria and particularly confusing for most clinicians are commonly associated emotional symptoms such as tearfulness, expressions of sorrow, sadness, depression, or any change from the patient's mood or affect baseline. Notably, the disturbance in level of consciousness can present as either agitation or quiet confusion, the latter being particularly likely to be missed in medical floors and ICUs.

It is critical for physicians and nurses to fully appreciate that delirium is generally, in this country and others, poorly recognized and yet very common in general hospital

TABLE 27-1	Diagnostic and Statistical Manual of Mental Disorders 5th Edition: Delirium Criteria

1. Disturbance in attention (i.e., reduced ability to direct, focus, sustain, and shift attention) and orientation to the environment.
2. Disturbance develops over a short period of time (usually hours to a few days) and represents an acute change from baseline that is not solely attributable to another neurocognitive disorder and tends to fluctuate in severity during the course of a day.
3. A change in an additional cognitive domain, such as memory deficit, disorientation, language disturbance, or perceptual disturbance that is not better accounted for by another preexisting, established, or evolving neurocognitive disorder.
4. Disturbances in Nos. 1 and 3 must not occur in the context of a severely reduced level of arousal, such as coma.

settings. This is especially the case in ICU patients and in patients over 65 where delirium rates are estimated to range from 50% to 70%.[9] Improved identification and more systematic management of delirium could potentially improve hospital and posthospital mortality and morbidity rates across gender, age, and race. Delirium is also notoriously associated with higher health care costs, which could perhaps be moderated as well.[10]

Delirium comprises a set of behavioral, emotional, and cognitive symptoms that is ironically often considered "medical" by psychiatrists and "psychiatric" by other physicians. This common misinterpretation increases the risk of inadequate management of delirious patients by everyone! Delirium is (i) a serious syndrome, with high morbidity and mortality; (ii) not caused directly by primary psychiatric disturbances; and (iii) nonspecific, similar to a fever. Delirium requires urgent medical, nonpsychiatric workup and management because of its significant association with adverse outcomes. Psychiatrists are often consulted to evaluate the agitation or hallucinations of delirious patients either because they are thought to suffer from primary psychiatric disturbances or because they need symptomatic management.

The pathophysiology of delirium is complex and multifactorial; an exploration of the contemporary theories of causation exceeds the scope of this chapter. It is commonly summarized and remembered with the ominous mnemonic "I WATCH DEATH" (see Table 27-2), a stern reminder of the serious nature of delirium and also a quick guide to a comprehensive workup to identify, correct, or mitigate underlying problem(s).

The difficulty in recognizing delirium further increases risk to patients. Adverse outcomes include terror or discomfort, preventable falls, injuries to self or others, and worsening medical conditions. A useful tool to methodically assess for delirium is the Confusion Assessment Method (CAM) (see Table 27-3).[10] The CAM is superior

---

TABLE 27-2 | I WATCH DEATH: A Mnemonic Commonly Used to Remember Delirium Risk Factor Categories

I	Infection (CNS—central nervous system—or other)
W	Withdrawal (alcohol, benzodiazepines, or other sedatives)
A	Acute metabolic (electrolyte imbalance, acidemia, alkalosis, hepatic or renal)
T	Trauma (brain, surgery, burns, hyper- or hypothermia)
C	CNS (tumor, hematoma, ictal or postictal, encephalitis, vasculitis)
H	Hypoxia (respiratory or cardiac failure, anemia, hypotension, carbon monoxide poisoning)
D	Deficiencies: vitamins
E	Endocrinopathies (cortisol, glucose, thyroid, parathyroid)
A	Acute vascular (stroke, shock, arrhythmia, hypertension)
T	Toxins (pesticides, solvents, licit or illicit CNS active drugs, vitamins, many medications)
H	Heavy metals

Adapted from Bienvenu OJ, Neufeld K, Needham DM. Treatment of four psychiatric emergencies in the intensive care unit. *Crit Care Med.* 2012;40:2662–70.

TABLE 27-3 Confusion Assessment Method (CAM)

Acute onset

1. Is there evidence of an acute change in mental status from the patient's baseline?

Inattention

2. A. Did the patient have difficulty focusing attention, e.g., being easily distractible or having difficulty keeping track of what was being said?
Not present at any time during interview/Present at some time during an interview, but in mild form/Present at some time during interview, in marked form/Uncertain
(If 2 present or abnormal continue with evaluation of inattention, otherwise proceed to 3)

   B. Did this behavior fluctuate during the interview, i.e., tend to come and go or increase and decrease in severity?
Yes/No/Uncertain/Not applicable

   C. Please describe this behavior:

Disorganized thinking

3. Was the patient's thinking disorganized or incoherent, such as rambling or irrelevant conversation, unclear or illogical flow of ideas, or unpredictable switching from subject to subject?
Yes/No/Uncertain/Not applicable

Altered level of consciousness

4. Overall, how would you rate this patient's level of consciousness?
Alert (normal)/Vigilant (e.g., hyperalert, overly sensitive to environmental stimuli, startled very easily)/Lethargic (e.g., drowsy, easily aroused)/Stupor (difficult to arouse)/Coma (unarousable)/Uncertain

Disorientation

5. Was the patient disoriented at any time during the interview, such as thinking that he or she was somewhere other than the hospital, using the wrong bed, or misjudging the date or time of day?
Yes/No/Uncertain/Not applicable

Memory impairment

6. Did the patient demonstrate any memory problems during the interview, such as inability to remember events in the hospital or difficulty remembering instructions?
Yes/No/Uncertain/Not applicable

Perceptual disturbances

7. Did the patient have any evidence of perceptual disturbances, e.g., hallucinations, illusions, or misinterpretations (such as thinking something was moving when it was not)
Yes/No/Uncertain/Not applicable

TABLE 27-3 Confusion Assessment Method (CAM) (*Continued*)

Psychomotor activity

8. A. Agitation
   At any time during the interview, did the patient have an unusually increased level of motor activity, such as restlessness, picking at bedclothes, tapping fingers, or making frequent sudden changes of position?
   Yes/No/Uncertain/Not applicable

   B. Retardation
   At any time during the interview, did the patient have an unusually decreased level of motor activity, such as sluggishness, staring into space, staying in one position for a long time, or moving very slowly?
   Yes/No/Uncertain/Not applicable

Altered sleep–wake cycle

9. Did the patient have evidence of disturbance of the sleep–wake cycle, such as excessive daytime sleepiness with insomnia at night?

Delirium diagnosis by CAM (need 10 AND 11 to be true)

10. There is acute onset of change in mental status, and inattention and a fluctuating course.
11. Disorganized thinking or an altered level of consciousness.

Adapted from Inouye SK, van Dyck CH, Alessi CA, et al. Clarifying confusion: the confusion assessment method. A new method for detection of delirium. *Ann Intern Med.* 1990;113(12):941–8.

to using clinical acumen, which will often convince physicians that they are in the presence of a mentally disturbed patient rather than a medically impaired one. The CAM has been validated more than other existing instruments.[11,12] Steps involved in the management of delirium are outlined in Figure 27-1. Importantly, delirium can be hypo- or hyperactive and it can be multifactorial. Also, recovery can be progressive and slow even after correction of triggering agent(s). Morbidity can occur either because of uncorrected underlying problems or because of the higher prevalence of erratic behaviors in delirious patients.

AGGRESSION

Aggression by patients or visitors in health care settings is a common and potentially dangerous phenomenon. It is often directed toward nurses and also experienced by physicians and other professionals. Aggression in general hospitals and elsewhere does not just originate from patients or visitors with psychiatric disorders. However, several psychiatric, behavioral, and personality disorders predispose to aggression in stressful acute care settings. The health care costs of aggression, or its threat, are high because of absenteeism and staff work stress.

We should first note that (i) research into the scope of the problem of health care setting aggression is more advanced than the research on its prevention and management and (ii) the research so far often lumps qualitatively distinct aggressive acts ranging from verbal aggression to assault. What is relatively well known from a recent systematic review is (i) of known risk factors for aggression, none is as predictive as

A: MANAGING DELIRIUM

Step 1: Treat agitation: haloperidol PO or IV (*If intractable consider Dexmedetomidine for ventilated patients*)

Step 2: Use Sedatives very carefully and minimize Anticholinergics

Step 3: Manage any pain which risks further disrupting sleep

Step 4: Attempt to normalize the Sleep–Wake cycle

Step 5: If appropriate, consider physical therapy and occupational therapy

Step 6: Actively reduce sensory deprivation and disorientation

B: MANAGING NEUROLEPTIC MALIGNANT SYNDROME

Step 1: Discontinue all dopamine blockers

Step 2: (Only for mild cases) Consider IV Benzodiazepines, particularly in the presence of catatonic symptoms

Step 3: Provide supportive care including hydration, monitoring of electrolytes abnormalities, external cooling for severe hyperthermia, and monitoring and management of any cardiopulmonary, renal, or hematological complications.

Step 4: Consider dopaminergic agents such as Bromocriptine and Amantadine

Step 5: Consider dantrolene (not if patient is receiving calcium channel blockers)

Step 6: Consider electroconvulsive therapy (ECT) after 2 days of failure to respond to pharmacotherapy

C: MANAGING SEROTONERGIC SYNDROME

Step 1: Discontinue serotonergic agents

Step 2: Provide supportive care including IV hydration, hyperthermia control, vital signs stabilization, and avoiding β-blockers, which increase hypotensive risk in autonomically unstable patients

Step 3: Manage agitation and avoid restraints, which can worsen acidosis and hyperthermia

Step 4: Consider serotonin$_{2A}$ antagonists, avoid Bromocriptine and Dantrolene

Step 5: Control autonomic instability, avoiding dopamine, which can precipitate exaggerated hemodynamic response

Figure 27-1. Key steps in managing delirium, NMS, and SS. (Adapted from Bienvenu OJ, Neufeld K, Needham DM. Treatment of four psychiatric emergencies in the intensive care unit. *Crit Care Med.* 2012;40:2662–70.)

a previous history of aggression; (ii) staff training appears critical for prevention and management of aggression, in part because it mediates improved team functioning; (iii) chemical restraints are widely used with efficacy of certain agents or combination of agents better established for patients with aggression related to psychosis; and (iv) mechanical restraints if applied appropriately, carefully, and parsimoniously can be useful and relatively safe in the management of aggression.[13,14] Regarding the prevention and management of aggression, because of the paucity of randomized clinical trials, the evidence is currently only preliminary. Much of the research on aggression comes from psychiatric inpatient settings, which does not translate well to other settings given systematic differences between their patient and staff populations. Findings from research in nonpsychiatric settings have well documented the typical absence of preparedness of many health care workers in preventing or managing aggression. Notably, there are no prevention algorithms applicable to every setting because health care settings differ importantly across key variables (e.g., types of patients or visitors, spatial variables, served communities, systems, or on-site resources) so that the establishment of multidisciplinary teams is highly recommended when a hospital or a unit prioritizes quality improvement efforts in this domain. One recommendation, however, can be made emphatically: firearms or weapons in a hospital, including those carried by security or law enforcement officers, significantly increase the risk of very serious aggression injury to patients and others.[15]

The use of chemical restraints highly depends on the setting, which will often dictate whether an agent like midazolam can or cannot be used safely. Similarly, each clinical situation will dictate whether an oral agent is feasible or if an agent with a less rapid onset of action like an atypical antipsychotic is preferable to a relatively faster-acting agent like haloperidol or lorazepam. Familiarity with dosage recommendations, potential side effects, and interactions of better-studied agents used to mitigate aggression is essential (e.g., droperidol, haloperidol, midazolam, lorazepam). Mechanical restraints are also widely used especially in emergency departments (EDs) and intensive care units (ICUs), and when used appropriately and ethically, they can have an important role. A 1-year long prospective study of mechanical restraint use, with or without adjunctive use of chemical restraints, in a busy inner-city American ED, suggested a 7% rate of mostly minor complications. Most of the complications stemmed from patients getting out of restraints, but there were few injuries to self or others.[16] Notably, this low rate of complications occurred in the context of mindful use (e.g., using checklists, monitoring patients and tracking time spent in restraints).

Expert consensus points to the prevention of aggression in health care settings as an area ripe for further research in quality improvement. For instance, staff harmony may be more efficacious at preventing aggression in health care settings than a show of force by physically intimidating male staff.[13]

SUICIDE

Suicide is defined as a sentinel event by the Joint Commission with the stated goal of zero suicides in health care settings. Suicide in and out of hospitals remains a vexing problem: there are now many well-known suicide risk factors but that knowledge has not successfully led to significant prevention at the population level. The latest National Strategy for Suicide Prevention is extremely ambitious.[17] This plan recognizes that a strategy piecing together many prevention and intervention networks, cumulatively highly sensitive to the major suicide risk factors, is necessary to combat this enormous public health problem. This plan also states explicitly that the battle for suicide prevention can only be won by transcending the bounds of psychiatric management: suicide needs interdisciplinary solutions.

What about suicide in health care settings? Despite being defined as a sentinel event, the global burden of suicide in medical settings remains unknown.[18] There is some overlap between suicide risk factors for psychiatric inpatients and the general hospital inpatients such as male gender, a history of suicide attempt including suicide attempt leading to admission for medical clearance, lack of social or familial support, and depression. Some factors are unique to general medical inpatients, such as being middle aged, poor adjustment to catastrophic or chronic medical illness, and agitated delirium leading to erratic mood and behavior.[19] Prevention of inpatient suicide requires a multidisciplinary approach, including an environmental evaluation, mental health screening for inpatients, treatment of psychiatric disease, staff training, and establishment of policies regarding suicide risk monitoring.[19] Reports of success following systematic depression care have been impressive; the Henry Ford Health System noted a 75% decrease in patient suicide after implementation of the "perfect depression care program."[20] Targeted training in Suicide Risk Assessment (SRA) has been demonstrated as feasible and can increase confidence of nonpsychiatrist physicians, but the systematic deployment of SRA (beyond depression care) across many hospital settings could be premature.[21,22] More research is needed to understand how to implement Suicide Risk Assessment tools across different health care settings and with different patient populations.

MEDICATION-RELATED PSYCHIATRIC EMERGENCIES

ED and general hospital physicians are relatively familiar with some medication-related psychiatric emergencies such as suicide attempt or inadvertent drug overdose, which will not be discussed extensively here. Some general hospitals choose to employ dedicated teams to manage overdoses. Such teams can include toxicology, critical care, and mental health or substance use experts. Notably, prescription opiate overdoses have become epidemic. Nearly two million people in the US are dependent or abusing opioids, and deaths from prescription pain killers have quadrupled since 1999.[23] Examination, monitoring, and improvement of physician prescribing practices, which contribute to those partially iatrogenic deaths, could be greatly facilitated by state prescription registries or drug monitoring programs, now available in almost all states.

Two syndromes merit further discussion: neuroleptic malignant syndrome (NMS), which occurs in patients who are taking dopamine antagonists such as typical or atypical antipsychotics or other dopamine blockers, and serotonergic syndrome (SS), which occurs in patients on serotonergic drugs such as selective serotonin reuptake inhibitors (SSRIs) or serotonin–norepinephrine reuptake inhibitors (SNRIs). These syndromes are important because they are highly lethal if unrecognized or poorly managed and because they have a relatively good prognosis if recognized and managed appropriately. NMS has a variably acute onset of about 3 days, whereas SS tends to be even more acute with an onset of about 12 hours. As noted in a review by Bienvenu et al.,[12] NMS and SS share identical features of serious autonomic instability with hypertension, tachycardia, tachypnea, and hyperthermia, severe hypersalivation and diaphoresis. They have overlapping features of variably altered mental states and abnormal muscle findings; NMS patients typically exhibit "lead-pipe" rigidity contrasting with SS patients, who typically exhibit hypertonia, particularly in lower extremities. The two syndromes are distinguished by hyporeflexia, normal pupils, and normal or decreased bowel sounds in NMS and hyperreflexia or clonus, dilated pupils, and hyperactive bowel sounds in SS. It is very critical to not confuse the two syndromes while toxicology results are pending but management needs to be initiated. Bromocriptine or dantrolene, which can help manage NMS, can exacerbate symptoms or be lethal in SS patients. The Hunter Serotonin Toxicity Criteria should be used to diagnose SS in patients on a serotonergic agent who have spontaneous clonus, inducible clonus, agitation, diaphoresis, tremor, hyperreflexia, high temperature (>38°C), and hypertonicity/rigidity; the criteria have excellent sensitivity and specificity compared to diagnosis by an expert toxicologist.[24] Figure 27-1 illustrates the steps that should be considered for management of NMS and SS.

CONCLUSION

An important subtext, not developed in this chapter, is that advocacy for improving access to psychiatrist care is highly encouraged. Optimal interdisciplinary collaborations to improve psychiatric care of patients in every setting would greatly benefit from the psychiatric field's development of mental health quality indicators. Such indicators are currently not commonly used to evaluate psychiatric or mental health services. Healthcare workers should be prepared to encounter patients with psychiatric symptoms and to be able to initially manage these patients. For some of issues such as delirium, aggression, and the management psychiatric medication adverse effects, empirical evidence suggests that patient care and safety would improve if awareness, knowledge, expertise, and specific algorithms were disseminated outside the bounds of psychiatric circles.

KEY POINTS

- Delirium is a serious medical problem, which is often confused with primary psychotic or mood disorders. It is associated with high morbidity and mortality and high health care costs.
- Especially for nonpsychiatrists, the use of the Confusion Assessment Method (CAM) to diagnose delirium, is highly recommended.
- Staff training is critical to prevent and manage aggression in health care settings.
- The 2012 National Strategy for Suicide Prevention calls for dissemination of suicide prevention efforts and expertise outside of mental health bounds.
- Medical systems, which have comprehensively implemented better networks for depression identification, management, and care, have successfully decreased the number of patient suicides.
- The development of training paradigms and collaborative models to improve patient safety around psychiatric issues is needed.

ONLINE RESOURCES

1. AFSP: American Foundation for Suicide Prevention: http://www.afsp.org/
2. AVERT: Electronic suicide risk assessment system: https://www.ert.com/suicide-risk/
3. Center for Aggression Management: http://www.aggressionmanagement.com/

REFERENCES

1. Ramsawh HJ, Chavira DA, Stein MB. Burden of anxiety disorders in pediatric medical settings. *Arch Pediatr Adolesc Med.* 2010;164:965–72.
2. Mehnert A, Koch U, Schulz H, et al. Prevalence of mental disorders, psychosocial distress and need for psychosocial support in cancer patients – study protocol of an epidemiological multi-center study. *BMC Psychiatry.* 2012;12:70–9.

3. Wu LT, Swartz MS, Wu Z, et al. Alcohol and drug use disorders among adults in emergency department settings in the United States. *Ann Emerg Med.* 2012;60:172–80.

4. Kessler RC, Merikangas KR, Wang PS. Prevalence, comorbidity and service utilization for mood disorders in the United States at the beginning of the twenty-first century. *Annu Rev Clin Psychol.* 2007;3:137–58.

5. Lawrence D, Hancock KJ, Kisely S. The gap in life expectancy from preventable physical illness in psychiatric patients in Western Australia: retrospective analysis of population based registers. *BMJ.* 2013;346:f2539.

6. Accreditation Council for Graduate Medical Education (ACGME) training requirements in Pediatrics. Available at: http://www.acgme.org/acgmeweb/Portals/0/PFAssets/2013-PR-FAQ-PIF/320_pediatrics_07012013.pdf. Cited August 7, 2013.

7. Center for Diseases Control (CDC) suicide briefs. Available at: http://www.cdc.gov/ViolencePrevention/suicide/youth_suicide.html. Cited December 22, 2015.

8. American Psychiatric Association. *Diagnostic and Statistical Manual of Mental Disorders.* 5th ed. Arlington, VA: American Psychiatric Publishing; 2013.

9. Khan BA, Zawahiri M, Campbell NL, et al. Delirium in hospitalized patients: implications of current evidence on clinical practice and future avenues for research – a systematic evidence review. *J Hosp Med.* 2012;7:580–9.

10. Inouye SK, van Dyck CH, Alessi CA, et al. Clarifying confusion: the confusion assessment method. A new method for detection of delirium. *Ann Intern Med.* 1990;113(12):941–8.

11. Wei LA, Fearing MA, Eliezer J, et al. The confusion assessment method (CAM): a systematic review of current usage. *J Am Geriatr Soc.* 2008;56(5):823–30.

12. Bienvenu OJ, Neufeld K, Needham DM. Treatment of four psychiatric emergencies in the intensive care unit. *Crit Care Med.* 2012;40:2662–70.

13. Kynoch K, Wu CJ, Chang AM. Interventions for preventing and managing aggressive patients admitted to an acute hospital setting: a systematic review. *Worldviews Evid Based Nurs.* 2011;8(2):76–86.

14. Hahn S, Muller M, Hantikainen V, et al. Risk factors associated with patient and visitor violence in general hospitals: results of a multiple regression analysis. *Int J Nurs Stud.* 2013;50:374–85.

15. Kelen GD, Catlett CL, Kubit JG, et al. Hospital-based shootings in the United States: 2000 to 2011. *Ann Emerg Med.* 2012;60:790–8.

16. Zun LS. A prospective study of the complication rate of use of patient restraint in the emergency department. *J Emerg Med.* 2003;24:119–24.

17. US DHSS—Department of Health and Senior Services: 2012 National Strategy for Suicide Prevention. Available at: http://www.surgeongeneral.gov/library/reports/national-strategy-suicide-prevention/full_report-rev.pdf. Cited August 7, 2013.

18. Ballard ED, Pao M, Henderson D, et al. Suicide in the medical setting. *Jt Comm J Qual Patient Saf.* 2008;34:474–81.

19. Tishler CL, Reiss NS. Inpatient suicide: preventing a common sentinel event. *Gen Hosp Psychiatry.* 2009;31:103–9.

20. Coffey CE. Building a system of perfect depression care in behavioral health. *Jt Comm J Qual Patient Saf.* 2007;33:193–9.

21. Fallucco E, Hanson M, Glowinski AL. Teaching pediatric residents to assess adolescent suicide risk with a standardized patient module. *Pediatrics.* 2010;125:953–9.

22. Fallucco EM, Colon M, Gale G, et al. Use of a standardized patient paradigm to enhance proficiency in risk assessment for adolescent depression and suicide, 2012. *J Adolesc Health.* 2012;51:66–72.

23. CDC Drug Overdose in Home & Recreational Safety in Injury Center. Available at: http://www.cdc.gov/homeandrecreationalsafety/poisoning/. Cited August 7, 2013.

24. Dunkley EJ, Isbister GK, Sibbritt D, et al. The Hunter Serotonin Toxicity Criteria: simple and accurate diagnostic rules for serotonin toxicity. *QJM.* 2003;96:635–42.

28 Laboratory, Transfusion Medicine, and Pathology Services

Charles S. Eby

CLINICAL VIGNETTE

A hypotensive patient arrived in the emergency department bleeding from internal injuries after a car accident. She received multiple units of type O red blood cells until her blood type was determined on a pretransfusion sample. Subsequently, the patient received B⁺ red cells. Bleeding was surgically controlled, and the patient's condition stabilized except for acute kidney injury, hematuria, and anemia. Seventy-two hours later, the blood bank required a new blood specimen for repeat typing, and now, the patient's blood tested positive for both type A⁺ and B⁺ red cells, indicating her true blood type was A⁺ and she had been erroneously transfused with B⁺ red cells. Further investigation showed that the patient treated in the trauma room prior to this patient was blood type B⁺. The conclusion of a root cause analysis was that an unlabeled tube of blood from the previous patient was labeled as the next patient's blood leading to release of B⁺ incompatible red cells, an acute hemolytic transfusion reaction, and possibly contributing to the patient's kidney failure. Emergency department staff was informed of the consequences of the mislabeled specimen error, and they participated in revising processes and procedures for labeling blood specimens on trauma patients.

- How can the collection, labeling, and handling errors of laboratory and pathology samples be minimized?
- What are some of the other important safety and quality issues that are unique to clinical laboratory, transfusion medicine, and anatomic pathology services?

INTRODUCTION

Most medical diagnostic and management decisions depend upon information provided by clinical laboratories or pathology services. In order to avoid sentinel patient safety errors like the one described in the clinical vignette, quality systems must be in place, monitored, and supported to minimize the risk of preanalytical, analytical, and postanalytical errors. This chapter first reviews the principles of quality assurance as they apply to clinical laboratory services and then provides specific guidance for transfusion medicine and anatomic pathology services.

A QUALITY SYSTEM APPROACH TO CLINICAL LABORATORY SERVICES

The principles of quality management and improvement introduced in Chapters 2–6 also apply to clinical laboratory services.

TABLE 28-1	Laboratory Testing: A Multistep Process

Prior to specimen arrival to laboratory
    Decision to order a test
    Test ordering process
    Specimen collection
    Specimen transportation

Specimen in laboratory
    Specimen processing
    Specimen testing
    Time to test results
    Critical value reporting
    Corrected reports
    Interpretations

Postrelease of test results
    Medical decisions
    Informing patient

Laboratory leaders participate in a wide range of primarily operational quality and safety activities to ensure tests are done correctly[1] (Table 28-1). However, laboratory medicine quality indicators should be expanded to include all activities, which contribute to ordering the most clinically useful tests and to interpreting the results appropriately[2] (Table 28-2). There are two types of medical errors, and the laboratory testing process is vulnerable to both of them: knowledge-based and rule-based mistakes and execution errors when a repetitive task is done incorrectly.

PRELABORATORY PROCESSES

Test Ordering Decisions: Primarily Cognitive Errors

How clinicians decide which tests to order for a patient's condition is extremely complex, but there is wide acceptance that the number of ordered tests does not correlate with the quality of patient care and may be associated with adverse outcomes

TABLE 28-2	Comprehensive Laboratory Medicine Quality Indicators

Increase medical school and postgraduate laboratory medicine education

Analytical validity: Document errors and corrective actions, perform external proficiency testing, adhere to recognized guidelines for test calibration and result units, monitor quality of point of care testing by other health care providers

Clinical utility: Retire out-of-date tests, with input from appropriate clinical specialists, do not offer new tests lacking credible utility, ensure stability of methods for chronic disease monitoring, follow laboratory components of recognized diagnostic and therapeutic guidelines

Adapted from Barth JH. Selecting clinical quality indicators for laboratory medicine. *Ann Clin Biochem.* 2012;49(Pt 3):257–61, with permission.

including patient dissatisfaction from frequent phlebotomies, iatrogenic anemia, and potentially harmful tests and procedures to "follow-up" on unexpected, often false-positive, results. Motivations for excessive testing include time pressure to evaluate multiple diagnoses simultaneously rather than sequentially, unselective testing due to knowledge deficits, and insecurity, in the presence of uncertainty, about relying on clinical judgment and experience. These are long-term challenges for medical educators and clinical mentors, but informatics tools can provide immediate assistance:

- **Benefits of computer provider order entry (CPOE)**
  - Standardized test menu prevents vague, illegible written orders.
  - Customized order sets for common clinical conditions improve efficiency.
  - Improved utilization of diagnostic tests[3]:
    - Online aids: laboratory test handbook, algorithms for sequential testing of common diagnostic pathways, and decision support tools (dosing algorithms, evidence-based guidelines, general medical information).
    - Display cost of selected tests.[4]
    - Noninterruptive alerts and advice: for example, duplicate test warning while providing most recent result.[5]
    - Interruptive alerts: require action to complete order: provide indication and contact laboratory to request exemption from institutional rules.
- **Potential problems with CPOE**
  - Pop-up fatigue from alerts: ignored or bypassed.
  - Ordering convenience causes excess testing: checking every box on an order set and automatic routine daily tests.
  - Order sets require maintenance to keep up with changes in practice standards.[6]
  - Confusing test names without key word search functionality leads to incorrect test selection.[7]
- **Specimen collection and processing errors primarily slipups:** Specimen collection and labeling mistakes are the major sources of laboratory errors.[8]
- **Phlebotomy-related needlestick injuries** are a major risk for transmission of infectious diseases for health care workers.[9]
  - Included in the Federal Needlestick Safety Prevention Act (NSPA) of 2000 was a requirement for employers to provide safety-engineered devices to those performing activities such as phlebotomy, inserting venous and arterial lines, obtaining body fluid and tissue samples, and surgical procedures.
  - NSPA is enforced by the Occupational Safety and Health Administration (OSHA).
  - In post-NSPA enactment in 2001, annual rates of percutaneous injuries (PI) dropped nearly in half to 1–2.5/100 full-time employees.[10,11]
  - In 2002, a prospective survey of house staff reported an overall PI rate of 2.9/100 first year residents/month. Highest PI rates were for OB-GYN (9.7), surgery (7.2), and pathology (5.3) first year residents. Forty percent of PIs were from needlesticks.[12]
  - Among the first year residents, PIs occurred approximately twice as often at night or after overnight call (extended hours) and were more likely to be attributed to fatigue compared to PIs occurring during nonextended hours.[12]
- **Collection errors**
  - Hemolysis due to collecting blood in a syringe from an IV; accessing small distal veins, using small-bore needle (gauge < 21).[13]
  - Blood contamination from IV fluid, heparin, or skin flora causing chemistry, coagulation, and microbiology artifacts.

- ○ Incorrect collection tube, quantity not sufficient (QNS), and inadequate mixing with anticoagulant causing a clotted sample.
- **Specimen mislabeling** is the most serious type of specimen collection errors. A survey of US clinical laboratories identified 379 specimen identification errors per million billable tests, which is an underestimate due to insensitive detection methods.[14]
  - ○ Many labeling errors are identified before releasing test results: during laboratory processing or when results are different from previous results for the same patient (δ checks).
  - ○ Other labeling errors are identified after releasing results due to clinician inquiries.
  - ○ Clinical consequences of undetected specimen labeling errors are difficult to quantify, except for fatalities due to blood typing labeling errors, but given the billions of orderable tests performed annually, there must be adverse consequences due to treatment decisions based on incorrect information.
  - ○ Bedside technology can reduce specimen labeling errors. Bar code technology for electronic positive patient identification (ePPID) reduces mislabeled specimen rates.[15] However, staff can create work-arounds for any technological improvement unless there is a supportive culture for process improvement, patient safety, and regular competency assessment.
- **Specimen transportation:** Time, temperature, and trauma can cause ex vivo changes in cellular and chemical parameters.[8] Some pneumatic tube system designs produce physical forces causing platelet activation[16] and hemolysis causing clinically significant changes in potassium, phosphate, lactate dehydrogenase, and aspartate aminotransferase.[17] Laboratories should compare results from split samples transported by walkers and via pneumatic tube system to rule out these preanalytical sources of errors before accepting "tubed" specimens.

In-Laboratory Processes and Errors: Primarily Slipups, Rarely Analytical Mistakes

Laboratory automation reduces "slipup" processing errors and improves turnaround times in proportion to the number of steps that are performed by machines. However, even the most automated clinical laboratory relies on manual processes for some test methods, handling urgent testing (code specimens), sending out esoteric tests to reference laboratories, and calling and documenting critical value alerts to clinicians.

- **Analytical step:** High-volume tests are performed using federal Food and Drug Administration (FDA) licensed automated instruments and reagents with excellent precision and accuracy specifications.[18] Quality metrics include the following:
  - **Quality control (QC):** frequently testing stable, normal, and abnormal materials whose results must be within established narrow ranges.
  - Periodic validation of instrument calibration and linearity for quantitative methods.
  - External proficiency testing: comparing analyte results to results from other laboratories testing identical specimens and using the same instruments and reagents (peer group).
  - Accuracy surveys: comparing analyte results to an international standard method (available for a growing number of tests).
  - Sporadic QC outliers or unacceptable deviations from proficiency or accuracy external survey results require process review and reagent/instrument troubleshooting.

- **Reporting test results:** Automated instruments directly transmit most results to the laboratory information system (LIS) software, which relays them to electronic medical record (EMR) systems, reducing turnaround times and the risk of postanalytical manual transcription errors. Establishing and periodically validating the fidelity of instrument to LIS and LIS to EMR electronic interfaces require considerable informatics support.
- **Test result enhancements and interpretations:** Most test results are accompanied by reference ranges derived from a small sample of healthy individuals, and the ordering clinician must determine the meaning of an "outlier" result.
  - For some tests, standard interpretive comments, therapeutic ranges, or automated calculations assist clinicians with test interpretation, therapeutic drug monitoring, assessing renal function, or following a diagnostic algorithm.
  - Tests requiring customized interpretations by a pathologist or clinical scientist are limited: examples include blood smear morphology, urine sediment microscopy, hemoglobin and protein electrophoresis, hypercoagulation panels, selected molecular diagnostic tests, and blood bank serology workups; they require selective peer review to ensure professional competency and to minimize incorrect, ambiguous, or delayed test interpretations, which can cause adverse clinical events.
  - Clinical laboratories issue corrected reports for preanalytical, analytical, or interpretation errors. Electronic and printed reports must be revised, clearly showing the original and corrected result. Monitoring the frequency and causes of corrected reports and effectiveness of process improvement actions are crucial quality management goals.

Post–Laboratory Test Result Errors

Clinicians can commit both slipup and cognitive errors after laboratory results are released.

- Ignoring test results: Other than for critical results, laboratories do not ensure clinicians review test results, which are available to them via electronic or printed reports. Yet, ignoring results, failing to act upon them, or not informing patients of their test results are important postanalytical errors. One safeguard is to provide patients with online access to some of their test results as many health systems are now doing.
- Cognitive errors based on incorrect interpretation of test results are difficult to quantify but are probably common given the continuously expanding complexities of diagnosis and treatment of human illnesses. Rapid access to electronic medical decision support resources can mitigate these errors and can be embedded within an EMR. For example, warfarindosing.org is a Web-based algorithm for predicting a patient's therapeutic warfarin dose based on clinical, demographic, and, if available, pharmacogenetic information.

BLOOD TRANSFUSION SAFETY AND QUALITY MANAGEMENT

Collection, processing, and administration of blood products from volunteers are closely scrutinized with oversight of all or selected activities by the Joint Commission, American Association of Blood Banks (AABB), FDA, and, if blood products are irradiated, the Nuclear Regulatory Commission and Homeland Security.

Blood Donors

Approximately 16 million volunteer blood donations are collected annually. They may occur at a free-standing facility or at a hospital transfusion department. Procedures range from simple phlebotomy to collect whole blood to apheresis to collect single components. Processing of whole blood usually includes removal of white cells by filtration to reduce intracellular pathogens like cytomegalovirus (CMV) and reduces febrile transfusion reactions and separation of plasma from red cells by centrifugation.

Donor Safety and Satisfaction

Donating blood involves risks (hematoma, vasovagal reactions, seizure, and, extremely rarely, death), requires informed consent, and requires that the donor meets specific eligibility criteria.[19] A positive donor experience encourages repeat donations, which are important to maintain an adequate and safe blood supply.

Protecting Recipients from Harm

Donors undergo direct questioning to identify medical and travel histories, and behaviors, which could increase the risk of adverse events to a recipient. Deferrals are based on FDA regulations and AABB standards.[20]

Donated blood is tested for at least seven pathogens using serologic and molecular methods (Table 28-3). Units with positive test results are destroyed, and donors are contacted, instructed not to donate again, and provided initial counseling. Rare cases of transfusion-transmitted dengue fever and babesiosis in the US are examples of emerging infectious disease risks requiring quantitative risk assessment before making policy decisions to add additional testing and expense to the blood collection process.[22]

TABLE 28-3	FDA Required Testing of Donated Blood for Seven Pathogens to Prevent Infectious Disease Transmission to Recipients	
Pathogen	Detection Methods	Estimated Risk of Transmission[21]
HIV-1/HIV-2	HIV-1 nucleic acid testing HIV-1, HIV-2 antibodies	1:2,300,000
HCV	Nucleic acid testing HCV antibody	1:1,800,000
HBV	Nucleic acid testing Hepatitis B surface antigen Antibodies to hepatitis B core antigen	1:352,000
HTLV-I/HTLV-II	HTLV-I, HTLV-II antibodies	1:641,000
Syphilis	Antitreponemal antibody or heterophile antibodies	
West Nile virus	Nucleic acid testing	Seasonal and regional variation
Trypanosoma cruzi	IgG antibodies to *T. cruzi*	

From Roback J, Grossman B, Harris T, et al., eds. *Technical Manual.* 17th ed. Bethesda, MD: AABB; 2011.

The risks of transmission of HIV, HCV, and HBV are extremely low but will never be zero due to narrow window periods (7–10 days for HIV and HCV, and 38 days for HBV) when viral loads are below detection and donors remain asymptomatic.[21]

Bacterial contamination of a blood product can occur if a donor has bacteremia and is asymptomatic or if bacteria are introduced into the collection bag. Sepsis and death due to contaminated blood products are rare events.[21] Freezing plasma prevents bacterial multiplication. Refrigeration of red cells restricts growth to certain gram-negative pathogens—*Yersinia enterocolitica* and *Serratia marcescens* most commonly. Platelet units are stored at room temperature and have the highest relative risk of causing transfusion-related sepsis, due to both gram-positive and gram-negative organisms. To reduce this risk, platelets expire 5 days after collection and a sample of the unit is cultured after 24 hours and quarantined from 12 to 24 hours prior to its release.[20]

Blood collection centers perform ABO and Rh typing and antibody screens of donor blood and discard units with clinically important alloantibodies to other red cell antigens, which could cause hemolytic reactions in a recipient.

Blood Recipient

Approximately 5 million patients receive blood transfusions each year. Despite low risks of contracting HIV, hepatitis C or B, or other infections (i.e., blood safety), transfusion of red blood cells, plasma, and platelets involves other short-term and potentially fatal risks (Table 28-4). The most common cause of fatalities from transfusion is transfusion-related acute lung injury (TRALI). TRALI typically occurs when patients with underlying inflammatory or infectious conditions are transfused with a blood product from a multiparous female donor whose plasma contains HLA antibodies recognizing recipient neutrophils and inducing cytokine-mediated lung injury. Blood centers no longer provide plasma from women and reduced exposure to platelets containing HLA antibodies, which has decreased TRALI fatalities (Table 28-4).

TABLE 28-4	Transfusion-Related Mortalities and Associated Mechanisms Reported to the FDA: 2007 and 2011	
Complication	2007, *N* (%)	2011, *N* (%)
TRALI	34 (65)	10 (33)
HTR (non-ABO)	2 (4)	6 (20)
HTR (ABO)	3 (6)	3 (10)
Microbial infection	6 (12)	4 (13)
TACO	5 (10)	4 (13)
Anaphylaxis	2 (4)	2 (7)
GVHD	0	1 (3)
Total	52	30

http://www.fda.gov/downloads/BiologicsBloodVaccines/SafetyAvailability/ReportaProblem/TransfusionDonationFatalities/UCM300764.pdf
FDA, Food and Drug Administration; GVHD, graft versus host disease; HTR, hemolytic transfusion reaction; TACO, transfusion-associated cardiac overload; TRALI, transfusion-related acute lung injury.

Errors can occur at many points from donor blood collection to transfusion into the recipient (Table 28-5). Special attention is given to questionable decisions to transfuse, suboptimal informed consent process, mislabeled blood samples for blood typing, and transfusion of the wrong blood product into a patient.

Blood Management

Avoidance of unnecessary blood transfusions optimizes patient safety, making the decision to transfuse a critically important step. Comprehensive blood management programs focus on correction and prevention of anemia prior to major surgery, minimizing blood loss with preoperative hemodilution and red cell salvage, restoration of coagulopathies during surgery, and using evidence-based guidelines for hemoglobin nadir thresholds for transfusion of hemodynamically stable anemic medical patients when appropriate.[23]

TABLE 28-5	Major Types of Transfusion-Related Errors from Blood Donor to Recipient	
Location/Step	Error	Prevention
Donor center	Collect from infected donor Bacterial contamination Leukoreduction failure False-negative pathogen test Incorrect ABO/Rh type False-negative screen for other red cell antibodies	Good manufacturing processes Infectious disease testing Quality management program
Decision to transfuse	Based on routine/habit Placebo effect Unproven benefits Ignore evidence-based guidelines	Comprehensive blood management program[a] Surgical procedure specific type and cross requirements Robust IT support
Obtaining informed consent	Incomplete explanation of benefits, risks, alternatives Embedding transfusion in consent for surgery, invasive procedures	Oversight by hospital transfusion committee Education level appropriate consent form and supplemental information[a] Processes to identify and manage patients refusing blood[a]
Collection of blood for typing	"Wrong blood in tube" Wrong tube Hemolyzed/clotted blood	Independent collection of 2nd sample to confirm blood type[a] Bar code system to ID patient, label, order, and phlebotomist[a]

Location/Step	Error	Prevention
TABLE 28-5	**Major Types of Transfusion-Related Errors from Blood Donor to Recipient (Continued)**	
Blood bank laboratory	Incorrect confirmatory typing of donor blood or typing of patient Failure to ID clinically important patient red cell alloantibodies Failure to provide safest product to immunodeficient patient (irradiated, leukoreduced, CMV) Crossmatching errors Product-labeling errors Delayed release of uncrossmatched red cells, plasma, platelets for massive transfusion protocol Placing returned, expired blood back into inventory	Follow AABB standards Rigorous quality management program[a] Robust informatics system and support
Transport and storage	Improper storage temperature	Inventory control Satellite storage + distribution kiosks
Transfusion	"Wrong blood into patient" Rapid infusion Inadequate monitoring Not suspecting a transfusion reaction	Bar code ID of patient, unit, infusionist, and physical locks on blood units requiring positive patient ID to open[a] Nursing education and auditing[a]

[a]Indicates roles for Blood Safety Officer.

Informed Consent

Prior to blood transfusions in nonemergent situations, it is mandatory to obtain a patient's informed consent. AABB minimum standards are description of risk, benefits, and treatment alternatives to transfusion, opportunity to ask questions, and the right to accept or refuse transfusions.[24] However, what physicians say and what patients understand during the consent process may be insufficient to ensure true informed consent.[25] Hospital transfusion practice committees should ensure that consent forms for surgical and invasive procedures do not substitute for a separate transfusion consent form, that a person with limited education can comprehend the consent form, and that other resources are available and used to help patients understand the risks, benefits, and alternatives to transfusion and should audit the consent process by direct observation.

Mislabeled Type and Screen Samples

In order to protect patients from acute or delayed hemolytic transfusion reactions by providing type-specific red cells, plasma, and platelets, blood banks have zero tolerance for receiving a mislabeled type and screen specimen for the intended recipient, that is, "wrong blood in tube (WBIT)," which occurs once in every 2000–3000 collections.[26] Requiring a second signature on the type and screen tube from a caretaker who witnessed patient identification, blood collection, and tube labeling does not prevent WBIT incidents.[27] Successful efforts to reduce this critical error include:

• Independent collection of a second tube of blood and requiring identical type results before issuing nonemergent blood requests.[28]
• Using bar code and radiofrequency technology and software to identify the patient, identifiers on the tube label, and the person collecting the blood.[26]

Blood Bank Mistakes

Errors can occur at many points within the blood bank, but surveys consistently show that most clinically important errors are preanalytical and postanalytical.[29] Blood bank managers and directors monitor many quality metrics (Table 28-6), including turnaround times to deliver blood products to operating rooms and trauma patients. FDA-licensed software products are critical tools for efficient and safe blood bank operations and must have the capability of linking to LIS and EMRs to provide blood utilization reports by service and clinician to support a comprehensive blood management program.

After blood products leave the blood bank, there are specific storage and transportation QC requirements to maintain quality and safety.

Transfusing a Patient

Ensuring the right blood product is transfused into the right patient is critically important. Yet, this is another step where human errors occur due to incorrect identification of patients and blood product labels. Successful error reduction interventions include bar code and radiofrequency tag technologies to prompt and document necessary identification steps[26,30] and containers for blood units with mechanical barrier systems that require a code to unlock.[26]

TABLE 28-6 Quality Metrics for Transfusion Medicine Service
Mislabeled type and screen samples
Transfusion reactions
Wasted blood products
Surgery crossmatch to transfusion ratio
Massive transfusion protocol turnaround time
Customer feedback
Blood utilization trends
Monitoring physician ordering and transfusion effectiveness

Nursing and transfusion medicine policies and procedures provide guidance and instructions for patient identification, rate of transfusion, monitoring intervals, and suspecting and managing a transfusion reaction, beginning with stopping the transfusion if not complete and returning the residual product to the blood bank for confirmatory typing, inspection for hemolysis, and possible culturing for bacterial contamination. All transfusion reactions are reviewed by a pathologist or blood bank director to determine likely causes and steps to prevent recurrent reactions (Table 28-7).

Total Quality Management

In order to monitor and achieve safety and quality management goals, many hospital clinicians and administrators:

• Provide leadership and resources to support blood management programs.
• Employ transfusion safety officers, typically nurses with transfusion therapy experience, to educate, audit, and report on quality and safety indicators encompassing the entire blood transfusion chain.
• Use standardized quality indicators and reports to share performance and identify opportunities for improvement through multicenter hemovigilance programs.

TABLE 28-7	Types of Transfusion Reactions	
Presenting Signs, Symptoms	Likely Cause	Management/Prevention
Fever +/− chills or rigors	Cytokines from donor leukocytes	Leukoreduced red cells, pre-tx acetaminophen
Urticaria	Allergic reaction to antigen in donor plasma	Antihistamines
Anaphylaxis	First transfusion possible IgA deficiency	Supportive therapy Measure IgA level; if absent, obtain blood products from IgA-deficient donor
Hypotension, tachycardia, fever	Possible bacterial contamination	Culture residual blood product Empiric antibiotic treatment supportive therapy
Shock, back pain, hematuria	Possible acute hemolytic tx reaction	Confirm patient and blood unit types Urine and serum hemoglobin testing Hydrate/diuresis
Dyspnea, hypoxia, bilateral pulmonary infiltrates	Possible TACO or TRALI	Assess cardiac/fluid status Supportive therapy If TRALI highly suspected, contact blood supplier— screen donor for HLA antibodies

Anatomic Pathology: Specimen Integrity and Diagnostic Accuracy

By examining cytology, biopsy, and surgical resection specimens, anatomic pathologists produce diagnostic and prognostic information to guide patient management decisions. Unlike the quantitative data from other clinical laboratories, the output from anatomic pathologists is the result of a complex qualitative process involving interpretation of clinical and morphologic information and consisting of three components: diagnostic accuracy, complete and clear reporting, and timely delivery. Pathologists apply quality management systems to monitor the preanalytical, analytical, and postanalytical stages of their diagnostic services to prevent, detect, and correct both individual and process errors. Some quality metrics are mandated by regulatory and accreditation organizations[31] while others are defined by local practice performance and case mix.[32,33]

SOURCES OF PREANALYTICAL ERRORS

Collaboration and communication between pathologists and clinical staff are crucial to identify and correct preanalytical deficiencies.

- Collection
  - Pathologists rely on clinical colleagues to obtain adequate specimens, to correctly label specimen containers and requisitions, and to place them in the correct transport medium.
  - Direct communication between pathologists and clinicians during specimen collection minimizes errors.
  - Pathologists need sufficient anatomic and clinical information from clinicians accompanying specimens in order to provide optimal diagnostic information.
- Delivery: Delays or temperature extremes during transport of specimens from patient to the pathology department can degrade biologic material and diminish its diagnostic usefulness.
- Accession: Handling and labeling errors in the pathology department during gross specimen identification and preparation for analysis are uncommon but grievous since most specimens are irreplaceable. The introduction of bar coding tracking systems can reduce many in-laboratory errors.[34]

SOURCES OF ANALYTICAL ERRORS

Specimen Processing

Specimens undergo multiple preparation steps prior to analysis by pathologists, which require quality monitoring. The major functions include the following:

- Frozen section preparation for intraoperative consultation: to distinguish benign from malignant for a mass, tissue margins, or regional lymph node
- Histology: embedding tissue in paraffin blocks and subsequent cutting and staining of tissue sections
- Cytology: fixation and staining of Pap smear, non-GYN fluid, or fine-needle aspiration specimens
- Special processing: immunohistochemical staining, molecular diagnostic testing, and whole slide digital imaging[35]

Diagnostic Accuracy

Long-term clinical follow-up to confirm many pathologic diagnoses is impractical.

Interobserver agreement between pathologists (precision) is an acceptable substitute for monitoring the accuracy of diagnoses and is a crucial component of a pathology department quality improvement program. When pathologists reviewed surgical pathology cases they signed out >1 year ago, the intraobserver major error rate was 0.9%,[35] which can serve as a benchmark for comparison of interobserver disagreement rates.

There is no consensus on the optimal system for pathologist peer review of cytology and surgical pathology diagnoses or on definitions for types of interobserver disagreements. Nevertheless, recent retrospective studies have reported disagreement rates of 7–9%[32,33] and an estimate that 1% of diagnostic discrepancies could cause patient harm.[33]

Surgical pathology groups develop diagnostic accuracy quality assurance policies customized to their case mix and past experience. Components of quality assurance programs for pathologic diagnostic accuracy can include:

- Random review of a percentage of all cases.
- Selective review of paired GYN cytology and subsequent excised tissue diagnoses, paired frozen section and permanent section diagnoses, all cancer specimens, all specimens from tissues with recognized higher diagnosis discordant rates (breast, GYN, prostate).
- Blind review to prevent knowledge of the original diagnosis from biasing the reviewer.
- Rapid review prior to or <48 hours after sign out to reduce potential clinical consequences.
- Inclusion of negative (normal) cases to identify false-positive errors.
- The frequency and types of corrected pathology reports must be monitored. The reasons for corrections may be minor (typographical error) or major (benign diagnosis changed to malignant diagnosis after review or additional stains). Keep in mind that even "minor" errors such as mistaking right for left can have catastrophic consequences for the patient.

Postanalytical Sources of Errors

- Completeness of pathology reports: This is critical for cancer staging and must meet the standards set by the American College of Surgeons Commission on Cancer. The quality assurance benchmark is ≥90% of cancer-related reports will contain all required elements for optimal pathologic diagnosis and staging.
- Timeliness of results: For intraoperative pathology consultation review of a frozen section, the benchmark is completion of 90% of cases within 20 minutes.
- Surgical pathology sign-out times are highly dependent on the type and complexity of the case, the need for special testing (decalcification, immunohistochemistry), and the practice setting (private practice vs. academic practice). The College of American Pathologists has not mandated specific turnaround time guidelines, but diagnoses should be available in a sufficient time to provide optimal patient care for a specific medical community.
- Clarity of report: Pathologists must provide information in a format which will be unambiguous to clinicians.
- Fidelity of electronic transmission of anatomic pathology results: Pathology departments must periodically confirm reports in downstream EMR repositories are complete and accurate, as well as rapidly investigate of feedback from clinicians about "dropped" reports indicating an interface failure.
- Surveys indicate clinicians are confident in the diagnostic accuracy of their anatomic pathology colleagues while areas cited for improvement include delays in reporting results.[36]

KEY POINTS

While clinical laboratory medical directors, managers, and technologists are solely responsible for performance, interpretation, and reporting of laboratory tests, they must also be champions for quality management of pre- and postanalytical processes, which is where the majority of errors occur, and optimal utilization of laboratory resources.

While blood safety has improved dramatically due to donor selection and testing strategies, transfusion safety risks persist due to both biologic complications and human errors—especially mislabeling of type and screen specimens and transfusing blood products to the wrong patient. While technologic advances are reducing human errors, patient safety will be further improved by minimizing transfusions through effective blood management programs.

In addition to the quality metrics that apply to clinical laboratories, anatomic pathologists must continuously monitor the accuracy of their cytology and surgical pathology diagnoses thru peer review of selected cases.

ONLINE RESOURCES

1. Preanalytical laboratory issues: http://www.specimencare.com/
2. Clinical laboratory test information for patients from American Association of Clinical Chemistry (AACC): http://labtestsonline.org
3. Reference laboratory clinical test selection resources for clinicians:
   • Mayo Medical Laboratories: http://www.mayomedicallaboratories.com/test-catalog/
   • Associated and Regional University Laboratories (ARUP): http://www.aruplab.com/
4. Improving Diagnosis in Healthcare. Institute of Medicine Report September 2015: http://iom.nationalacademies.org/Reports/2015/Improving-Diagnosis-in-healthcare

REFERENCES

1. Shahangian S, Snyder SR. Laboratory medicine quality indicators: a review of the literature. *Am J Clin Pathol.* 2009;131(3):418–31.
2. Barth JH. Selecting clinical quality indicators for laboratory medicine. *Ann Clin Biochem.* 2012;49(Pt 3):257–61.
3. Baron JM, Dighe AS. The role of informatics and decision support in utilization management. *Clin Chim Acta.* 2014;427:196–201.
4. Feldman LS, Shihab HM, Thiemann D, et al. Impact of providing fee data on laboratory test ordering: a controlled clinical trial. *JAMA.* 2013;173(10):903–8.
5. Nies J, Colombet I, Zapletal E, et al. Effects of automated alerts on unnecessarily repeated serology tests in a cardiovascular surgery department: a time series analysis. *BMC Health Serv Res.* 2010;10:70.
6. Leu MG, Morelli SA, Chung OY, et al. Systematic update of computerized physician order entry order sets to improve quality of care: a case study. *Pediatrics.* 2013;131(Suppl 1):S60–7.
7. Passiment E, Meisel JL, Fontanesi J, et al. Decoding laboratory test names: a major challenge to appropriate patient care. *J Gen Intern Med.* 2013;28(3):453–8.

8. Lippi G, Chance JJ, Church S, et al. Preanalytical quality improvement: from dream to reality. *Clin Chem Lab Med.* 2011;49(7):1113–26.

9. Knapp MB, Grytdal SP, Chiarello LA, et al. Evaluation of institutional practices for prevention of phlebotomy-associated percutaneous injuries in hospital settings. *Am J Infect Control.* 2009;37(6):490–4.

10. Phillips EK, Conaway M, Parker G, et al. Issues in understanding the impact of the needle-stick safety and prevention act on hospital sharps injuries. *Infect Control Hosp Epidemiol.* 2013;34(9):935–9.

11. Sohn S, Eagan J, Sepkowitz KA, et al. Effect of implementing safety-engineered devices on percutaneous injury epidemiology. *Infect Control Hosp Epidemiol.* 2004;25(7):536–42.

12. Ayas NT, Barger LK, Cade BE, et al. Extended work duration and the risk of self-reported percutaneous injuries in interns. *JAMA.* 2006;296(9):1055–62.

13. Heyer NJ, Derzon JH, Winges L, et al. Effectiveness of practices to reduce blood sample hemolysis in EDs: a laboratory medicine best practices systematic review and meta-analysis. *Clin Biochem.* 2012;45(13–14):1012–32.

14. Valenstein PN, Raab SS, Walsh MK. Identification errors involving clinical laboratories: a College of American Pathologists Q-Probes study of patient and specimen identification errors at 120 institutions. *Arch Pathol Lab Med.* 2006;130(8):1106–13.

15. Morrison AP, Tanasijevic MJ, Goonan EM, et al. Reduction in specimen labeling errors after implementation of a positive patient identification system in phlebotomy. *Am J Clin Pathol.* 2010;133(6):870–7.

16. Hubner U, Bockel-Frohnhofer N, Hummel B, et al. The effect of a pneumatic tube transport system on platelet aggregation using optical aggregometry and the PFA-100. *Clin Lab.* 2010;56(1–2):59–64.

17. Streichert T, Otto B, Schnabel C, et al. Determination of hemolysis thresholds by the use of data loggers in pneumatic tube systems. *Clin Chem.* 2011;57(10):1390–7.

18. Hawkins R. Managing the pre- and post-analytical phases of the total testing process. *Ann Lab Med.* 2012;32(1):5–16.

19. Shaz BH, Demmons DG, Hillyer CD. Critical evaluation of informed consent forms for adult and minor aged whole blood donation used by United States blood centers. *Transfusion.* 2009;49(6):1136–45.

20. Roback J, Grossman B, Harris T, et al., eds. *Technical Manual.* 17th ed. Bethesda, MD: AABB; 2011.

21. Lindholm PF, Annen K, Ramsey G. Approaches to minimize infection risk in blood banking and transfusion practice. *Infect Disord Drug Targets.* 2011;11(1):45–56.

22. Gallagher LM, Ganz PR, Yang H, et al. Advancing risk assessment for emerging infectious diseases for blood and blood products: proceedings of a public workshop. *Transfusion.* 2013;53(2):455–63.

23. Marques MB, Polhill SR, Waldrum MR, et al. How we closed the gap between red blood cell utilization and whole blood collections in our institution. *Transfusion.* 2012;52(9): 1857–67.

24. AABB. *Standards for Blood Banks and Transfusion Services.* Bethesda, MD: AABB; 2011:41.

25. Friedman M, Arja W, Batra R, et al. Informed consent for blood transfusion: what do medicine residents tell? What do patients understand? *Am J Clin Pathol.* 2012;138(4):559–65.

26. Dzik WH. New technology for transfusion safety. *Br J Haematol.* 2007;136(2):181–90.

27. Ansari S, Szallasi A. 'Wrong blood in tube': solutions for a persistent problem. *Vox Sang.* 2011;100(3):298–302.

28. Goodnough LT, Viele M, Fontaine MJ, et al. Implementation of a two-specimen requirement for verification of ABO/Rh for blood transfusion. *Transfusion.* 2009;49(7):1321–8.

29. Fastman BR, Kaplan HS. Errors in transfusion medicine: have we learned our lesson? *Mt Sinai J Med.* 2011;78(6):854–64.

30. Miller K, Akers C, Magrin G, et al. Piloting the use of 2D barcode and patient safety software in an Australian tertiary hospital setting. *Vox Sang.* 2013;105(2):159–66.

31. Brainard JA, Birdsong GG, Elsheikh TM, et al. Prospective and retrospective review of gynecologic cytopathology: findings from the College of American Pathologists Gynecologic Cytopathology Quality Consensus Conference working group 2. *Arch Pathol Lab Med.* 2013;137(2):175–82.
32. Renshaw AA, Gould EW. Comparison of disagreement and amendment rates by tissue type and diagnosis: identifying cases for directed blinded review. *Am J Clin Pathol.* 2006;126(5):736–9.
33. Raab SS, Nakhleh RE, Ruby SG. Patient safety in anatomic pathology: measuring discrepancy frequencies and causes. *Arch Pathol Lab Med.* 2005;129(4):459–66.
34. Pantanowitz L, Mackinnon AC Jr, Sinard JH. Tracking in anatomic pathology. *Arch Pathol Lab Med.* 2013;137(12):1798–810.
35. Bauer TW, Schoenfield L, Slaw RJ, et al. Validation of whole slide imaging for primary diagnosis in surgical pathology. *Arch Pathol Lab Med.* 2013;137(4):518–24.
36. Zarbo RJ. Determining customer satisfaction in anatomic pathology. *Arch Pathol Lab Med.* 2006;130(5):645–9.

29 Medication Safety

Thomas M. De Fer

CLINICAL VIGNETTE

A thin and frail 76-year-old woman with a history of coronary artery disease and prior stent placement at an outside hospital is admitted via the emergency department after a 25-minute episode of chest pain. It is decided that a cardiac catheterization should be performed. She also reports a vague history of contrast allergy and cannot provide further details due to poor memory. The contrast allergy pretreatment order set is prescribed by the cardiologist, and it consists of prednisone 50 mg at 13, 7, and 1 hour preprocedure, diphenhydramine 50 mg at 7 and 1 hour preprocedure, and ranitidine 150 mg at 7 and 1 hour preprocedure. She receives all of the premedications as ordered, but at 5:00 PM the catheterization is canceled due to an emergency case. She is rescheduled for tomorrow at 10:00 AM; therefore, the pretreatment protocol is ordered again. Transport arrives at 10:00 AM and finds the patient lying on the floor mumbling about having to go to the bathroom and with a 5-cm laceration on her forehead. A cause mapping analysis determines that the multiple doses of diphenhydramine over a short period of time were the primary contributing factor of this adverse event.

- What other factors contributed to this error?
- How should this error be categorized?
- How might this error have been prevented?

GENERAL PRINCIPLES

Medication errors are defined as "any preventable event that may cause or lead to inappropriate medication use or patient harm while the medication is in the control of the health care professional, patient, or consumer. Such events may be related to professional practice, health care products, procedures, and systems, including prescribing, order communication, product labeling, packaging, and nomenclature, compounding, dispensing, distribution, administration, education, monitoring, and use."[1] About 1% of medication errors result in patient harm.[2]

Adverse drug events (ADEs) are any adverse occurrence related to the administration of medication, whether or not an error occurred. **Preventable ADEs are those that reach the patient and are due to medical error**. Potential ADEs are those errors that were discovered **before** reaching the patient. They are frequently called near misses.

Those ADEs that are not due to medical error and are nonpreventable are typically called **adverse drug reactions** (ADRs). A colloquial term for ADRs is side effects, though this implies that they are all negative and unintended. **Type A** ADRs are the most common. They are predictable, due to the pharmacologic properties of the drug in question, and are often dose dependent. For example, anticholinergics cause sleepiness and nonsteroidal anti-inflammatory drugs cause dyspepsia. **Type B** ADRs are less common and are unpredictable. Idiosyncratic and immunologically mediated (allergic) reactions are included here. There are some idiosyncratic reactions for which the mechanism is known (e.g., hemolytic anemia in a patient treated with nitrofurantoin due to glucose-6-phosphate dehydrogenase deficiency), but more often, it is unclear (e.g., clozapine-induced agranulocytosis). Type B ADRs usually produce signs and symptoms that are unrelated to the pharmacologic properties of the drug. An exception, also included in this group, is patients with unique intolerance to a drug even at low doses; the classic example being one aspirin pill causing tinnitus. Figure 29-1 illustrates the relationship between medication errors, ADEs, and ADRs.[3–9]

The magnitude and scope of medication errors are troublingly large, and they contribute very significantly to the overall rate of medical errors. ADEs are thought to account for about 700,000 emergency department visits and result in 100,000 hospitalizations per year.[8,9] At least 400,000 ADEs occur during hospitalizations yearly and are estimated to cost \$3.5 billion (in 2006 dollars).[10,11] The overall inpatient preventable ADE rate is approximately 2.4–6.5 per 100 admissions.[10–12] One study did report a much higher rate of 52 per 100 admissions.[13] ADE rates may be higher in intensive care unit settings.[14] Likewise, over half a million ADEs occur in the ambulatory setting and upward of 800,000 in long-term care facilities annually.[10,15,16]

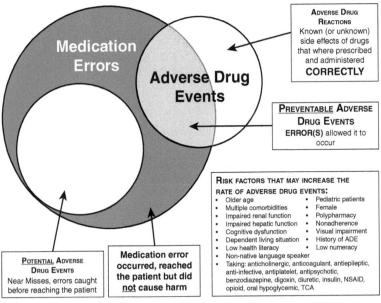

Figure 29-1. Medication errors, ADEs, and ADRs. ADE, adverse drug event; NSAID, nonsteroidal anti-inflammatory drug; TCA, tricyclic antidepressant. (Adapted from Gandhi TK, Seger DL, Bates DW. Identifying drug safety issues from research to practice. *Int J Qual Health Care.* 2000;12:69–76.)

One out of 131 (0.8%) outpatient deaths and 1 out of 854 (0.1%) inpatient deaths are attributable to medication errors—this amounts to more than 7000 deaths per year.[17] Overall, data suggest that the rate of fatal medication errors has increased; this is particularly true in the domestic setting and when alcohol and street drugs are involved.[18] Rates may increase significantly at the beginning of the academic year in counties with teaching hospitals as opposed to those without.[19]

Multiple patient-based risk factors for ADEs have been identified by various studies. Increasing age is a consistent finding. Taking multiple medications has also frequently been associated with ADEs. Commonly cited medications include anticoagulants, antiplatelet agents, insulin, and oral hypoglycemics. **High-risk medications** designated by the Institute for Safe Medication Practices (ISMP) are presented in Table 29-1.[20] Other suggested risk factors are listed in Figure 29-1.[3–9,15,16]

TABLE 29-1	Institute for Safe Medication Practices High-Alert Medications
Class/Category/Drug	Examples/Notes
Adrenergic agonists (IV)	Dopamine, epinephrine (also including SC), norepinephrine, phenylephrine
Adrenergic antagonists (IV)	Esmolol, labetalol, metoprolol, propranolol
Anesthetics (inhaled and IV)	Etomidate, fentanyl, sufentanil, remifentanil, ketamine, propofol
Antiarrhythmics (IV)	Amiodarone, bretylium, ibutilide, lidocaine, procainamide
Antithrombotics	Unfractionated and low molecular weight heparin Warfarin Direct thrombin inhibitors (e.g., argatroban, bivalirudin, dabigatran, desirudin) Factor Xa inhibitors (e.g., apixaban, edoxaban, fondaparinux, rivaroxaban) Thrombolytics (e.g., alteplase, reteplase, streptokinase, tenecteplase) Glycoprotein IIb/IIIa inhibitors (e.g., abciximab, eptifibatide, tirofiban)
Cardioplegia solutions	High concentration magnesium and potassium (e.g., cardioplegic, Plegisol)
Chemotherapy	Oral and parenteral For oncologic and nononcologic use Small molecules and biologics
Dextrose and saline, hypertonic	≥20% or >0.9% concentration, respectively
Dialysis solutions	Commercial or compounded, all with potentially dangerous concentrations of solutes (e.g., sodium, potassium, calcium, magnesium, bicarbonate, glucose)
Epidural and intrathecal medications	Anesthetics, chemotherapy, glucocorticoids

(Continued)

TABLE 29-1	Institute for Safe Medication Practices High-Alert Medications (Continued)

Class/Category/Drug	Examples/Notes
Epoprostenol	Risk of sudden cardiopulmonary decompensation with abrupt cessation
Hypoglycemics, oral	Sulfonylureas (e.g., chlorpropamide, glyburide, glipizide, glimepiride, gliclazide) Metformin (lactic acidosis, particularly in those with renal impairment and acute or progressive heart failure) Meglitinide (e.g., nateglinide, repaglinide)
Inotropes (IV)	Digoxin, dobutamine, milrinone
Insulin	All forms U-500 insulin particularly high risk
Liposomal formulations vs. conventional formulations	Liposomal amphotericin B vs. amphotericin B deoxycholate, bupivacaine, cytarabine, daunorubicin, morphine, vincristine
Magnesium sulfate (IV)	Risk of injurious or fatal overdose
Sedation agents (IV, moderate)	Dexmedetomidine, etomidate, fentanyl, ketamine, midazolam, propofol
Opioids	All formulations, oral, IV, transdermal Includes opium tincture
Oxytocin	Risk of fetal harm may outweigh potential benefits when used unnecessarily or in unnecessarily high doses
Potassium chloride (IV)	Risk of injurious or fatal overdose
Potassium phosphate (IV)	Risk of calcium precipitation and injurious of fatal potassium overdose
Neuromuscular blockers	Atracurium, cisatracurium, pancuronium, rocuronium, succinylcholine, vecuronium
Nitroprusside	Risk for cyanide toxicity, particularly in those with renal impairment and/or prolonged administration
Parenteral nutrition solutions	Potentially dangerous concentrations of solutes
Promethazine (IV)	Risk of severe tissue injury/gangrene, particularly with perivascular extravasation
Radiocontrast (IV)	Risk of hypersensitivity reactions and acute kidney injury
Sterile water for injection	For inhalation, injection, and irrigation in containers ≥100 mL (potential for injurious or fatal hypotonicity)
Vasopressin	Underrecognized or appreciated risk of typical vasoconstrictor complications

Adapted from Institute for Safe Medication Practices (ISMP). *List of High-Alert Medications in acute Care settings.* Horsham, PA: Institute for Safe Medication Practices; 2014. Available at: www.ismp.org. Last accessed 10/1/15.

CATEGORIZING MEDIATION ERRORS

Medication errors can be categorized in multiple ways including psychological domain, harm score, type of error, process step involved, and proximal causes. Each has its advantages and disadvantages. **Psychological theory** attempts to explain the way adverse events occur and has been applied to a broad range of medical errors.[21] Some medication errors are termed **mistakes** and result from **knowledge-based** errors or **rule-based** errors. Others are **skill-based errors**, which result from **action-based errors (slips)** or **memory-based errors (lapses)**. Understanding the psychological basis of an error informs the process of reducing its recurrence.

A commonly used **harm scoring** system is that of National Coordinating Council for Medication Error Reporting and Prevention. This scale (Fig. 29-2) ranges from the potential for error, no harm, temporary harm, permanent harm, and death across nine-lettered categories, A to I.[22] The regular use of a clear, consistent, and workable harm scoring system is critical to the tracking of medication errors.

The administration of any type of medication to patients takes place over multiple **process steps** (Fig. 29-3):

1. **Prescribing**: The prescription process is complex and involves all of the cognitive effort of the prescriber to determine whether to prescribe (or not), what precisely to prescribe, the dose, formulation, route, timing, and frequency of the chosen drug, and the process of formulating this information into a verbal, written, or

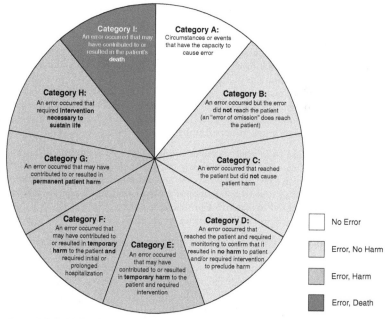

Figure 29-2. Medication error categories. (Adapted from National Coordinating Council for Medication Error Reporting and Prevention. *NCC MERP Index for Categorizing Medication Errors.* 2001. Available at: http://www.nccmerp.org/types-medication-errors. Last accessed 10/1/15.)

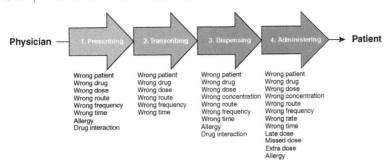

Figure 29-3. Potential error types by process step.

electronic prescription. Individual patient factors such as renal and hepatic function, allergies, and drug–drug interactions must also be taken into account.

2. **Transcribing**: Transcription happens at any point where an order/prescription, be it electronic or handwritten, is interpreted by another health care professional and handwritten or electronically entered into a different system. Poor handwriting contributes greatly to errors in this step.

3. **Dispensing**: Medication dispensing is largely a function of the pharmacy staff. Interpretation of prescriptions, rechecking for allergies and drug–drug interaction, retrieval of the medication from its place of storage, counting, bottling, labeling, and, sometimes, compounding are all involved. In the inpatient setting, the process may also involve stocking unit-based medication storage and dispensing devices.

4. **Administration**: The administration step is also multifaceted. Nurses must determine who requires what medication when using the medication administration record (MAR). Medications must be retrieved from storage and safely transported to the site of administration. The patient must be positively identified and the opportunity to check for allergies presents itself once again. The medication is then given to the patient. If the medication is IV, for example, more steps are involved and, therefore, there are more opportunities for error.

Each one of these surprisingly complex process steps can be broken down into multiple subprocesses—this is often necessary in order to design less error-prone systems. Other important steps that do not necessarily fit into a chronological sequence are storage, monitoring, and documentation. **Problems at any point in the process chain have the potential to result in a preventable ADE**.

Commonly accepted **types of medication errors** are as follows:

- **Missed dose**: Standards vary from institution to institution as to what constitutes a missed dose. A stringent inpatient definition would be >0.5–1 hour past the scheduled admiration time. A more realistic definition, particularly in the outpatient setting, would be greater than half the prescribed dosing interval. Of course, some medications are quite time sensitive, while others are not. Some institutions will have an intermediate category called **late dose**.
- **Extra dose**: Typically, an extra dose occurs when a provider is not aware that a preceding provider has already given the intended dose, which could be due to a handoff and/or documentation issue.
- **Wrong dose**: Incorrect quantity of the medication is given.

- **Wrong rate** is a variation of wrong dose that applies to IV medications, which occurs when the wrong volume (quantity) per unit time is entered into the pump.
- Likewise, **wrong concentration** is also a variation of wrong dose and can result in under- or overdosing.
- **Wrong form**: For example, an order for IV morphine is entered and oral morphine gel is drawn into a syringe and given IV.
- **Wrong route**: An extended release tablet is intended to be given PO; instead, it is crushed and administered via a gastrostomy tube.
- **Wrong frequency/timing**: An intravenous antibiotic is prescribed as every 18 hours but is given every 24 hours.
- **Wrong drug**: A particular medication is intended for a patient, but during removal from storage, the incorrect medication is retrieved and subsequently given to the patient. In other words, the wrong drug is given to the right patient. This can occur at either the dispensing or administration step.
- **Wrong patient**: This occurs when the correct medication is obtained and intended to be given to the corresponding patient, but at the point of administration, the patient is misidentified resulting in the right medicine being given to the wrong patient.
- **Known allergy**: A medication to which the patient has a documented allergy is nonetheless given. This technically excludes a conscious, reasoned decision by the clinician to disregard an allergy, for example, cefazolin is purposefully prescribed for a patient with a documented penicillin allergy.

A Food and Drug Administration (FDA) study found that between 1993 and 1998, the most common types of fatal ADEs were wrong dose (41%), wrong drug (16%), and wrong route (9.7%). Nearly half of these fatal events happened in patients >60 years old.[23] Extrapolating these data to nonfatal ADEs and across all care settings is difficult. The most common errors seen depend on the severity of harm and the characteristics of caregivers and patients in a given environment. As an example, the most common medication error overall in acute care inpatient settings is likely to be missed/late dose, which results in no harm to the patient the large majority of the time. In the outpatient setting, patient-driven errors (e.g., missed doses, extra doses, wrong doses) will be more prominent. Types of errors according to process step are presented in Figure 29-3.

CAUSES OF MEDICATION ERRORS

Regardless of the process step or type of error, health care providers are often most interested in the so-called **proximal causes**.[24,25] Determining cause can be challenging in individual situations, and most often, there are multiple causes and contributing factors. As with any other type of medical error, some factors are active while others are latent. Proximal causes crosscut process steps and health care provider roles. The following is not intended to be an exhaustive list:

- **Lack of knowledge regarding a drug** and lack of readily available, accurate drug/prescribing information. This can be a limitation for both the prescriber and the individual administering the medication. It is simply not possible for physicians, pharmacists, and nurses to be familiar with all of the >16,000 FDA-approved prescription drug products available in the US (including all dosages, forms, and generics).[26]

- **Failure to consider patient-specific factors** that alter pharmacokinetics and pharmacodynamics, such as renal function, hepatic function, obesity, and age. In older adults, absorption may be slower, the ratio of fat to lean mass increases, phase I metabolism is slower, excretion may be slower, and the pharmacodynamics of some drugs are altered.
- **Lack of immediate availability of patient-specific information** that may alter prescribing such as laboratory results concerning renal and hepatic function or parameters such as weight and body mass index.
- **Patient mis-/nonidentification.**
- **Lack of monitoring**, for example, coagulation parameters in patients receiving anticoagulants and certain antibiotic or anticonvulsant levels.
- Use of **ambiguous abbreviations**, be they in handwritten or electronic format (Table 29-2).[27]
- **Sound-alike/look-alike** medications can easily be confused (Table 29-3).[28]
- **Illegible handwriting** remains an issue as computerized order entry has not been deployed in many care settings.
- **Failure of communication** and teamwork.
- **Medication mis-/nonreconciliation** at care transitions, which are known to be vulnerable times for medication errors. Reconciliation is "the process of creating the most accurate list possible of all medications a patient is taking—including drug name, dosage, frequency, and route—and comparing that list against the physician's admission, transfer, and/or discharge orders, with the goal of providing correct medications to the patient at all transition points."[29] Studies have demonstrated high rates of unintended variances (approximately 50–60%) and potential ADEs (approximately 20–30%).[30–33]
- **Medication mis-/nonidentification.** Many pills and much packaging look very similar.
- **Improper storage**, for example, visually very similar bags of dopamine and dobutamine solutions being stored in immediate physical proximity or lack of refrigeration where required.
- **Lack of standardization**, such as failing to have an enforce standard concentrations of IV vasopressors and heparin solutions.
- **Supply chain changes**, which can result in drug packaging appearing suddenly different from prior resulting in confusion during dispensing and administration.
- **Environmental factors** such as noise, lighting, physical layout of the pharmacy, cluttered work areas, interruptions, high patient acuity, and staffing.
- **Provider factors** such as fatigue, long work hours, stress, hunger, illness, boredom, and substance use.
- **Lack of competence/training** operating new and/or complex administration devices. The newest, most sophisticated, and expensive delivery devices are useless (or worse) without proper training.
- **Lack of administration device standardization** and administration **device failure**. If, for example, patient-controlled analgesia delivery devices differ across care units in the same institution, it is unlikely that any single nurse will be competent in operating all of them.
- **Computer system inadequacy and malfunction** are likely to become more significant factors as the US health care system continues to become more and more dependent on electronic documentation, prescribing, and administration systems.
- Inadequate, conflicting, or **lack of allergy documentation.**

TABLE 29-2	Prohibited Abbreviations
Unacceptable	**Acceptable**
AU, AS, AD	Both ears, left ear, right ear
BT	Bedtime
cc	mL
D/C	Discharge, discontinue
HS/hs	Half-strength, bedtime
IJ	Injection
IN	Intranasal
IU	Units
µg	mcg
MgSO$_4$	Magnesium sulfate
MS/MSO$_4$	Morphine
OU, OS, OD	Both eyes, left eye, right eye
OD/od	Daily
OJ	Orange juice
Per os	PO
q1d	Daily
q6PM, etc.	Daily at 6 PM or 6 PM daily
QD/qd	Daily
qhs	Nightly, at bedtime
qn	Nightly, at bedtime
QOD/qod	Every other day
SC, SQ, subq	Subcutaneously or subcut
SS/SSI	Sliding scale insulin
i/d	1 daily
TIW/tiw	3 times weekly
U/u	Unit
UD	As directed
Trailing zero, 1.0 mg	No trailing zero, 1 mg
No leading zero, .1 mg	Leading zero, 0.1 mg

Adapted from Institute for Safe Medication Practices (ISMP). *List of Error-Prone Abbreviations, symbols, and Dose Designations.* Horsham, PA: Institute for Safe Medication Practices; 2014. Available at: www.ismp.org. Last accessed 10/1/15.

TABLE 29-3 Sound-Alike, Look-Alike Medications with Tall Man Lettering	
acetaZOLAMIDE	acetoHEXAMIDE
buPROPion	busPIRone
chlorproMAZINE	chlorproPAMIDE
clomiPHENE	clomiPRAMINE
cycloSERINE	cycloSPORINE
DAUNOrubicin	DOXOrubicin
dimenhyDRINATE	diphenhydrAMINE
DOBUTamine	DOPamine
glipiZIDE	glyBURIDE
hydrALAZINE	hydrOXYzine
medroxyPROGESTERone	medroxyPREDNISolone
methylTESTOSTERone	medroxyPROGESTERone medroxyPREDNISolone
niCARdipine	NIFEdipine
prednisoLONE	predniSONE
sulfADIAZINE	sulfiSOXAZOLE
TOLAZamide	TOLBUTamide
vinBLAStine	vinCRIStine

Adapted from U.S. Department of Health and Human Services, Food and Drug Administration, Office of Generic Drugs. *Name Differentiation Project.* Silver Spring, MD: Food and Drug Administration; 2013. Available at: http://www.fda.gov/Drugs/DrugSafety/MedicationErrors/ucm164587.htm. Last accessed 10/1/15.

- **Poor/nonexistent patient education**. It is worth remembering that patients administer their own medications at home and that process is directly analogous to what happens in the hospital; therefore, it is vulnerable to similar causes of error. In this context, patient education is vital.

DETECTING AND TRACKING MEDICATION ERRORS

Systematic methods to detect, track, and investigate medication errors are critical components of an overall plan to maximize medication safety. In order to capture as many medication errors as possible, multiple methods of detection are required including[25]:

1. **Voluntary anonymous self-reports**. One possible advantages of this method is that anonymity circumvents reporter concerns of disciplinary action/reprisal, whether he or she committed or witnessed the error. Anonymity greatly inhibits subsequent follow-up and investigation of the error. On the other hand, an anonymous report is better than no report at all. A robust culture of safety should theoretically reduce the perceived need for anonymous reporting.

2. **Voluntary nonanonymous reports/incident reports**. In an ideal culture of safety, all medication errors (including potential ADEs) would be reported voluntarily and nonanonymously. As previously noted, however, medication errors are very underreported. Reports of error (including anonymous ones) should contain at minimum: identifying patient information, the drug involved, what happened, speculation as to why it happened, any additional monitoring or testing required, and any additional therapy needed to prevent or treat patient harm. In most organizations, this process is electronic and leads reporters through a standard template.

3. **Computer-assisted monitoring**.[34-36] Many institutions use computer systems to monitor for errors at multiple points in the process including prescribing, order verification, dispensing, and administration. For example, measures of renal function can be used as triggers with regard to use of specified renally cleared medications. Any order for naloxone can alert to a possible error in the use of an opiate. Likewise, any severe hypoglycemia may indicate inappropriate use of insulin or oral hypoglycemics. Many potential drug–drug interactions can be tracked in this way. While currently imperfect, computerized ADE monitoring detects more errors than voluntary reporting and has the potential to intercept significant ADEs.

4. **Chart review** is more often a research technique, but individuals who routinely review charts (e.g., billing/coding and health information management personnel) can be trained to detect medication errors.

5. **Direct observation** is also generally a research technique. It can detect more errors but is time consuming and expensive.

Medication error data should be compiled and analyzed systematically, and this is often done by safety and quality professionals along pharmacy personnel. Very clear lines of communication and involvement of physicians and staff are also necessary. Overall error rates (e.g., events per 1000 patient days) are typically followed using standard run charts. Different charts can be scaled to best display rates and control limits of potential errors (A), errors with no harm (B, C, D), errors with harm (E, F, G, H), and errors with death (I). Rates can vary quite a bit over time and are often due to variations in reporting rather than true changes in rate. More complex graphical representations that display numbers of types of errors (e.g., missed dose, wrong dose, etc.) by process step can be very helpful (Fig. 29-4). For example, missed dose errors due to dispensing or administration issues will likely require rather different strategies to ameliorate.

MITIGATION STRATEGIES

No individual mitigation strategy is capable of addressing all sources of error. Therefore, meaningful reductions in medication error rates require strategies that involve the individual providers (physician, pharmacist, pharmacy technician, nurse, and patient) and the system as a whole. A sound culture of safety is an absolutely necessary foundation for these strategies to have their maximal impact.

Health Care Provider Strategies

The rights of safe prescribing remain entirely relevant and are presented in Table 29-4. These include the right patient, drug, dose, route, frequency, and duration. Right monitoring implies, for example, coagulation testing for patients taking

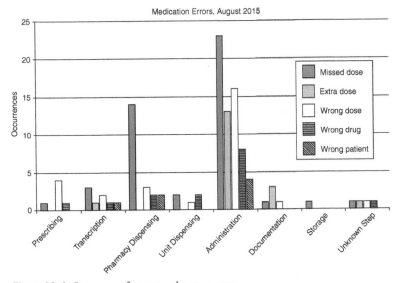

Figure 29-4. Occurrence of error types by process step.

certain anticoagulants, drug level monitoring when appropriate, awareness of and observation for known side effects, etc. Right cost asks the prescriber to consider if an equally efficacious drug is available for a lower price. Extra care and vigilance are necessary whenever prescribing an ISMP-designated **high-risk medication** (Table 29-1).[20] **Drug–drug interactions** should always be considered and the possibility of such an interaction increases with number of medications prescribed. Prescribers should be educated regarding commonly implicated medications (e.g., warfarin, macrolide

TABLE 29-4	The Rs of Safe Prescribing and Administration
Right patient	
Right drug	
Right indication	
Right dose/concentration	
Right route/form	
Right frequency/rate	
Right duration	
Right monitoring	
Right documentation	
Right cost	

antibiotics, sulfa drugs, amiodarone, azole antifungals, protease inhibitors, etc.) and use interaction software liberally. Appropriate dose adjustments should be made for **renal and hepatic dysfunction** when necessary. Where electronic prescribing is not available, it is clearly the prescriber's responsibility to **write legibly and avoid the use of disallowed abbreviations** (Table 29-2).[27]

Particular attention should be paid to prescribing for children and the elderly. **Dosing in children** very frequently requires dosage calculations based on patient-specific parameters (e.g., weight, height, body mass index, body surface area). Such information must be readily available in a standardized format (e.g., always kilograms instead of pounds), and prescribers should have easy access to methods of calculating dose. Difficult or high-risk calculations should be verified by others. Additionally, many medications commonly used in adults are not approved and/or unsafe for children.

The elderly are subject to more ADEs as well and mindfulness in prescribing is necessary. Certain medications have been designated as potentially inappropriate for older adults, the most well-known list being the American Geriatrics Society **Beers Criteria** (Table 29-5).[37-41] While not absolutely contraindicated in every situation, careful consideration should occur prior to starting any of them in older patients. The Screening Tool of Older Persons' potentially inappropriate Prescriptions (STOPP)

TABLE 29-5 American Geriatric Society 2012 Modified Beers Criteria[a]	
Class/Category/Drug	Examples/Notes
Anticholinergics, nonselective	Chlorpheniramine (in many OTC allergy/cold relief medications), diphenhydramine (in many OTC allergy/cold relief/motion sickness products, and sleep aids), doxylamine (e.g., NyQuil, Unisom), hydroxyzine (e.g., Vistaril, Atarax), promethazine Greater risk of significant anticholinergic side effects
Antiparkinson agents	Benztropine, trihexyphenidyl More effective antiparkinson drugs available and not recommended for the prevention of extrapyramidal effects with antipsychotics
Antispasmodics	Belladonna, clidinium, dicyclomine, hyoscyamine, scopolamine Very anticholinergic
Dipyridamole, oral short acting	Orthostatic hypotension May be given as extended release or IV for stress testing
Nitrofurantoin	Avoid use for long-term suppression or in those with CrCl <60 mL/min (ineffective concentration in urine) Risk of pulmonary toxicity
α_1-Blockers	Doxazosin, prazosin, terazosin for hypertension management More effective therapies available Risk of orthostatic hypotension

(Continued)

TABLE 29-5	American Geriatric Society 2012 Modified Beers Criteria (*Continued*)

Class/Category/Drug	Examples/Notes
α-Agonists, central	Clonidine, methyldopa Risk of CNS side effects, bradycardia, hypotension More effective first-line agents available
Antiarrhythmics	Amiodarone, disopyramide, dofetilide, dronedarone, flecainide, ibutilide, procainamide, propafenone, quinidine, sotalol Most older patients better served by rate control Amiodarone particularly associated with multiple toxicities Disopyramide is negatively inotropic and strongly anticholinergic
Digoxin >0.125 mg/day	Increased risk of toxicity without added benefit
Nifedipine, immediate release	Orthostatic hypotension
Spironolactone >25 mg/day	Or with concomitant NSAID, ACE inhibitor, ARB, or potassium supplements Hyperkalemia
Tricyclic antidepressants, tertiary	Amitriptyline, clomipramine, doxepin, imipramine Very anticholinergic Orthostatic hypotension
Antipsychotics	Increased mortality in those with dementia; avoid in these patients unless nonpharmacologic therapies have failed and patient presents a significant risk to self or others Increased risk of stroke,[38] anticholinergic effects (e.g., chlorpromazine, thioridazine, clozapine), and QT prolongation (e.g., thioridazine, ziprasidone)
Barbiturates	Butalbital (e.g., Fiorinal, Fioricet), phenobarbital Risk of overdose and dependence
Benzodiazepines	Increased risk of delirium, reduced cognition, and falls
Meprobamate	Sedating Risk of addiction
Other hypnotics	Eszopiclone, zaleplon, zolpidem Increased risk of delirium, reduced cognition, and falls
Androgens	Testosterone, methyltestosterone Contraindicated in prostate cancer Risk of cardiovascular effects

TABLE 29-5 American Geriatric Society 2012 Modified Beers Criteria (*Continued*)

Class/Category/Drug	Examples/Notes
Estrogens	With or without progestins Potential increased risk of breast and endometrial cancer Vaginal estrogen acceptable
Desiccated thyroid	Safer alternatives
Growth hormone	Acceptable for replacement postpituitary resection
Insulin, sliding scale	Risk of hypoglycemia in any care setting
Sulfonylureas, long acting	Chlorpropamide, glyburide Risk of hypoglycemia
Megestrol	Marginally effective Increased risk of thromboembolic events, potentially mortality[39,40]
Metoclopramide	Increased risk of extrapyramidal side effects
Mineral oil, oral	Risk of aspiration Multiple safer alternatives
Trimethobenzamide	Tigan Limited effectiveness for nausea Risk of extrapyramidal side effects
Nonselective NSAIDs	Avoid chronic use; if used, consider addition of a PPI[40] Increased risk of gastrointestinal bleeding, particularly in those >75 or taking steroids, anticoagulants, or antiplatelet agents
Meperidine	Demerol Limited oral analgesic effect Risk of neurotoxicity Safer alternatives available
Muscle "relaxants"	Carisoprodol, chlorzoxazone, cyclobenzaprine, metaxalone, methocarbamol Sedation, anticholinergic side effects Carisoprodol potentially more addictive

[a]Very uncommonly used medications excluded.
ACE inhibitor, angiotensin-converting enzyme inhibitor; ARB, angiotensin receptor blocker; CrCl, creatinine clearance; NSAID, nonsteroidal anti-inflammatory drug;OTC, over the counter; PPI, proton pump inhibitor.
Adapted from American Geriatric Society 2012 Beers Criteria Update Expert Panel. American Geriatrics Society updated Beers Criteria for potentially inappropriate medication use in older adults. *J Am Geriatr Soc.* 2012;60:616–31.

criteria may be more effective at preventing avoidable ADEs.[42] **Polypharmacy** is a particular problem in the elderly. Physicians should avoid prescribing an additional medication to counteract the side effects presumably due to another, leading to a so-called prescribing cascade.[43] Efforts should be made to discontinue drugs that do not have an evidence-based or reasonably valid indication, particularly when possible ADEs/side effects are not clearly outweighed.[44]

Other than the outpatient setting, nurses are the primary actors of the administration process step. It is the last opportunity to intercept errors that have occurred upstream and gone undetected. The rights are no less important here (i.e., right patient, drug, dose, route, and time). In many instances, there are other policy-based actions that must also occur at the time of administration (e.g., tracing the line for IV infusions). As discussed in Causes of Medication Errors, many factors may impact on an individual nurse's ability to perform flawlessly at this critical point.

System Strategies

Computerized provider order entry (CPOE) systems, sometimes accompanied by varying degrees of clinic decision support systems (CDSS), are now becoming much more common. Such systems may be a component of an all-encompassing electronic health record but sometimes not. Systems may be large commercial ventures or single institution-only locally developed ones. Either way, they are extraordinarily expensive and labor intensive to implement and maintain. Nevertheless, CPOE systems have the potential to substantially reduce ADEs. Individual studies of CPOE with or without CDSS have demonstrated reductions in medication error rates, and a smaller number have shown decreases in ADEs.[45–49] Results may not be broadly applicable across systems and sites of care. A few studies point to unintended negative consequences of CPOE.[50,51] The proper balance of number/types of alerts versus perceived positive effects of such alerts is a major issue for busy clinicians. Much remains to be learned in order to maximize the effectiveness of these systems.

Similarly, **smart pumps** have much potential. These devices have software allowing for drug-specific infusions, on-board rate calculations, alerts/warnings (soft stops), and hard stops. Some smart pumps have scanning technology to confirm the identity of IV solutions. They may have the capability of wirelessly updating libraries and downloading information regarding key strokes, bypassed alerts, etc. Unfortunately, this expensive technology has yet to live up to its potential. There are frequent and easy opportunities to bypass safeguards, particularly ignoring alerts/soft stops. Even hard stops can be bypassed, for example, by programming a pump as a normal saline solution rather than a heparin solution. At present, the typical smart pump is not assigned to a particular patient and does not interface with an electronic MAR. In other words, the pump is only smart enough to know that a provider has indicated which drug is to be given and the general administration rules that have been uploaded for that drug. Failures to standardize IV medication concentrations, update drug libraries, and implement hard stops are other important issues.[52] Notwithstanding, the potential remains and continued work is needed to realize the benefits of smart pumps.

Bar coding is also a technology that has a high degree of face validity. As would be expected, patients and medications are bar coded and these codes interface with the appropriate MAR. Patient and drug are scanned at the point of administration to confirm that drug X is on patient Y's MAR and is due at the present time. A study of over 14,000 medication administrations demonstrated a 41.4% relative reduction in medication errors and a 50.8% relative reduction in potential ADEs with the use of bar coding technology. These rates exclude timing errors and the absolute reduction in potential ADEs was 1.5%.[53] An earlier study by the same group also demonstrated significant reductions in potential ADEs with the use of bar code technology during pharmacy dispensing.[54]

Medication reconciliation issues are well known to be associated with medication errors.[30-33] The Joint Commission includes medication reconciliation in its current national patient safety goals, essentially requiring hospital organizations to demonstrate that it is occurring in a systematic and effect manner. This too remains a work in progress with substantial potential to reduce errors. Reviews on the subject have generally agreed that results have been mixed regarding clinically important outcomes and that more rigorously designed research is needed.[55-59] It is likely that medication reconciliation is just one component of effective care transitions. Having an accurate and readily accessible electronic repository of **allergy documentation** is also imperative. Ideally, it would cut across multiple sites of care and interact directly with CPOE, dispensing, and bar coding systems to alert providers at multiple process steps. Unfortunately, it is not rare for patients to unintentionally receive a medication to which they have a documented allergy.

The inclusion of **clinical pharmacists** on inpatient services is likely to improve patient care. More than half of studies have demonstrated reductions in errors, ADEs, and ADRs.[60] While it is entirely reasonable to suppose that pharmacists would be ideal individuals to perform medication reconciliations, at least one recent trial failed to show an effect.[61] Other pharmacy-based strategies include the use of **tall man lettering** for sound-alike/look-alike drugs (Table 29-3), automated storage and retrieval systems, unit-based storage and dispensing systems, IV compounding workflow management systems, and robotic prescription dispensing devices.[28]

KEY POINTS

- Medication errors and adverse drug events are common in all care settings, result in approximately 100,000 hospitalizations per year and are very costly.
- Medication errors are underreported.
- Medication errors can be categorized by psychological theory, process step, proximal cause, and degree of patient harm.
- Health care organizations must have functional and transparent methods of reporting, detecting, tracking, and analyzing medication errors.
- Multiple mitigation strategies exist, but no single strategy will eliminate all errors.

ONLINE RESOURCES

1. Institute for Safe Medical Practices: http://www.ismp.org. Last accessed 11/18/15.
2. National Coordinating Council for Medication Error Reporting and Prevention: http://www.nccmerp.org. Last accessed 11/18/15.
3. U.S. Food and Drug Administration MedWatch: http://www.fda.gov/Safety/MedWatch/. Last accessed 11/18/15.
4. U.S. Department of Health and Human Services, National Action Plan for Adverse Drug Event Prevention: http://health.gov/hcq/ade.asp. Last accessed 11/18/15.

REFERENCES

1. National Coordinating Council for Medication Error Reporting and Prevention. *About Medication Errors*. Rockville, MD: National Coordinating Council for Medication Error Reporting and Prevention; 2015. Available at: http://www.nccmerp.org/about-medication-errors. Last accessed 10/1/15.
2. Bates DW, Boyle DL, Vander Vliet MB, et al. Relationship between medication errors and adverse drug events. *J Gen Intern Med*. 1995;10:199–205.
3. Gandhi TK, Seger DL, Bates DW. Identifying drug safety issues from research to practice. *Int J Qual Health Care*. 2000;12:69–76.
4. Leendertse AJ, Egberts AC, Stoker LJ, et al. Frequency of and risk factors for preventable medication-related hospital admissions in the Netherlands. *Arch Intern Med*. 2008;168:1890–6.
5. Davies EC, Green DF, Taylor S, et al. Adverse drug reactions in hospital in-patients: a prospective analysis of 3695 patient-episodes. *PLoS One*. 2009;4:e4439.
6. Al Hamid A, Ghaleb M, Aljadhey H, et al. A systematic review of hospitalization resulting from medicine-related problems in adult patients. *Br J Clin Pharmacol*. 2014;78:202–17.
7. Kaufman CP, Stämpfli D, Hersberger K, et al. Determination of risk factors for drug-related problems: a multidisciplinary triangulation process. *BMJ Open*. 2015;5:e006376.
8. Budnitz DS, Pollock DA, Weidenbach KN, et al. National surveillance of emergency department visits for outpatient adverse drug events. *JAMA*. 2008;296:1858–66.
9. Budnitz DS, Lovegrove MC, Shehab N, et al. Emergency hospitalizations for adverse drug events in older Americans. *N Engl J Med*. 2011;365:2002–12.
10. Institute of Medicine. *Preventing Medication Errors*. Washington, DC: National Academy Press; 2006.
11. Bates DW, Cullen DJ, Laird N, et al. Incidence of adverse drug events and potential adverse drug events. Implications for prevention. ADE Prevention Study Group. *JAMA*. 1995;274:29–34.
12. Classen DC, Pestotnik SL, Evans RS, et al. Adverse drug events in hospitalized patients. Excess length of stay, extra costs, and attributable mortality. *JAMA*. 1997;277:301–6.
13. Nebeker JR, Hoffman JM, Weir CR, et al. High rates of adverse drug events in a highly computerized hospital. *Arch Intern Med*. 2005;165:1111–6.
14. Wilmer, Louie K, Dodek P, et al. Incidence of medication errors and adverse drug events in the ICU: a systematic review. *Qual Saf Health Care*. 2010;19:e7.
15. Gurwitz JH, Field TS, Harrold LR, et al. Incidence and preventability of adverse drug events among older persons in the ambulatory setting. *JAMA*. 2003;289:1107–16.
16. Gurwitz JH, Field TS, Judge J, et al. The incidence of adverse drug events in two large academic long-term care facilities. *Am J Med*. 2005;118:251–8.
17. Institute of Medicine. *To Err Is Human: Building a Safer Health System*. Washington, DC: National Academy Press; 2000.
18. Phillips DP, Barker GE, Eguchi MM. A steep increase in domestic fatal medication errors with use of alcohol and/or street drugs. *Arch Intern Med*. 2008;168:1561–6.
19. Phillips DP, Barker GE. A July spike in fatal medication errors: a possible effect of new medical residents. *J Gen Intern Med*. 2010;25:774–9.
20. Institute for Safe Medication Practices (ISMP). *List of High-Alert Medications in Acute Care Settings*. Horsham, PA: Institute for Safe Medication Practices; 2014. Available at: www.ismp.org. Last accessed 10/1/15.
21. Aronson JK. Medication errors: what they are, how they happen, and how to avoid them. *QJM*. 2009;102:513–21.
22. National Coordinating Council for Medication Error Reporting and Prevention. *NCC MERP Index for Categorizing Medication Errors*. Rockville, MD: National Coordinating Council for Medication Error Reporting and Prevention; 2001. Available at: http://www.nccmerp.org/types-medication-errors. Last accessed 10/1/15.
23. Phillips J, Beam S, Brinker A, et al. Retrospective analysis of mortalities associated with medication errors. *Am J Health Syst Pharm*. 2001;58:1835–41.

24. Leape LL, Bates DW, Cullen DJ, et al. Systems analysis of adverse drug events. ADE Prevention Study Group. *JAMA*. 1995;274:35–43.

25. Cohen MR, ed. *Medication Errors*. 2nd ed. Washington, DC: American Pharmacists Association; 2007.

26. U.S. Department of Health and Human Services, Food and Drug Administration, Office of Medical Products and Tobacco, Center for Drug Evaluation and Research, Office of Generic Drugs. *Approved Drug Products with Therapeutic Equivalence Evaluations*. 35th ed. Cumulative Supplement 8, August 2015. Silver Spring, MD: Food and Drug Administration; 2015.

27. Institute for Safe Medication Practices (ISMP). *List of Error-Prone Abbreviations, Symbols, and Dose Designations*. Horsham, PA: Institute for Safe Medication Practices; 2014. Available at: www.ismp.org. Last accessed 10/1/15.

28. U.S. Department of Health and Human Services, Food and Drug Administration, Office of Generic Drugs. *Name Differentiation Project*. Silver Spring, MD: Food and Drug Administration; 2013. Available at: http://www.fda.gov/Drugs/DrugSafety/MedicationErrors/ucm164587.htm. Last accessed 10/1/15.

29. Institute for Health Care Improvement. *Medication Reconciliation to Prevent Adverse Drug Events*. Cambridge, MA: Institute for Health Care Improvement; 2015. Available at: http://www.ihi.org/topics/adesmedicationreconciliation/Pages/default.aspx. Last accessed October 1, 2015.

30. Cornish PL, Knowles SR, Marchesano R, et al. Unintended medication discrepancies at the time of hospital admission. *Arch Intern Med*. 2005;165:424–9.

31. Vira T, Colquhoun M, Etchells E. Reconcilable differences: correcting medication errors at hospital admission and discharge. *Qual Saf Health Care*. 2006;15:122–6.

32. Wong JD, Bajcar JM, Wong GG, et al. Medication reconciliation at hospital discharge: evaluating discrepancies. *Ann Pharmacother*. 2008;42:1373–9.

33. Lee JY, Leblanc K, Fernandes OA, et al. Medication reconciliation during internal hospital transfer and impact of computerized prescriber order entry. *Ann Pharmacother*. 2010;44:1887–95.

34. Classen DC, Pestotnik SL, Evans RS, et al. Computerized surveillance of adverse drug events in hospital patients. *JAMA*. 1991;266:2847–51.

35. Jha AK, Kuperman GJ, Teich JM, et al. Identifying adverse drug events: development of a computer-based monitor and comparison with chart review and stimulated voluntary report. *J Am Med Inform Assoc*. 1998;5:305–14.

36. Handler SM, Altman RL, Perera S, et al. A systematic review of the performance characteristics of clinical event monitor signals used to detect adverse drug events in the hospital setting. *J Am Med Inform Assoc*. 2007;14:451–8.

37. American Geriatric Society 2012 Beers Criteria Update Expert Panel. American Geriatrics Society updated Beers Criteria for potentially inappropriate medication use in older adults. *J Am Geriatr Soc*. 2012;60:616–31.

38. Maher AR, Maglione M, Bagley, et al. Efficacy and comparative effectiveness of atypical antipsychotic medications for off-label uses in adults: a systematic review and meta-analysis. *JAMA*. 2011;306:1359–69.

39. Bodenner D, Spencer T, Riggs AT, et al. A retrospective study of the association between megestrol acetate administration and mortality among nursing home residents with clinically significant weight loss. *Am J Geriatr Pharmacother*. 2007;5:137–46.

40. Thomas DR. Incidence of venous thromboembolism in megestrol acetate users. *J Am Med Dir Assoc*. 2004;5:65–6.

41. Rostom A, Dube C, Wells G, et al. Prevention of NSAID-induced gastroduodenal ulcers. *Cochrane Database Syst Rev*. 2002;(4):CD002296.

42. Hamilton H, Gallagher P, Ryan C, et al. Potentially inappropriate medications defined by STOPP criteria and the risk of adverse drug events in older hospitalized patients. *Arch Intern Med*. 2011;171:1013–9.

43. Rochon PA, Gurwitz JH. Optimising drug treatment for elderly people: the prescribing cascade. *BMJ*. 1997;315:1096–9.

44. Garfinkel D, Mangin D. Feasibility study of a systematic approach for discontinuation of multiple medications in older adults: addressing polypharmacy. *Arch Intern Med.* 2010;170:1648–54.
45. Bates DW, Leape LL, Cullen DJ, et al. Effect of computerized physician order entry and a team intervention on prevention of serious medication errors. *JAMA.* 1998;280:1311–6.
46. Kaushal R, Shojania KG, Bates DW. Effects of computerized physician order entry and clinical decision support systems on medication safety: a systematic review. *Arch Intern Med.* 2003;163:1409–16.
47. Eslami S, Abu-Hanna A, de Keizer NF. Evaluation of outpatient computerized physician medication order entry systems: a systematic review. *J Am Med Inform Assoc.* 2007;14:400–6.
48. Wolfstadt JI, Gurwitz JH, Field TS, et al. The effect of computerized physician order entry with clinical decision support on the rates of adverse drug events: a systematic review. *J Gen Intern Med.* 2008;23:451–8.
49. Georgiou A, Prgomet M, Paoloni R, et al. The effect of computerized provider order entry systems on clinical care and work processes in emergency departments: a systematic review of the quantitative literature. *Ann Emerg Med.* 2013;61:644–53.
50. Koppel R, Metlay JP, Cohen A, et al. Role of computerized physician order entry systems in facilitating medication errors. *JAMA.* 2005;293:1197–203.
51. Strom BL, Schinnar R, Aberra F, et al. Unintended effects of a computerized physician order entry nearly hard-stop alert to prevent a drug interaction: a randomized controlled trial. *Arch Intern Med.* 2010;170:1578–83.
52. Ohashi K, Dalleur O, Dykes PC, et al. Benefits and risks of using smart pumps to reduce medication error rates: a systematic review. *Drug Saf.* 2014;37:1011–20.
53. Poon EG, Keohane CA, Yoon CS, et al. Effect of bar-code technology on the safety of medication administration. *N Engl J Med.* 2010;362:1698–707.
54. Poon EG, Cina JL, Churchill W, et al. Medication dispensing errors and potential adverse drug events before and after implementing bar code technology in the pharmacy. *Ann Intern Med.* 2006;145:426–34.
55. Bayoumi I, Howard M, Holbrrok AM, et al. Interventions to improve medication reconciliation in primary care. *Ann Pharmacother.* 2009;43:1667–75.
56. Mueller SK, Sponsler KC, Kripalani S, et al. Hospital-based medication reconciliation practices: a systematic review. *Arch Intern Med.* 2012;172:1057–69.
57. Christensen M, Lundh A. Medication review in hospitalised patients to reduce morbidity and mortality. *Cochrane Database Syst Rev.* 2013;(2):CD008986.
58. Kwan JL, Lo L, Sampson M, et al. Medication reconciliation during transitions of care as a patient safety strategy: a systematic review. *Ann Intern Med.* 2013;158:397–403.
59. Lehnbom ED, Stewart MJ, Manias E, et al. Impact of medication reconciliation and review on clinical outcomes. *Ann Pharmacother.* 2014;48:1298–312.
60. Kaboli PJ, Hoth AB, McClimon BJ, et al. Clinical pharmacists and inpatient medical care: a systematic review. *Arch Intern Med.* 2006;166:955–64.
61. Kripalani S, Roumie CL, Dalal AK, et al. Effect of a pharmacist intervention on clinically important medication errors after hospital discharge: a randomized trial. *Ann Intern Med.* 2012;157:1–10. Available at: http://www.accessdata.fda.gov/scripts/cder/ob/. Last accessed 10/1/15.

30 Transitions in Care and Readmissions

Emily Fondahn and Elna Nagasako

CLINICAL VIGNETTE

Mrs. H is a 72-year-old widowed woman with type 2 diabetes, hypertension, and hyperlipidemia who initially presented to the hospital with severe chest pain. She was diagnosed with a non–ST elevation myocardial infarction and underwent a coronary catheterization with placement of two drug-eluding stents. She tolerated the procedure well and had no complications during her hospital stay. She went home with a list of new prescriptions, including clopidogrel. She was unable to drive to the pharmacy for 3 days due to feeling weak and had no one at home to help her. When she went to pick up her new medications, she was unable to afford clopidogrel. She was too embarrassed to call her physician and tell him that she was not taking the medication. Ten days after she was discharged, she again began experiencing severe chest pain and returned to the hospital. She was readmitted and diagnosed with an ST elevation myocardial infarction and new heart failure due to in-stent stenosis from not taking her clopidogrel.

- What factors led her to being readmitted to the hospital?
- How could her readmission for a myocardial infarction and heart failure have been prevented?

INTRODUCTION

Recently, hospital readmissions have been highlighted as an indicator of poor quality of care and high costs within the health care system. Currently, 1 out of 5 Medicare beneficiaries are readmitted within 30 days with an estimated cost of 17.5 billion dollars![1] While some readmissions reflect worsening of disease, many are a result of an uncoordinated and confusing discharge process for patients or incomplete treatment of an illness. Increased emphasis is being placed on hospitals to redesign their models for transitions of care into a more patient-centered process. Centers for Medicare and Medicaid Services (CMS) have begun penalizing hospitals with an excess rate of readmissions. Hospitals are currently being penalized based on readmission rates for congestive heart failure, pneumonia, acute myocardial infarction, chronic obstructive pulmonary disease exacerbation, elective total hip arthroplasty, and elective total knee arthroplasty.[2]

CMS defines a transition of care as "The movement of a patient from one setting of care (hospital, ambulatory primary care practice, ambulatory specialty care practice, long-term care, home health, rehabilitation facility) to another." These care transitions usually mean a change of health care providers which predisposes patients to fragmentation of care. Especially in elderly or chronically ill patients, multiple providers and care settings may be involved, which can quickly become confusing and overwhelming for a patient or caregiver to navigate. Currently, there are few incentives for providers to take on the task of care coordination and no specific person or group in the health care setting is responsible for coordinating postdischarge care. Patients are often discharged into a "gray zone" where no one provider will assume responsibility for their care. The current gaps in the system can be viewed as hospital care systems issues, patient-related issues, and clinician-related issues.[3] The deficiencies within the hospital system include poor communication to the outpatient provider, inadequate patient information, medication errors, lack of timely follow-up, and lapse in home services. Patient-specific factors consist of development of new medical problems, worsening of previous problem, addiction issues, language and/or cultural issues, medication adherence, and follow-up. The clinician-specific issues consist of inappropriate discharge of a patient, inappropriate medications, inadequate home services, or errors in ordering, seeing, or acting upon a laboratory or test result. Each of these deficiencies represents as possible area to improve transitions of care and reduce preventable readmissions.

HIGH-RISK PATIENTS

Identifying patients at high risk for readmission and adverse events is a critical step in improving care transitions. Identification allows for better use of resources and tailored interventions. Risk assessment tools are available and generally include areas such as previous admissions, diagnoses, and age. Social and cultural factors can also play a key role in making a patient high risk, such as having a poor support system or not speaking English. In addition, cognitive impairment, poor health literacy, and low self-efficacy are other important nonclinical risk factors, which are often underrecognized by clinicians but impact a patient's ability to remember and follow discharge instructions.[4] These patients may be labeled as "noncompliant" by the health care team but really require simplification of traditional discharge materials and more support from family members or caregivers. Project BOOST (Better Outcomes for Older Adults Through Safe Transitions), a national initiative to improve care transitions led by the Society for Hospital Medicine, has developed the 8P screening tool as a quick, easy way to identify high-risk patients (Table 30-1).[5] These risk factors can be used in conjunction with targeted interventions.

COMMUNICATION DURING TRANSITIONS OF CARE

Communication with Primary Care Provider

Communication of a hospital course to the primary care provider is a critically important step in the discharge process. The hospital discharge summary serves as a traditional mode of communication between the inpatient and outpatient providers, which should provide a summary of the hospital course, significant findings, pending test results, and patient status (Table 30-2). However, adequate communication between inpatient and outpatient teams occurs infrequently. In one systematic review, Kripalani et al. found that direct communication between the hospital physician and primary care physicians was rare, occurring in between 3% and 20% of encounters, and that the primary care physicians had the discharge summary available at only 12–34% of postdischarge visits.[6] Additionally, even when a discharge summary was

TABLE 30-1	Project BOOST 8P Screening Tool
Problems with medications	Anticoagulants, insulin, oral hypoglycemics, aspirin and clopidogrel dual therapy, digoxin, narcotics or polypharmacy ≥10 routine medications)
Psychological	Depression screen positive or history of depression diagnosis
Principal diagnosis	Cancer, stroke, diabetic complications, COPD, heart failure
Physical limitations	Frailty, deconditioning, or other limitations that impair ability to help with own care
Poor health literacy	Inability to do teach-back
Poor social support	Absence of caregiver to assist with discharge and home care
Prior hospitalization	Nonelective hospitalization in the prior last 6 months
Palliative care	Would you be surprised if this patient died in the next year? Does this patient have an advanced or progressive illness?

(Adapted from Project BOOST. http://www.hospitalmedicine.org/Web/Quality_Innovation/ Implementation_Toolkits/Project_BOOST/Web/Quality___Innovation/Implementation_Toolkit/ Boost/BOOST_Intervention/Tools/Risk_Assessment.aspx. Accessed 12/21/15).

TABLE 30-2	Components of an Optimal Discharge Summary

Dates of admission and discharge

Reason for hospitalization

Significant findings from history and exam

Significant laboratory findings

Significant radiologic findings

Significant findings from other tests

List of procedures performed

Procedure report findings

Pathology report findings

Discharge diagnosis

Condition at discharge

Discharge medications

Follow-up issues

Pending test results

Information provided to the patient and/or family

(Adapted from O'Leary KJ, Liebovitz DM, Feinglass J, et al. Creating a better discharge summary: improvement in quality and timeliness using an electronic discharge summary. J Hosp Med. 2009;4:219–25.)[7]

available for a provider, key information was often missing. Improving information exchange leads to improved continuity of care, hospital use, patient status, primary care use, and decreases errors, near misses, or adverse events.[8] These gaps in communication lead to confusion for the patient and the providers and could be a potential course of adverse events and readmissions.

COMMUNICATING WITH PATIENTS

Discharge Instructions

Traditional discharge instructions can be confusing and overwhelming for patients. Even patients with adequate health literacy may not be able to process all the information provided due to illness, stress, or excitement about going home. In one study of patients 70 years or older interviewed 3 days after discharge, over half (54.2%) did not recall having someone talk to them about how to care for themselves after hospitalization and only 27% had a telephone name or number to call if they needed help after returning home.[9] Patients then leave the hospital confused about how to manage their care when they arrive home. Additionally, the patient may not be the ideal learner in the hospital environment. It is imperative to identify the best person to receive the teaching, then provide him or her with the essential information that they need. Some patients and caregivers may not learn the best with written instructions; in those cases, it is important to ask how the patient or caregiver learns best and tailor the discharge education. Furthermore, the written discharge instructions should be provided in a patient-centered format. General principles include using large font (at least 12 point), writing in a sixth grade or below reading level, using upper- and lowercase text, using bulleted lists or short paragraphs, and avoiding information overload.[10]

These are the key components of discharge instructions:
- Reason for hospitalization (written in patient-friendly terminology)
- Medication list
- Potential side effects of medications
- Name and phone number of a person to call if problems arise
- Symptoms to watch out for
- How to keep health problems from getting worse
- Follow-up appointments for tests and clinical visits with dates, times, location, and contact number
- Diet
- Activity level
- Disease-specific instructions

Medication errors are one of the most common problems seen when patients leave the hospital. While inpatient, medications are frequently stopped, started, and changed. Patients need an accurate medication list upon discharge. Ideally, this medication list includes brand and generic names; dose of each medication; time to take medication; new medications, changed medications, and stopped medications; and indication for the medicine. One effective way to communicate this information is to create a personalized pill card or schedule (Fig. 30-1).

Teach-Backs

Teach-backs have been identified as one effective model to educate patients and check for understanding. Patients often do not understand or remember what is explained to them by clinicians. In essence, a teach-back helps "close the loop" to ensure that

Name: Sarah Smith					Date Created: 12/15/2015	
Pharmacy phone number: 123-456-7890						

Name	Used For	Instructions	Morning	Afternoon	Evening	Night
Simvastatin 20mg	Cholesterol	Take 1 pill at night				
Furosemide 20mg	Fluid	Take 2 pills in the morning and 2 pills in the evening				
Insulin 70/30	Diabetes (Sugar)	Inject 24 units before breakfast and 12 units before dinner	24 units		12 units	

Figure 30-1. Personalized pill card. (Adapted from How to Create a Pill Card. Rockville, MD: Agency for Healthcare Research and Quality; 2008. http://www.ahrq.gov/patients-consumers/diagnosis-treatment/treatments/pillcard/index.html. Accessed 12/21/15).

effective communication about disease and self-care has been communicated to the patient and/or caregivers.[11] The purpose of a teach-back is to have patients explain, in their own words, what the clinician told them. It is not a test of patient's understanding; rather, it is a method to check the clinician's ability to explain a concept clearly to a patient. If a patient is unable to verbalize a correct answer, the clinician needs to reteach the concept to the patient. Teach-back is more effective than asking a patient "Do you understand?" since patients will often reply "Yes," even if they are still confused. Clinicians should also remember to use plain language, a caring tone, and short statements when talking to patients.

Examples of teach-back questions:

- "I want you to explain to me how you will take your medication, so I can be sure I have explained everything correctly."
- "Please show me how you will use the asthma inhaler, so I can be sure I have given you clear instructions."
- "When you get home, your spouse will ask you what the doctor said; what will you tell your spouse?"

IMPROVING TRANSITIONS OF CARE

With the new focus on reducing readmissions and improving transitions of care, health care systems have started scrutinizing the discharge process and implementing novel approaches to improve transitions of care. A variety of strategies have been used, such as increasing the use of teach-backs, clarifying discharge instructions, comprehensive discharge planning, standardizing the discharge process with the use of templates or checklists, and creating transitional care teams. Several large widescale models have shown the use of these strategies to be effective in reducing readmission rates.

DISCHARGE PLANNING

With current attempts to shorten the inpatient length of stay and increase care provided in the ambulatory setting, more emphasis has been placed on discharge planning. Discharge planning is creating an individualized discharge plan for a patient prior to the patient leaving the hospital. A recent Cochrane Review reported that tailored discharge planning can reduce length of stay and readmission rates for individuals.[12] Discharge planning starts at admission and should be addressed throughout the hospital stay. A multidisciplinary group, with physicians, nurses, social workers, and case managers, can work together to identify barriers to discharge and identify solutions to those potential barriers. Common mistakes made by the care team in the hospital include having a poor understanding of a patient's ability to perform self-care in the home environment, not including patients and/or caregivers in the discharge process, transfer to a care venue that does not meet the patient's needs, medication errors and polypharmacy, worsening clinical status, and discharging a patient too early.[13] Hospitals often employ case managers, social workers, or dedicated discharge planners who can screen patients that will need support with discharge planning and assist with arranging complex discharge services. Discharge specialists can also navigate different insurance plans to help provide coverage for services and help arrange home services.

Components of discharge planning include:

- Where patient will go after discharge (home, rehabilitation facility, skilled nursing facility)
- Any special care that will be needed (home health, home physical therapy, hospice)
- Medication reconciliation, including new and changed medications and how a patient will obtain medications
- Durable medical equipment (walkers, supplemental oxygen, hospital bed)
- Activity level
- Follow-up appointments with primary care provider, specialists, and any needed laboratory or imaging studies
- Transportation home and to follow-up appointments (cabs, ambulances, private transportation, public transportation)

Some institutions are beginning to incorporate discharge checklists for the health care team and/or patient to ensure that all the key components of discharge are met. These discharge checklists may be disease specific (i.e., congestive heart failure, acute myocardial infarction) or universal for all patients discharged, regardless of their admitting diagnosis.

TRANSITIONAL CARE TEAMS

In order to assist patients through a smooth transition from the hospital to home, many health care systems are developing transitional care teams. These teams can be multidisciplinary and often led by nurses or case coordinators. These programs are tailored to identify and monitor high-risk patients. The transitional care nurse acts as the key contact person for the patient. The nurse meets the patient in the hospital, coordinates discharge care, and then follows up with the patient in the home and via telephone calls. The transitional care nurse will also accompany the patient to physician appointments and assist the care coordination between multiple providers. The goal of these programs is to address a patient's concerns and changes in health while in the outpatient setting to avoid unnecessary visits to the emergency department or inpatient hospitalization. The transitional care nurse can also identify and correct possible adverse events or errors, such as noticing that a patient does not have an important medication. Research for these programs has generally been promising in showing a reduction in readmission rates and longer lengths of time out of the hospital for patients.

SPECIFIC MODELS

BOOSTing Care Transitions (Better Outcomes by Optimizing Safe Transitions) has been developed by the Society for Hospital Medicine to provide a framework and support to improve care transitions.[5] The goals of Project BOOST were to:

1. Reduce 30-day readmission rates for general internal medicine patients
2. Improve patient satisfaction and HCAHPS scores
3. Improve information flow between inpatient and outpatient providers
4. Identify high-risk patients and target-specific interventions
5. Improve patient and family preparation for discharge

Project BOOST has developed specific tools to identify high-risk patients and standardize the discharge process. The BOOST toolkit includes a risk stratification process (8P tool, Table 30-1), a risk-specific intervention plan, the universal checklist, and the general assessment of preparedness (GAP) to evaluate the readiness of patients to leave the hospital. The TARGET tool is designed to be filled out by a multidisciplinary group, but a specific individual should have ultimate ownership. Initial data on Project BOOST at the six pilot sites showed a reduction in readmission rates from 14.2% to 11.2%.[14]

Project Re-engineered Discharge (RED) was created at Boston University with support from the Agency for Healthcare Research and Quality (AHRQ) and National Institutes of Health (NIH).[15] Project RED identified 12 key components for discharge and presents them in a patient-centered manner (Table 30-3). Patients are provided with an "After Hospital Care Plan" when they leave the hospital, which contains key information about medications, follow-up, contact information of the primary care physician and discharge advocate, pending lab results, reason for hospitalization, and a calendar with scheduled tests and appointments. A "virtual patient advocate" named Louise was invented to assist with the discharge process. Louise simulates the patient–nurse interaction and helps teach patients about medications, follow-up appointments, and diagnoses through a computer touch screen display on a wheeled kiosk. In the pilot study for Project RED, the readmission rate was reduced by 30% in the

TABLE 30-3 Components of Project RED

Ascertain need for and obtain language assistance.

Make appointments for follow-up medical appointments and postdischarge tests/labs.

Plan for the follow-up of results from lab tests or studies that are pending at discharge.

Organize postdischarge outpatient services and medical equipment.

Identify the correct medicines and a plan for the patient to obtain and take them.

Reconcile the discharge plan with national guidelines.

Teach a written discharge plan the patient can understand.

Educate the patient about his or her diagnosis.

Assess the degree of the patient's understanding of the discharge plan.

Review with the patient what to do if a problem arises.

Expedite transmission of the discharge summary to clinicians accepting care of the patient.

Provide telephone reinforcement of the discharge plan.

(Adapted from Boston University School of Medicine. Project RED (Re-Engineered Discharge). http://www.bu.edu/fammed/projectred/. Accessed 3/5/13).

intervention group. Patients in the intervention group also had higher rates of follow-up with primary care physicians and reported being more prepared for discharge.[16]

Transitional Care Model (TCM) was created by Mary Naylor, RN, PhD, at the University of Pennsylvania.[17] This model utilizes advanced practice nurses called Transitional Care Nurses (TCNs) to coordinate pre- and postdischarge care in high-risk, elderly patients with chronic illness. The TCNs are in charge of discharge planning, then follow the patients when they return home. The TCN acts as a link between the inpatient and outpatient setting and provides home support, close follow-up with patients, and engagement of the patient and family. The goal is to interrupt patterns of frequent hospital or emergency department use and prevent health decline. Randomized trials evaluating this model have shown significant reductions in hospital readmissions, lengthened time to first readmission, and decreased cost of care.[18]

Care Transitions Program was developed by Eric Coleman, MD, MPH. This model is a 4-week program, which focuses on improving self-management skills with the help of a Transition Coach. The Transition Coach follows the patient from the inpatient hospitalization to the outpatient setting. Their role is assisting the patient in learning self-management skills and improving patient–provider communication. The Transition Coach teaches patients and caregivers how to respond to problems that may occur during and after transitions. This model showed a significant reduction in readmission rates in elderly people at 30, 90, and 180 days after discharge and a longer time until readmission.

The four components of the program are defined as the four pillars:

- Medication self-management
- Patient-centered record
- Follow-up with physician
- Knowledge of "red flags" or warning signs/symptoms and how to respond

KEY POINTS

- High readmission rates are an indicator of poor care coordination and an area of unnecessarily high costs in medicine.
- Comprehensive discharge planning is complex and requires a multidisciplinary team approach.
- Identification of patients at high risk for readmission should start at admission.
- High-risk patients need discharge planning throughout hospital stay to identify potential barriers for a smooth discharge.
- Communication with outpatient providers, patients, and caregivers is vital.
- Patients need clear discharge instructions and benefit from teach-back to ensure understanding of clinical instructions.
- Multiple models have shown multidisciplinary discharge planning and follow-up can reduce readmissions.

ONLINE RESOURCES

1. CMS Readmissions Reductions Program: https://www.cms.gov/medicare/medicare-fee-for-service-payment/acuteinpatientpps/readmissions-reduction-program.html
2. Project BOOST: http://www.hospitalmedicine.org/Web/Quality_Innovation/Implementation_Toolkits/Project_BOOST/Web/Quality___Innovation/Implementation_Toolkit/Boost/Overview.aspx?hkey=09496d80-8dae-4790-af72-efed8c3e3161
3. Project RED: http://www.bu.edu/fammed/projectred/
4. Transitional Care Model: http://www.transitionalcare.info/home
5. Care Transitions Model[19]: http://www.caretransitions.org/

REFERENCES

1. Jencks SF, Williams MV, Coleman EA. Rehospitalizations among patients in the Medicare fee-for-service program. *N Engl J Med.* 2009;360:1418.
2. https://www.cms.gov/medicare/medicare-fee-for-service-payment/acuteinpatientpps/readmissions-reduction-program.html. Accessed 12/21/15.
3. Greenwald JL, Denham CR, Jack BW. The hospital discharge: a review of a high risk care transition with highlights of a reengineered discharge process. *J Patient Saf.* 2007;3:97–106.
4. Coleman EA, Chugh A, Williams MV, et al. Understanding and execution of discharge instructions. *Am J Med Qual.* 2013;28(5):383–91.
5. Project BOOST. http://www.hospitalmedicine.org/Web/Quality_Innovation/Implementation_Toolkits/Project_BOOST/Web/Quality___Innovation/Implementation_Toolkit/Boost/Overview.aspx?hkey=09496d80-8dae-4790-af72-efed8c3e3161. Accessed 12/21/15.
6. Kripalani S, LeFevre F, Phillips CO, et al. Deficits in communication and information transfer between hospital-based and primary care physicians. *JAMA.* 2007;297(8):831–41.

7. O'Leary KJ, Liebovitz DM, Feinglass J, et al. Creating a better discharge summary: improvement in quality and timeliness using an electronic discharge summary. *J Hosp Med.* 2009;4:219–25.

8. Hesselink G, Schoonhoven L, Barach P, et al. Improving patient handovers from hospital to primary care. *Ann Intern Med.* 2012;157(6):417–28.

9. Flacker J, Park W, Sims A. Hospital discharge information and older patients: do they get what they need? *J Hosp Med.* 2007;2(5):291–6.

10. Weiss BD. *Health Literacy and Patient Safety: Help Patients Understand. Manual for Clinicians.* 2nd ed. Chicago, IL: AMA Foundation; 2007.

11. Schillinger D, Piette J, Grumbach K, et al. Closing the loop: physician communication with diabetic patients who have low health literacy. *Arch Intern Med.* 2003;163(1):83–90.

12. Shepperd S, Lannin NA, Clemson LM, et al. Discharge planning from hospital to home. *Cochrane Database Syst Rev.* 2013;(1):CD000313. DOI: 10.1002/14651858.CD000313. pub4.

13. Nielsen GA, Bartely A, Coleman E, et al. *Transforming Care at the Bedside How-to Guide: Creating an Ideal Transition Home for Patients with Heart Failure.* Cambridge, MA: Institute for Healthcare Improvement; 2008. http://www.IHI.org

14. Society of Hospital Medicine. BOOST Fact Sheet. http://www.hospitalmedicine.org/Web/Quality_Innovation/Implementation_Toolkits/Project_BOOST/Web/Quality___Innovation/Implementation_Toolkit/Boost/First_Steps/Fact_Sheet.aspx. Cited 12/21/15.

15. Boston University School of Medicine. Project RED (Re-Engineered Discharge). http://www.bu.edu/fammed/projectred/. Cited 3/5/13.

16. Jack BW, Chetty VK, Anthony D, et al. The re-engineered discharge: a RCT of a comprehensive hospital discharge program. *Ann Intern Med.* 2009;150:178–88.

17. Transitional Care Model. http://www.transitionalcare.info/index.html. Cited 3/5/13.

18. Naylor MD, Brooten D, Campbell R, et al. Comprehensive discharge planning and home follow-up of hospitalized elders: a randomized clinical trial. *JAMA.* 1999;281:613–20.

19. Coleman E. http://www.caretransitions.org/. Cited 3/6/13.

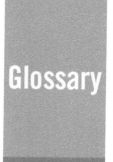

Glossary

Introduction to Patient Safety Terminology

Tina Doshi, Aaron J. Norris, and Andrea Vannucci

CLINICAL VIGNETTE

Mr. S, a 78-year-old man with ischemic cardiomyopathy, was admitted to the hospital for congestive heart failure exacerbation. At the time of his initial medical evaluation, he informed his medical team that he wished to have a "do not resuscitate/do not intubate" (DNR/DNI) status. Accordingly, DNR/DNI status was documented in both the paper chart and the electronic medical record (EMR). Later that evening, the EMR was down and paper charting was used. During that time, Mr. S was found unresponsive and in respiratory distress. The code team was called. Mr. S was resuscitated, intubated, and transferred to the intensive care unit, where he was sedated and received invasive respiratory support by mechanical ventilation. When the medical team contacted the patient's family, Mr. S's son stated that his father "did not want to be on life support." The family arrived and requested that the patient be taken off sedation, life support stopped, and comfort measures provided. Mr. S died shortly thereafter. You are on the committee reviewing the case and have been assigned to write a report of the findings.

- What are the appropriate terms to describe this scenario? Error, injury, harmful incident, adverse event? Is this a sentinel event?
- Was there a system failure?
- What is a root cause analysis?

INTRODUCTION

Patient safety and the related field of quality improvement in health care have a vocabulary that borrows from a variety of disciplines, including engineering, industry, business, cognitive psychology, and government regulatory agencies. Patient safety and quality improvement initiatives in health care have also generated a number of terms unique to those fields. The World Health Organization (WHO) conceptual framework for the International Classification for Patient Safety attempts to organize and schematize relationships between various broad concepts within the field of patient safety (Fig. G-1).[1] This framework is part of an extensive technical document that attempts to delineate "standardized sets of concepts with agreed definitions, preferred terms and the relationships between them."[1] Although the WHO framework provides a systematic approach to classifying patient safety

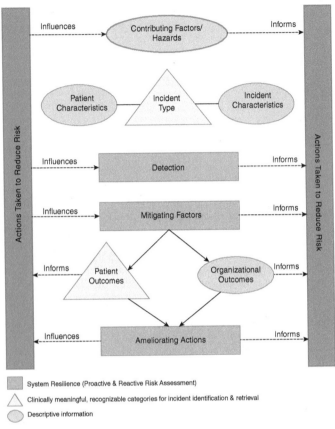

System Resilience (Proactive & Reactive Risk Assessment)

Clinically meaningful, recognizable categories for incident identification & retrieval

Descriptive information

The solid lines represent the semantic relationships between the classes. The dotted lines represent the flow of information.

Figure G-1. The conceptual framework for the international classification for patient safety. (Reproduced with permission from the World Health Organization.)

events, it also highlights the complexity of the many concepts and terms used in the field of patient safety. Moreover, it illustrates the difficulty in reaching standardized definitions for specific terms that are valid across various disciplines and geographic boundaries.

A number of groups have attempted to develop standard definitions for the most commonly used terms in patient safety, but these often vary between sources and may be inconsistent, depending on the context. Terms and definitions relating to quality of care and patient safety come from health care providers, professional societies, health care administrators, regulatory agencies, and public health organizations at the local, regional, national, or international levels, and they are used in medical, legal, regulatory, economic, and even sociologic settings. This array of sources and uses creates a considerable challenge to offering concise, widely accepted, and specific definitions for many important terms in patient safety and quality. For example, the term "sentinel event" has a number of definitions with potentially different medical, legal, and ethical implications (Table G-1). (Note that the WHO lists multiple definitions from multiple sources for its entry on "sentinel event."[1]) It is generally agreed that a sentinel event is an unexpected and possibly preventable adverse event in which serious harm has occurred. However, not all sources agree on (or even address) what constitutes serious harm, what types of events would be considered unexpected, whether such an event requires investigation, or whether the occurrence of a sentinel event is indicative of "serious problems in current policies or procedures." Thus, it can be difficult to determine the appropriate response to a potential sentinel event or even to establish whether or not a sentinel event occurred.

Given the challenges described above and ongoing debates surrounding the exact definitions of many terms, this chapter provides only a brief introduction to common terms used in the fields of patient safety and quality, beginning with several "core" terms that aid in providing context and framework for the broader vocabulary. Because a complete listing of terms is beyond the scope of this chapter, selected terms and definitions are subsequently listed. For more extensive lists of terms and definitions, we encourage the reader to explore the references provided at the end of this chapter, many of which have been used to create the definitions in this glossary.

CORE TERMS

Patient Safety

This term was first used in a manner consistent with its modern usage in a 1960 article addressing the relative safety of regional versus general anesthesia in obstetric patients.[7] Since that time, the term has continued to evolve and grow. Narrowly considered, patient safety refers to freedom from preventable or accidental injury during the course of medical care.[1,8,9] In a broader context, patient safety can also denote the discipline that applies safety science to the processes of health care delivery to minimize errors, injuries, and adverse outcomes.[1,8–10]

Quality

Prior to its usage in health care, the concept of quality came into popular use in industry, particularly manufacturing. W. Edwards Deming famously conceptualized the term as "Quality = (Results of work efforts)/(Cost)."[8] In health care, the results of work efforts are the diagnosis and treatment of patients as well as the extent to which health services provide the desired outcomes. However, on a more practical level, defining, quantifying, and improving quality of health care is a source of ongoing discussion and debate, and multiple frameworks have been proposed. The IOM defines quality by six adjectives that describe care: safe, effective, patient centered, timely, efficient, and equitable.[11] Multiple measures of quality in health care (quality metrics) have been developed in an effort to quantify the quality of care delivered. Quality metrics often rely on administrative data and readily available clinical information to assess quality at every level of care, from prevention to treatment, outpatient to inpatient, or patient to population. Various tools used to improve quality metrics in health care have been adapted from manufacturing and include Total Quality Management, Six Sigma, Lean methodology, and Continuous Quality Improvement.

Table G-1 Definition of "Sentinel Event"

	The Joint Commission[2]/Committee of Experts on Management of Safety and Quality in Health Care (SP-SQS)[3]/WHO[1]	Agency for Healthcare Research and Quality (AHRQ)[4]	National Quality Foundation (NQF)[5]/WHO[1]	Institute of Medicine (IOM)[5]/WHO[1]
Definition	A sentinel event is an unexpected occurrence involving death or serious physical or psychological injury, or the risk thereof. Serious injury specifically includes loss of limb or function. The phrase "or the risk thereof" includes any process variation for which a recurrence would carry a significant chance of a serious adverse outcome. Such events are called "sentinel" because they signal the need for immediate investigation and response. The Joint Commission requires each accredited organization to define sentinel event for its own purposes and to communicate this definition throughout the organization (LD.04.04.05, EP7).	An adverse event in which death or serious harm to a patient has occurred; usually used to refer to events that are not at all expected or acceptable—e.g., an operation on the wrong patient or body part. The choice of the word sentinel reflects the egregiousness of the injury (e.g., amputation of the wrong leg) and the likelihood that investigation of such events will reveal serious problems in current policies or procedures.	Any event that has resulted in an unanticipated death or major permanent loss of function, not related to the natural course of the patient's illness or underlying condition.	An unexpected occurrence or variation involving death or serious physical or psychological injury or the risk thereof.

Key aspects of definition

"Adverse event"	X	X	Not explicitly stated	Not explicitly stated

"Unexpected"	X	X	X	X
Includes "death"	X	X	X	X
"Serious" harm or injury	Not explicitly defined but "includes loss of limb or function" and includes "physical or psychological injury, or the risk thereof"	Not explicitly defined; single example of "amputation of the wrong leg" is given to reflect "egregiousness" of incident	Not explicitly stated or defined but includes "major permanent loss of function, not related to the natural course of the patient's illness or underlying condition"	Not explicitly defined; no examples given but does include "physical or psychological injury or the risk thereof"
Investigation and response	"Signal[s] the need for immediate investigation and response"	Not specifically mandated	Not addressed	Not addressed
Implications	Not addressed	"Investigation... will reveal serious problems in current policies or procedures"	Not addressed	Not addressed
Other aspects	Includes phrase "or the risk thereof" to indicate circumstances that would create a significant chance of a serious adverse outcome			Does not define phrase "or the risk thereof"

System(s)

Systems are composed of multiple, interconnected, interacting, and/or interdependent components (e.g., personnel, equipment, and processes). Health care providers function within and as part of systems in their daily work. Individual components may affect the function of the system as whole as well as the functioning of other components. Characteristics of a system include structure (components and the manner in which they are organized), behavior (conversion of input to output), and interconnectivity (relationships and connections between components). Understanding health care outcomes, positive or negative, as the result of a system represents a departure from the traditional model that focused almost exclusively on individuals. With the traditional model, organizations frequently responded to negative outcomes and errors through punishment of often well-intending individuals (i.e., blame and shame). Systems thinking goes beyond the level of the individual and provides an alternative framework to understand and alter factors that contribute to the occurrence of errors.

Error

As with many terms in health care, the definition of error overlaps with other terms (e.g., mistake, adverse event, negligence), and its precise meaning is actively debated. The landmark report "To Err is Human" defines medical error as "failure of a planned action to be completed as intended or the use of a wrong plan to achieve an aim."[9] Errors can result from either commission or omission and may be divided into the following types based on system and cognitive approaches:

Systems-Based Classification
- *Active errors* are unsafe acts committed by personnel in direct contact with the patient or system. They take a variety of forms: slips, lapses, fumbles, or mistakes.
- *Latent errors* are attributes of the system placed by designers or management that provoke further errors or create an inherent weakness in the system.

Cognitive Classification
- *Skill-based errors* are those when the action made is not the intended one.
- *Rule-based errors* occur when the action and intention match, but the desired outcome is not attained due to misapplication of a predetermined response pattern ("if X, then do Y").
- *Knowledge-based errors* are those in which the actions taken are intended but do not have the desired outcome due to a deficiency of information.[9]

KEY TERMS

Adverse event: An undesired injury cause by medical care (i.e., diagnosis or therapy) rather than the underlying disease or condition of the patient; it does not imply "error," "negligence," or poor care.

Ameliorating actions: Steps taken or circumstances altered to improve or compensate for any harm after an incident.

Benchmark: Attribute or achievement that serves as a point of reference or standard by which the performance of providers or institutions may be compared or judged.

Best practice: A technique, practice, or method that has been shown to achieve consistently better results than alternatives. Best practice also functions as a benchmark by which other methods can be measured.

Briefing: A conversation sharing relevant information prior to a procedure or activity (e.g., surgical "time-out").

Close call: An event or situation that may have resulted in patient injury, but did not, either due to chance or timely intervention (also known as *near miss*).

Closed-loop communication: Dialogue in which the recipient of an instruction repeats or clarifies the task in order to affirm that he or she understands and will complete the task and to notify the team leader when the task has been completed.

Contributing factors: A circumstance, action, or influence that may have increased the risk or led to the development of an incident. (See also *error.*)

Core measures: Quality metrics used to determine health care organization performance and compare quality of health care delivery across institutions. The most commonly used core measures are those developed by The Joint Commission (TJC) and the Centers for Medicare and Medicaid Services (CMS), which are national, evidence-based quality indicators for various settings and disease processes. Examples of core measurement areas include acute myocardial infarction, tobacco treatment, and childhood immunization. (See also "Quality" section in "Core Terms in Patient Safety.")

Crew resource management (CRM): Also called "crisis resource management." A range of approaches, developed initially in the aviation industry, for training groups to function as teams rather than as collections of individuals. CRM emphasizes the role of "human factors," management styles, and organizational cultures on high-stress, high-risk environments. (See also *human factors.*)

Critical language: Key phrases understood by all team members to mean "Stop and listen, we have a potential problem." Specific phrases may differ from one institution or unit to another.

Debriefing: A conversation sharing relevant information following a procedure or activity; identifies what went well, what could have been done differently, and what was learned.

Disclosure (error disclosure): Notification of an adverse event to the affected patient or patient advocate. Elements of disclosure may include statement of all harmful errors, an explanation of the error(s), possible effects of the error, how the error's effects will be minimized, steps taken to prevent recurrences, acknowledgement of responsibility, and/or an apology. Disclosure is often a process and not a single event.

Error: See above entry in "Core Terms in Patient Safety."

Failure to rescue: Shorthand for "failure to rescue from a complication of an underlying illness or complication of medical care." In other words, it is an inability to prevent or adequately respond to an important clinical deterioration, such as death or permanent disability (e.g., cardiac arrest in a patient with acute myocardial infarction or major hemorrhage after thrombolysis for acute myocardial infarction).

Forcing function: An aspect of a design that prevents a behavior from continuing until the problem has been corrected.

Handoffs, handovers, sign-outs: The process of exchanging information about a patient's health status (e.g., condition, care, treatment, medications, services, and any recent or expected changes) from one health care professional to another for the purpose of taking over the patient's care. In general, handoffs should be accurate, clear, and complete, but this can be challenging due to the need to be concise, unstructured handoff procedures, and attending to other demands of patient care. Handoffs are areas of particular concern in patient safety, as important details may be missed or information may be misinterpreted during the handover process.

Health Insurance Portability and Accountability Act (HIPAA): Federal regulations first introduced in 1996 to increase patient privacy and security during transmission of "protected health information" among providers, payors, or other health care entities. "Protected health information" includes medical records and health care payment history.

Health literacy: Individuals' ability to find, process, and comprehend basic health information necessary to act on medical instructions and make decisions about their health.

Heuristics: Informal rules (i.e., "rules of thumb") developed through trial and error that are used to complete a judgment or make a decision. Although heuristics are important tools that allow providers to respond promptly to urgent or complex situations, they may also be wrong or applied inappropriately, leading to medical errors.

High-reliability organizations (HROs): Organizations or systems that operate in high-risk environments yet have fewer adverse events than expected. Features of HROs include (1) preoccupation with failure, which acknowledges the error-prone nature of the organization's activities and strives to achieve consistent safety; (2) commitment to resilience, developing mechanisms within the system to detect, contain, mitigate, or recover from unexpected threats; (3) sensitivity to operations, in which frontline workers are attentive to potential issues and are empowered to respond to such threats; and (4) a culture of safety.

Hindsight bias: The tendency to regard past occurrences as expected or obvious, while in real time, they may have been unexpected or confusing. In the context of patient safety, it refers to the tendency to judge the events leading up to a negative outcome as errors because the negative outcome is already known. As a result, those reviewing an adverse event after the fact may deem an outcome as more foreseeable and more preventable than if they had been observing the event in real time.

Human-centered design, human factors, human factors engineering: A discipline that attempts to support or enhance human performance by identifying and addressing safety problems that occur in the interactions between humans, the tools and equipment they use, and the environments in which they live and work.

Iatrogenic: Pertaining to illness or injury resulting from medical care rather than from an underlying disease process.

Informed consent: The process in which a physician or physician representative presents to a patient the risks and benefits of a proposed therapy or test and then allows the patient to decide whether or not to undergo the procedure discussed. The term can also be used to mean the patient's authorization to perform a proposed therapy or test after such a discussion.

Just culture: An environment in which individuals feel comfortable reporting errors (including their own), balanced by the need to maintain professional accountability. In such an environment, there is recognition that even competent individuals make mistakes, and moreover, they should not be held responsible for systemic problems over which they have no control. However, individuals in a just culture should still be responsible for their own actions, and reckless behavior or misconduct is not tolerated.

Mistake: An error in which the intended action is performed, but the desired outcome is not achieved, either due to lack of knowledge or misinterpretation (i.e., a knowledge-based error) or through misapplication of a rule (i.e., a rule-based error).

All mistakes are errors, but not all errors are mistakes. Mistakes may be addressed by improving education or increasing supervision, but other types of errors, such as slips or fumbles caused by lapses in concentration, or latent errors within the system, must be addressed through different mechanisms. (See also "Error" section in "Core Terms in Patient Safety.")

Mitigating factor: An action or circumstance that prevents or diminishes the progression of an incident toward harming a patient.

Near miss: See *close call.*

Patient safety: See above entry in "Core Terms in Patient Safety."

Quality: See above entry in "Core Terms in Patient Safety."

Resilience: In the context of systems engineering, the ability of a system to recover from or adapt to an unexpected event. Resilient systems strive to achieve safety by relying on human judgment to assess safety concerns and human adaptability to manage adverse events. In sharp contrast, "ultrasafe" systems strive to achieve safety by establishing constraints that simplify processes and limit worker autonomy.

Risk management: Self-protective activities and strategies meant to prevent real or potential threats of financial loss due to accident, injury, or medical malpractice strategies through actions that minimize potential risks that could lead to injury of patients, staff members, or visitors.[12]

Root cause: The most fundamental reason an event has occurred.

Root cause analysis: A systematic process for identifying the underlying cause or contributing factors for an adverse event or incident. (See also *root cause.*)

Safety culture: An integrated pattern of individual and organizational behavior that continuously seeks to minimize harm, which may result from the processes of care delivery. Safety culture permeates all levels of an organization, from frontline workers to management and executives. Features include (1) acknowledgment of the high-risk, error-prone nature of an organization's activities, (2) a blame-free environment where individuals are able to report errors or close calls without punishment, (3) an expectation of collaboration across ranks to seek solutions to vulnerabilities, and (4) a willingness on the part of the organization to direct resources to address safety concerns.

SBAR: Stands for "Situation, Background, Assessment, and Recommendation." A standard communication technique that provides a framework for conveying information between members of a health care team, particularly those requiring immediate attention and action.

Sentinel event: An unexpected adverse event in which death or serious harm to a patient has occurred (see Table G-1).

Six Sigma: A set of quality improvement techniques that seek to provide near-perfect outcomes. "Sigma" refers to the Greek letter used to refer to the standard deviation of a normally distributed population; 2 standard deviations ("2 sigma") encompass 95% of the population being considered. Six Sigma processes target a defect rate of 3.4 defects per million (99.99966% success without defect); in actuality, this is 4.5 sigma, but a 1.5 sigma "shift" has been introduced into the calculation to account for long-term process variations.

Standard of care: Often a term associated with medical legal issues, meaning the degree of skill and care that a competent practitioner would exercise under similar circumstances. More generally, the standard of care indicates a treatment strategy or regimen accepted by medical experts as appropriate treatment for diseases.

Standard work: A description of each work activity, specifying cycle time, rate of demand for the product of the activity, sequences of specific tasks, and the minimum inventory of supplies to complete the activity.

Systems, systems approach, system improvement: See above entry in "Core Terms in Patient Safety."

Ultrasafe: See *resilience*.

EXAMPLE GLOSSARIES

See references 1, 2, 3, 4, and 5.

See also:

VA National Center for Patient Safety. *Glossary of Patient Safety Terms* 2013 [updated 2013 July 18; cited 2013 July 30]. http://www.patientsafety.va.gov/professionals/publications/glossary.asp

Wachter RM. *Understanding Patient Safety*. New York, NY: McGraw-Hill Medical; 2008.

REFERENCES

1. World Health Organization. *Conceptual Framework for the International Classification for Patient Safety*. Geneva, Switzerland: World Alliance for Patient Safety. Project to Develop the International Classification for Patient Safety; 2009. http://www.who.int/patientsafety/implementation/taxonomy/icps_technical_report_en.pdf?ua=1. Accessed 12/22/15.
2. Joint Commission on Accreditation of Healthcare Organizations. *Lexicon: Dictionary of Health Care Terms, Organizations, and Acronyms for the Era of Reform*. 2nd ed. Oakbrook Terrace, IL: Joint Commission on Accreditation of Healthcare Organizations; 1998.
3. Committee of Experts on Management of Safety and Quality in Health Care. *Glossary of Terms Related to Patient and Medication Safety—Approved Terms*. Strasbourg, France: Council of Europe; 2005. http://www.who.int/patientsafety/highlights/COE_patient_and_medication_safety_gl.pdf. Accessed 12/22/15.
4. Agency for Healthcare Research and Quality. *Glossary*. [cited July 30, 2013]. https://psnet.ahrq.gov/glossary. Accessed 12/22/15.
5. National Quality Forum. *NQF Patient Safety Terms and Definitions*. 2010 [cited December 22, 2015]. http:// www.qualityforum.org/Topics/Safety_Definitions.aspx
6. Kohn LT, Corrigan J, Donaldson MS. *To Err is Human : Building a Safer Health System*. Washington, DC: National Academy Press; 2000.
7. Kreul W. Regional anesthesia for increasing obstetrical patient safety. *Wis Med J*. 1960;59:370–373.
8. Deming WE. *Out of the Crisis*. Cambridge, MA: Massachusetts Institute of Technology, Center for Advanced Engineering Study; 1986.
9. Reason JT. *Human Error*, Vol. xv. Cambridge, England: Cambridge University Press; 1990:302.
10. Emanuel L, Berwick D, Conway J, et al. *What Exactly Is Patient Safety? Advances in Patient Safety: New Directions and Alternative Approaches*. Rockville, MD: Agency for Healthcare Research and Quality; 2008.
11. Institute of Medicine (U.S.), Committee on Quality of Health Care in America. *Crossing the Quality Chasm : A New Health System for the 21st Century*. Washington, DC: National Academy Press; 2001.
12. Kuhn AM. The need for risk management to evolve to assure a culture of safety. *Qual Saf Health Care*. 2002;11(2):158–162.

Index

Note: Page numbers followed by *f* refer to figures and followed by *t* refer to tables